The Los Angeles
Healer's Guide

The Best of Holistic Care
2007

Raising Awareness
Changing the Future of Health Care

Healer's Guide
The Best Of Holistic Care 2007

United States Copyright © 2007
by Elissa Michaud and Milan Polak

First Edition: 2007

Published by Learn2heal
P.O. Box 6717
Pine Mountain Club, CA 93222
USA

For information regarding special discounts
for bulk purchases and for all orders contact Healer's Guide:
www.healerguide.com
1.800.495.7106
ISBN: 1-4276-0223-9

Illustrations & Graphic Design: Milan Polak
Editor-in-Chief: Nzingha Clarke
Cartoon Illustrations: Jason Love

Inquiries to the authors may be addressed to:
Learn2heal - Healer's Guide
P.O. Box 6717
Pine Mountain Club, CA 93222
www.healerguide.com, www.healers-guide.com
customerservice@healerguide.com

The concept of the Healer's Guide was born from years of studies, observations and follows nearly a decade of practicing a broad range of healing modalities. During our journey, we noticed that several elements were missing for an effective integration of healthcare. First it was obvious that far too many healers and healthcare professionals fostered a sectarian approach, maintaining that their approach was the only true and effective way. Secondly, we grew to understand that merely a handful of individuals within the new age, or alternative communities, were familiar with holistic healing practices and that key information was not easily available to the mainstream community. Thirdly, although the beginning stages to integrate western medical care and complementary therapies have occurred, this shift is slow. In addition, there has been little done to integrate western care, complementary therapies and the healing arts that work with subtle energies on the soul level. Many complementary and alternative medicines ("CAM") do not, in fact, address the body-mind-spirit and must be supported by esoteric healing practices. We believe that uniting these three aspects is the key. Unless they are united harmoniously, and practiced preventatively, massive improvements in our society's health are next to impossible. We have been fortunate and blessed to have had incredible teachers and in turn, the desire to share this information with as many people as possible. We strive to maintain balance between all healthcare practices, while sharing the philosophies and ideals that through our practice and observations we have come to embody. We hope that the information presented in Healer's Guide helps as many individuals as possible.

In love, light and service,

Milan Polak & Elissa Michaud

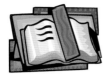

Table of Contents

PART 1

PART 2

PART 3

- ➢ **Acupuncture**
- ➢ **Ayurveda**
- ➢ **Biofeedback**
- ➢ **Chinese Medicine**
- ➢ **Chiropractic**
- ➢ **Colon Therapy**
- ➢ **Cranial Sacral Therapy**
- ➢ **Doula**
- ➢ **Energetic Balancing**
- ➢ **Feng Shui**
- ➢ **Holistic Dentistry**
- ➢ **Holistic M.D.**
- ➢ **Holistic Senior Care**
- ➢ **Homeopathy**
- ➢ **Hypnotherapy**
- ➢ **Integrated Energy Therapy**
- ➢ **Life Coaching**
- ➢ **Massage Therapy**
- ➢ **Naturopathy**
- ➢ **Neurofeedback**
- ➢ **Neuro Linguistic Prog.**
- ➢ **Nutritional Counseling**
- ➢ **Osteopathy**
- ➢ **Physical Therapy**
- ➢ **Pranic Healing**
- ➢ **Reiki**
- ➢ **Rolfing**
- ➢ **Spiritual Psychology**
- ➢ **Transitional Healing**

PART 4

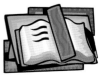

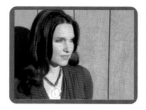

"Allopathic Medicine provides us with unparalleled knowledge and an understanding of the mechanics of the human body and the pathology of disease. Through experimentation, research and development, especially during the past century, we have witnessed a dramatic extension of the human life span and the cure or management of many previously life threatening infections and diseases. Effectively healing disease and achieving wellness requires a holistic approach from each and every one of us. Recognize, understand and address the many health-related aspects of your complex nature and combine allopathic and alternative medicine in an intelligent, integrative fashion. Together, we will revolutionize the future of healthcare and help take the evolution of humanity to the next level."

Elissa Michaud, Healer

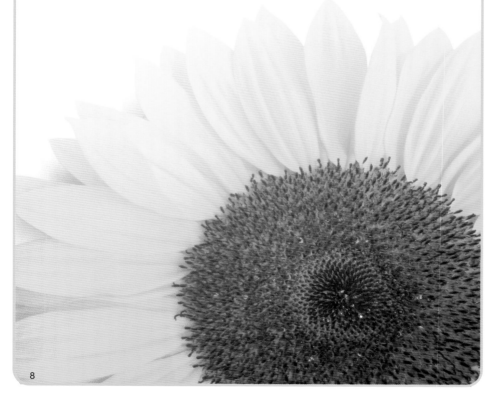

"We are blessed today with simple, inexpensive, accessible techniques that have the potential to revolutionize our sense of wellness, shift the patterns that trap us in chronic disease, and dramatically raise our thresholds of happiness. I challenge you to experiment with these methods and see what results they produce in your own life. And as you have the courage to travel the healing journey, I salute the divinity within you and trust God's blessings with you always."

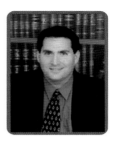

Eric B. Robins, M.D.

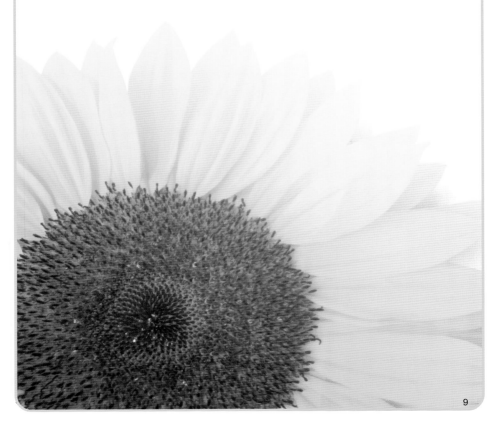

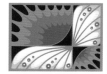

Part 1

Introduction

For the first time in the history of our western society, true health has the opportunity to prevail. More recently, society has been outwardly expressing concerns that Western Medicine, as we know it, is an incomplete system, and the belief that it is failing them in many ways. Although partially correct, it is unwise to rebel against the system in its entirety. One must acknowledge the outstanding benefits of conventional medicine. Certain medications and surgical procedures have saved, prolonged or improved millions of lives, globally. Complementary medicine is gradually becoming accepted and not a moment too soon. As its name states, complementary medicine complements western care and improves the overall quality of the service provided to patients. But progress is slow. It is tough to implement the necessary changes overnight. It is often easier to remain safe and comfortable in habits, than to undertake the difficult steps and the challenges they bring, required for growth.

Medication or surgical procedures are not at fault, but the abuse by professionals and patients alike is, not to mention the fact that sole reliance on these solutions is in many cases, impractical. Medications are often prescribed for health conditions, which may have required little more than rest, lifestyle changes or clean living. Surgeries are often recommended and consentually performed without prior attempts to find less invasive alternatives. Almost any practitioner of conventional medicine asked will agree that the practice of medicine does not address, treat or heal all aspects of the patient - the body, mind and spirit. Therefore, the root cause of the illness often remains, with the potential to re-create a similar or seemingly new pattern of disease.

Alternative or complementary healing systems are not perfect either, the difference is that alternative healthcare practitioners do not claim their treatments cure. Their emphasis is on holistic healing, which does not necessarily result in an immediate disappearance of symptoms. With this being said, often alternative medical systems are just as, if not more successful than conventional medicine to help patients regain

Each green box in the *Healer's Guide* 2007 book presents additional research and/or content to complement the information in the chapter and the topic being discussed.

"The visits to practitioners of alternative therapy exceeded projected number of visits to all primary care physicians in the United States by an estimated 243 million visits."
-
"Trends in Alternative Medicine Use in the United States 1990-1997", David Eisenberg, M.D.

health. The aim of most alternative treatments is to bring the body into a state of balance, rather than disharmony, without any harmful side effects.

Critics will argue that there is not enough scientific research or evidence to prove the effectiveness of alternative medicine. Appropriate research criteria or standards to qualify or quantify most healing arts or systems have not yet been developed, nor do we have the scientific equipment sensitive enough to accurately measure the velocities of the human energy field. Currently, through the field of quantum physics, systems are being developed, though more research and testing is needed before they become mainstream.

Each red box in the *Healer's Guide* 2007 book presents a suggested action which the reader can take. The action is related to the chapter and the topic being discussed.

Medical practices other than western allopathy have been used successfully for thousands of years. Medical systems, such as acupuncture and ayurveda are based on healing through the balancing of bio-energy. Historically healers have worked with this energy and soon, upon its validation, it will be labeled as the "Newest Scientific Discovery" in the West! Many are able to see subtle energies (auras, chakras) on which alternative healing systems are based. Those who possess clairvoyant abilities report seeing similar energy structures belonging to the human body.

Alternative healthcare places focus on healing persons through preventative wellness, herbs and nutrition, instructing patients on how to harmonize with the laws of nature and utilizing bio-energetic healing. Practitioners educate each patient regarding preventative, self-care and lifestyle management and place the responsibility for their health on them.

"The acceptance of natural cycles, obedience to their laws and the union between western medicine as we know it, prevention and uniquely tailored healing work done through the energetic anatomy of man, will eventually create the new face of health-care, resulting in the rapid healing of the individual and the whole of humanity"

-
Healer's Guide, 2007

Orthodox medicine prescribes medication for symptoms to ease suffering, operates on or removes the diseased body part, utilizing techniques formulated from scientific research and a thorough understanding of physical anatomy. The patient under orthodox care places the majority of the responsibility for decision making on the physician and are known to blame the result or outcome on the physician as well.

Both conventional and alternative systems are true expressions of divinity. Both are beneficial, therefore an integrative approach is sensible. Even though there are fundamental differences, their goal is the same, to restore the health of the patient and to serve humanity. The two, united in service, are more powerful and effective than one, alone.

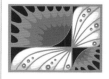

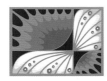

Until now, the attitude of so many conventional and alternative health care providers has been one of separation and exclusiveness. Those days are gone. No longer will the alternative or conventional practitioner be able to maintain that their approach is the only correct way. The decision no longer is whether to use alternative or orthodox methods, but how to take advantage of the best both have to offer. There is no single, correct way based on just one system, regardless of proof or the outcome of the research. The fact that conventional medicine is supported by modern scientific studies and alternative treatment is often not, does not necessarily mean it will result in a more effective healing in all cases. Medicine may suppress symptoms, or allow one to live a pain-free life, but this is not healing. The human body possesses the innate ability to heal itself. All outer help, practitioners included, simply facilitate healing by providing treatment and advice, uniquely tailored to each patient's needs, requests, goals and desires.

Every living creature has an inborn ability to heal itself. It is a principle which can not be overlooked. It is possible, however, to diminish this ability by misuse of medication, unhealthy lifestyle, toxic environment, etc. When the inner healing ability is lost, healing will not be possible, no matter how many doctors and healers we have at hand.

Healing cannot occur by only addressing the needs of the physical body. Bringing the body into a disease-free state, a state of optimum health, requires treating the person as a whole, taking into account the body, mind and spirit. Advice and treatment options must be given, based on proven diagnostic techniques and accurate up-to-date knowledge and education. Practitioners must honor limitations, but also be willing to hold the highest possible outcome and move beyond, whenever possible.

"The people who say they don't have time to take care of themselves will soon discover they're spending all their time being sick."

-
The Book of Comforts,
Patricia Alexander & Michael Burgos

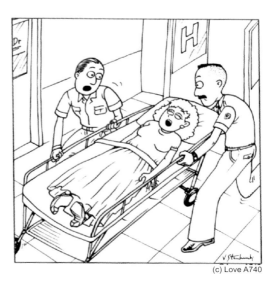

(c) Love A740

"One minute she was eyeing her hospital bill, and the next minute....."

The transition from conventional medicine to integrative care is a lengthy process for two reasons. First, many deeply ingrained, long standing beliefs regarding the origins and nature of illness must be disintegrated or altered. Secondly, we must learn to self-educate, not self medicate, and be responsible for our health, with a preventative, holistic approach to life.

This is where *Healer's Guide* can play an instrumental role by offering quality information, education and resources, not as this knowledge pertains to the reasons and solutions unique for each particular ailment, but as it pertains to preventative health care, general health and well-being and teaching the importance of identifying and addressing the potential reasons behind illness. Here, you will be introduced to new information, some of which may be hard to grasp depending on your background, education and beliefs and although you are not obligated to believe everything you read, you are encouraged to experiment and draw your own conclusions. The suggestions contained in *Healer's Guide* are not meant to replace orthodox medicine or cure. The body has its own wisdom and will heal itself as long as the cure selected is appropriate and harmonious with natural laws - described in detail in the chapters to follow.

> ☯
>
> **The *Healer's Guide* contains content which is not commonly known. All readers are encouraged to have an open mind. Experiment with new information and draw your own conclusions. Every-one grows and expands their abilities and under-standing at their own rate. Be patient when learning and give the process time.**

In general the Los Angeles lifestyle has little to do with following, or being in harmony with natural laws. Harmonious choices and the best intentions are often set aside by the family demands, lifestyle, career, paying the bills and the bureaucracy that surrounds us. The personal power residing within each and every one of us gives strength to set our own rules, guidelines, boundaries and standards for self care in order to live in a state of optimum health. *Healer's Guide* will help lead you to your personal power, to overcome the ever present external pressures and expectations of community, society and global influences.

**Disclaimer:
This publication contains research and the opinions, ideas and personal experience of its authors and is intended to provide informative material on the subject contained within. It is sold with the understanding that the authors and publisher are not engaged in providing medical or health services nor dispense, directly or indirectly, medical advice or prescribe the use of any technique as a form of treatment for physical or medical issues without the advice of a qualified physician. The authors and publisher specifically disclaim all responsibility for any liability, loss, or risk, personal or otherwise, that is incurred as a consequence directly or indirectly, from the application of any of the contents of this book. The reader should consult his or her medical or other health professional before following the suggestions and exercises in this book. The content of this book is not meant to replace orthodox medicine, diagnose diseases, prescribe any drugs/substances, or make any health claims or promises. The authors, publisher, and Healer's Guide are not responsible for the content of advertising materials.
The physicians, practitioners and businesses listed or referred to in editorial or advertisement sections are not responsible for the content and expressed views in this publication. The content is the sole responsibility of the authors and referenced resources.

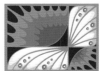

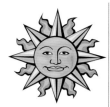

Healer's Guide Mission

Creating a Change

Wᵉ all have the ability to heal ourselves. The body's innate wisdom knows exactly what to do to maintain its balance. But with the pace and demands of this modern world, our bodies often lose their equilibrium and encounter health challenges that need professional care.

Healer's Guide introduces reputable healing modalities, successful techniques, validated resources and quality services for health maintenance and acute care. Should you need assistance, the tools and resources in this book are here, ready to help. *Healer's Guide* also empowers you to discover the healer within. Some have recently come to a decision to take personal responsibility for healing their chronic illness. Others are walking the road to wellness, already taking advantage of preventative healthcare. No matter how or what led you to select this book, *Healer's Guide* is your instruction manual for health. *Healer's Guide* offers information and education to help you navigate today's myriad of health related information. It will safely guide you through the healing process. The more knowledge, experience, supportive influences and resources are available, the faster you can heal. This book serves as inspiration and motivation, jump-starting you on the road to wellness.

Every event in our life can be considered a symptom of ease or disease. The ability to accept positive events with gratitude nurtures the ability to understand and learn the lesson of healing from any unpleasant events. By taking positive symptoms for granted and suppressing unpleasant ones, we loose the ability to follow the right direction towards a better life.

"As human beings, we are endowed with freedom of choice, and we cannot shuffle off our responsibility upon the shoulders of God or nature. We must shoulder it ourselves. It is our responsibility."

-
Arnold J. Toynbee, British Historian (1889 - 1975)

Many believe that the power to heal is beyond one's control and ability and that they must give the responsibility for healing to professionals. Conditioning tells everyone that healing must come from an outer source, so a pill or similarly easy solution is relied upon to quickly take troubles away. Well-intended, one-size-fits-all recommendations are made by the media, friends and health professionals alike.

" If you are not sleeping, why don't you try this medication? I take it and my friends recommended it. It will definitely work for you! Trust me, I saw it on TV! Ask your doctor!"

What if you were to replace the question, "What medication should I take?" with the question "What is the true cause of my sleeplessness?" Taking the first step to discover the root cause makes it possible for healing to begin. Instead of suppressing symptoms, apply this model to all disease or discomfort and see what happens! Symptoms manifest in several different ways.

Poor physical health, emotional imbalances, relationship and social problems, career stagnation, and financial challenges are all symptoms of underlying issues. Symptom suppression is not a cure! Symptoms are life's way of telling us there is a problem. Be grateful and appreciate the wisdom they offer, serving as pointers or indicators to the true illness behind. Suppression encourages the body to create a new, often more powerful symptom, to get attention. The new symptom may appear unrelated to the first, when in fact it is not.

The goal of *Healer's Guide* is to raise awareness and present a variety of solutions in an accessible format. We bring better understanding with regard to the most appropriate healing modalities for particular situations and the right place and time for their use, western medicine included. The *Healer's Guide* mission is not to discredit western medicine or medication, but to communicate a message of integration. There is a time and a place for everything. Ideally, approaches should work together synergistically.

Healer's Guide presents an opportunity to easily understand a holistic approach to life. It is suggested you read all the chapters, so the message of the interconnectedness of all levels - physical, emotional, mental and spiritual - can be understood.

Healer's Guide stresses a preventative lifestyle, through diet, exercise, meditation and stress redution, as well as regular preventative healing. Bodywork, acupuncture, energy healing, chiropractic and regular medical check-ups should be incorporated in a preventative manner, according to one's needs and lifestyle. *Healer's Guide* emphasizes the importance of building and strengthening the bridge between traditional medicine and alternative/complementary care. This is the true future of health care.

Healer's Guide creates a conscious link between the mainstream public, frustrated and disillusioned with the current healthcare system, and the purposeful integration of a holistic approach. After reading the following material you will have an understanding of how to implement holistic care. Guided self-analysis and introspection will lead you to a better understanding of areas in your life that demand attention and healing. The resource guide of professionals enables you to find the quality care providers you seek.

"The principle of self-recovery; *Healing* is the inborn ability of every living organism on this planet, humans included. Everyone is responsible for maximazing their self-healing power by not obstructing it."
-
Healer's Guide 2007

Taking the suggested actions, you will gain a deeper understanding of how important and precious your life is and how much personal power and control you have! You will gain priceless insight about your body-mind-soul connection and its care. Experience your maximum potential when it comes to your health. With a little willingness to follow simple instructions, the sky is the limit!

The Los Angeles Healer's Guide,
The Golden Middle Path Approach To Your Health & Wellness.
Raising Awareness,
Changing the Future of Health Care.

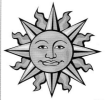

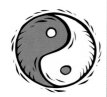

Raising Awareness

What is Holistic, Integrative or Alternative?

An introduction to Holistic Care brings a variety of foreign terms. What exactly is considered holistic? What is the difference between alternative and complementary? What is meant by integrative medicine?

Holistic Medicine - investigates and takes into consideration all aspects of the individual. Practitioners not only look for the physical symptoms of their clients, where illnesses is most apparent, but skillfully uncover the mental, emotional, environmental and sometimes spiritual aspects of disease, which often reveal more of the nature and actual root of the problem.

> The belief that alternative medicine is the same as holistic medicine is a misconception. Alternative medical systems commonly work with a unique healing approach which doesn't necessarily target all levels of human beings, while the holistic approach may use several different healing systems, taking care of each level - body, mind and spirit.

Physical symptoms are obvious, but not everyone is able to identify their true origin. For the holistic practitioner, trained to get to the root of illness, physical symptoms are simply the starting point. As the holistic practitioner determines the best healing method, harmonizing technique or antidote, no aspect - body, mind, emotions or spirit - is overlooked. The treatment is uniquely tailored to each patient. One solution is recommended for the physical body, another for mental or emotional aspects and one for spiritual health. This multi-level healing approach targets the underlying causes, bringing the system back to balance and reducing symptoms. These types of treatments or therapies reach beyond the techniques of conventional medicine.

The goal of holistic medicine is to facilitate healing, rather than suppressing symptoms. holistic medicine is typically practiced by a licensed medical professional who is able to identify the appropriate course of treatment. If the required method of treatment does not fall within the practitioner's range of abilities and must be addressed by other experts in the field, you will be referred to the appropriate holistic practitioner. holistic medical practitioners discuss the physical, emotional, mental, environmental and spiritual aspects with their patients, helping them to understand the complexity of their healing and recommending the most appropriate methods with the least side effects. Healing modalities are often referred to as alternative or complementary but this is not actually a label for a type of modality, but rather for the way the modality is being used. If the modality is used to replace conventional

"It is more important to know what sort of person has a disease than to know what sort of disease a person has."

\-
Hippocrates,
Greek physician
(460 - 377 B.C.)

medicine, it is called alternative. If it is used in conjunction with orthodox medicine, then it is called complementary. In the case of cancer, an example of this is:

Alternative - One patient chooses a combination of detox-ification, nutritional support, exercise, emotional therapy and proper diet to reverse cancer instead of undergoing surgery, radiation, or chemotherapy as recommended by a physician.

Complementary - A cancer patient uses Pranic (energy) Healing - one of the widely accepted forms of energy healing - before and after radiation treatment to support her allopathic treatments. This minimizes the damage which occurs to the healthy cells as a result of radiation, therefore hastening her recovery and minimizing the unpleasant side effects.

How many alternatives to conventional medicine are you familiar with? If you are able to name at least one, search through the *Healer's Guide,* Part 3 and discover what you do not know. It may be, to your surprise, that most alter-native modalities are in fact, complementary to conventional medicine and not a replacement.

Laboratory Study of Pranic Healing Using Contemporary Medical Imaging and Laboratory Method

Joie Jones, Ph.D., Professor of Radiological Sciences at the University of California, Irvine from a presentation at the Seventh World Pranic Healers' Convention:

"The study was to alter the effects of radiation and enhance the survival rates of the HeLa cells. In 520 experiments using 10 different Pranic Healers, typical survival rates increased from an expected 50% for untreated cells by Pranic Healing to over 90% for cells treated both before and after radiation."

Designation Survival Rate, 1 Day Post Radiation
A (control) ~ 100%
B (radiation only) ~ 50% (range: 49.4% - 50.7%)
C (PH after radiation) ~ 70% (range: 67.4% - 71.8%)
D (PH before radiation) ~ 80% (range: 78.1% - 82.9%)
E (PH before and after radiation) ~ 90% (range: 87.8% - 93.4%)

(find details at: www.pranichealing.bc.ca/articles2/hazelwardhal.pdf)

** "Pranic Healing is not intended to replace orthodox medicine, but rather to complement it."

"Miracles are fantastic events which utilize hidden laws of nature that most people are not aware of. Miracles do not break the laws of nature, they are actually based on them."
-
Master Choa Kok Sui, Modern founder of the ancient art and science of Pranic Healing

Integrative - the combination of a complementary modality with conventional care is considered integrative care. Integrative healthcare is growing rapidly and some medical clinics are already employing licensed acupuncturists, reflexologists, therapists trained in meditation, energy healers and herbalists or naturopaths to offer integrative services. You will find a partial list of integrative centers at the end of this chapter. The Consortium of Academic Health Centers for Integrative Medicine, *www.imconsortium.org* and The Bravewell Collaborative, *www.bravewell.org,* are two organizations dedicated to furthering the philosophy and implementation of integrative medicine. Both groups offer lists of centers in the U.S. and Canada on their website.

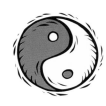

If suffering from a life threatening illness such as rapidly growing cancer or heart disease, a holistic approach is your best bet. It's simple. Your chances are increased when the effective tools of both worlds - orthodox and alternative - are implemented. If the illness is chronic in nature and requires medication, ask your doctor and alternative practitioner to work together. Many people have been able to reduce or even eliminate their prescription medication as their health improves. Remember, do not do this without consulting your physician, first. Begin only when it is considered medically safe. If your physician is not open to discussing this possibility, find another who is.

The National Center for Complementary and Alternative Medicine (NCCAM) of the National Institutes of Health (NIH) categorizes alternative modalities into seven fields:

The National Center for Complementary and Alternative Medicine (NCCAM) is a federal agency devoted to scientific research using advanced technologies to study complementary and alternative medicine (CAM).

The (NCCAM) is one of the institutes of The National Institutes of Health (NIH) within the U.S. Department of Health and Human Services.

www.nccam.nih.gov

• **Mind-body medicine** explores the ability of the mind to affect and, perhaps, heal the body. Examples are yoga, hypnosis, biofeedback and meditation.

• **Alternative medical systems** include therapies, such as Acupuncture, Ayurvedic Medicine, Homeopathy and Naturopathy. These systems are based on their individual and specific theories of health and disease.

• **Lifestyle and disease prevention** involves identifying and treating risk factors to prevent illness and maintain health. It includes making changes in diet and behavior, as well as exercise and stress management.

• **Biologically based therapies** use herbs, special diets - such as raw, vegan, vegetarian or macrobiotic - and other natural products to prevent and treat illnesses. These therapies also include drugs and vaccines not yet accepted or tested.

• **Manipulative and body-based systems** include chiropractic medicine, massage therapy, acupressure, reflexology and bodywork, in general.

• **Biofield medicine**, such as therapeutic touch, Pranic Healing and Reiki, which works with subtle energy fields and the energetic anatomy in and around the body for healing purposes.

"The greatest discovery of any generation is that human beings can alter their lives by altering the attitudes of their minds."

-
Albert Schweitzer, M.D.
(1875-1965)

• **Bioelectromagnetic applications** use the body's response to electromagnetic fields to heal the body.

Learning to apply holistic care involves learning a new habit. Unfortunately, this habit is usually acquired after health problems have developed. Holistic care requires regular attention and effort. It can be compared to dental care habits. From an early age everyone is taught to brush their teeth.

Flossing is often neglected until much later. After the teeth have a few cavities and suffering has befallen the individual, flossing then becomes important. But how often and why does the newly established flossing routine quickly fade away? The habit was not formed early on in life and therefore is not first nature. Similarly, everyone is taught to visit their conventional doctor, but so little advice is given regarding preventative and holistic health care. When an attempt is made to incorporate the new habit, it takes time before it becomes second nature.

Dentists emphasize the importance of dental hygiene. They educate and demonstrate, while making it clear that it is the patients' responsibility to implement a regular preventative program. They also encourage regular check-ups. Dentists will fix things after they have gone wrong, but are not responsible for the daily condition and health of your gums and teeth. Similarly, practitioners, medical doctors included, are not responsible for enforcing your health maintenance. A preventative lifestyle combined with regular check-ups and tune-ups using alternative modalities is the best insurance. If, after following a recommended treatment program, the healing has not happened as predicted, expected or in the time frame anticipated, try implementing a different appropriate healing modality. Remember that you maximize your body's innate healing ability by following a program of integrative care.

> ☯
> If you currently have a medical condition, take time to find out what the corresponding aspects of your illness are on all levels. How does it manifest physically? What are the possible underlying mental or emotional aspects? Is there a contributing environmental factor?

Holistic Medical Centers:

Agoura Hills

● Holistic Resource Center
Alan Schwartz, M.D.
29020 Agoura Rd. Suite A8
Agoura Hills, CA 91301
(818) 597-0966
www.holisticresourcecenter.com

Beverly Hills

● Ethos M.D. Integrative Med. Group
Lisa M. Schwartz, M.D.
9001 Wilshire Blvd. Suite 304
Beverly Hills, CA 90211
(310) 385-9432
www.ethosmd.com

● Khalsa Medical Clinic
Soram Singh Khalsa, M.D.
436 North Bedford Drive
Beverly Hills, CA 90210
(310) 274-6200
www.khalsamedical.com

● Holistic, Alternative, and Integrative Healthcare
Dr. Jafer, N.D.
9730 Wilshire Blvd, Ste 211
Beverly Hills, CA 90212
(310) 689-6599
www.drjafer.com

● Health Within Holistic Center
Thaddeus E. Jacobs, N.D., LAc
8601 Wilshire Blvd. Suite 1007
Beverly Hills, CA 90211
(310) 289-7872

● Lippman Center for Optimal Health
Cathie Lippman, MD
291 S. La Cienega Bl Suite 207
Beverly Hills, CA 90211
(310) 289-8430
www.cathielippmanmd.com

Burbank

● Wellness Center
Constance O'Reilly, D.C., N.D.
150 E. Olive Avenue, Suite 113
Burbank, CA 91502
(818) 955-9080

"No matter who you are, we are creatures of habit. The better your habits are, the better they will be in pressure situations."

Wayne Gretzky, professional hockey player

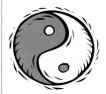

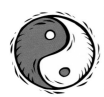

Holistic Medical Centers cont'd:

● Paramount Herbs   pg.271
Jon Buratti, N.D.
707A Main Street
Burbank, CA 91506
(818) 848-7414
www.paramountherbs.com

Costa Mesa
● Harmony Healing Naturopathic Clinic
Lena Kian, N.D.
234 E. 17th Street, Suite 210
Costa Mesa, CA 92627
(949) 910-6040
www.harmonyhealingclinic.com
(310) 809-2237 - learn2heal.com

El Segundo
● Body Doc Healing Center pg.234
1924 B East Maple Ave.
El Segundo, CA 90245
(310) 546-6863
www.bodydocchiropractic.com

Fulerton
● GMP Vitamins & Health Foods
Robert D. Kanter, N.D., M.H., C.N.C.
1319 S Harbor Blvd
Fullerton, CA 92832
(714) 879-5315

Irvine
● South Coast Medical Center For New Medicine
6 Hughes, Suite 100
Irvine, CA 92618
(949) 680-1880
www.scmedicalcenter.com

Los Angeles
● Joseph Sciabbarrasi, M.D.
2001 S. Barrington Avenue, Suite 208
Los Angeles, CA 90025
(310) 268-8466
www.drjosephmd.com

● Shiva Lalezar, D.O.
11611 San Vicente Blvd., Suite 650
Los Angeles, CA 90049
(310) 282-0455
www.computaid.com/shiva

● Heartfelt Medicine
Dana Churchill, N.M.D.
12665 Venice Blvd. # 4
Los Angeles, CA 90066
(310) 230-5228
www.heartfeltmedicine.com

● Tilo Medical and Acupuncture
Keegan Sheridan N.D.
2001 S Barrington Ave
Los Angeles, CA 90025
(310) 278-9050
www.tilomedical.com

● Lauren Feder, M.D. (pediatric)
6399 Wilshire Blvd., Ste 401
Los Angeles, California 90048
(323) 651-4454
www.drfeder.com

Newport Beach
● Pediatric Wellness Center
Pamela Middleton, M.D.
1501 Westcliff Drive #260
Newport Beach, CA 92260
(949) 631-5437
www.pediatricwellness.net

Pasadena
● Paracelsus Natural Family Health Ctr.
Simon Barker, N.D.
Daniel Brousseau, D.O.
740 N. Lake Avenue
Pasadena, CA 91104
(626) 794-4668
www.paracelsusla.com

Santa Monica
● Shera Raisen, M.D.
1260 15th Street, Suite 1006
Santa Monica, CA 90404
(310) 458-9200 www.doctorraisen.com

● Holistic, Complementary and Integrative Medicine pg.251
Wael Alomar, M.D.
1752 Ocean Park Blvd.
Santa Monica, CA 90405
(310) 433-5249
www.dralomar.com

● The Akasha Center for Integrative Medicine, Inc.
520 Arizona Avenue
Santa Monica, CA 90401
(310) 451-8880
www.akashacenter.com

Sherman Oaks
● Holistic Health Plus
Bruce Bielinski, W, M.D.
4419 Van Nuys Blvd Ste 400
Sherman Oaks, CA 91403
(818) 501-4202

Studio City

● **Sunrise Alternative Medicine Clinic**
Bena B. Won, L.Ac., Ph.D., R.N.
11239 Ventura Blvd., Suite 214
Studio City, CA 91604
(818) 508-6888
www.sunriseacupunctureclinic.com

Torrance

● **South Bay Total Health**
Arlan Cage, ND, MSOM, MS
2204 Torrance Blvd. Suite 104
Torrance, CA 90501
(310) 803-8803
www.southbaytotalhealth.com

● **Complete Wellness Foundation**
Trurina L. Cummings, C.T.N., Ph.D.
4001 Pacific Coast Hwy
Torrance, CA 90505
(310) 373-2250

● **Health Integration Center**
Eric I-Hung Lin, D.O.
3250 Lomita Blvd.,Suite 208
Torrance, CA 90505
(310) 326-8625

West Hollywood

● **Holistic Medical Center**
Emil Levin, M.D.   pg.29
8264 Santa Monica Blvd
West Hollywood, CA 90046
(323) 650-1789, (323) 650-9606

West Los Angeles

● **Kaya Wellness**
Poorvi Shah, D.O.
11925 Wilshire Boulevard, Suite 318
West Los Angeles, CA 90025
(323) 822-2901

Woodland Hills

● **Alternative Medicine Family Practice**
John Lynch, N.D.
23123 Ventura Blvd., Suite 210
Woodland Hills, CA 91364
(818) 259-0262
www.johnlynchnd.com

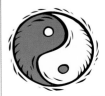

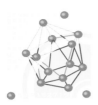

True Future of Healthcare

Uniting Alternative & Allopathic

Twenty years ago there was barely a glimmer of hope that conventional medicine would openly accept and share the limelight with complementary or alternative medicine. Alternative therapies were commonly labeled as quackery. A definition of quackery is *"the practice of fraudulent medicine for profit or for ego gratification and power,"* but the use of this term often points to something more general. It has been incorrectly and loosely used in the West to refer to any healthcare approach or modality that cannot be understood through the lens of allopathic training. Several organizations, created and supported by licensed medical doctors who distrust alternative medicine, broadcast their views on the internet, attempting to discredit the effectiveness of complementary modalities including acupuncture, ayurveda and chiropractic by using outdated, invalid scientific studies and conveniently forgetting to mention the most recent studies. The material is presented as fact and is written primarily by one opinionated M.D., attempting to create the illusion of mass opinion. Stuck in the past? Maybe, but things are beginning to change.

> Alternative medicine has an irreplaceable, positive role in our lives. Unfortunately it has been susceptible to the unjust "quackery" label. True quackery, however, still exists and caution must be taken in order to protect our wealth and health, which, in the hands of a quack is endangered. Quackery involves those with a medical degree as well as those without.

Western-oriented healthcare facilities throughout the US, frequently recommend, work with and even staff alternative healthcare professionals in their medical centers. More than one out of every four hospitals offer alternative and complementary therapies (CAM), such as acupuncture, homeopathy, or massage therapy. A new survey of nearly 1,400 U.S. hospitals shows that a great number of mainstream medical institutions are providing CAM therapies to meet the growing demand *[from: Hospitals Add Alternative Medicine, By Jennifer Warner WebMD Medical News, Reviewed By Louise Chang, MD, Thursday, July 20, 2006]* and it doesn't stop there. A survey of 18 HMOs and insurance providers, including Aetna, Medicare, Prudential, and Kaiser Permanente, found that 14 of the 18 covered at least 11 out of 34 alternative therapies. Chiropractic, massage therapy and acupuncture are the three most commonly covered therapies, followed by naturopathic care. *[from: 12 Common Questions About Insurance and Complementary / Alternative Medicine, From Cathy Wong, Your Guide to Alternative Medicine].*

"The art of healing comes from nature and not from the physician. Therefore, the physician must start from nature with an open mind."

-
Paracelsus,
Roman physician
(1493-1541)

When investigated closely, most of the alternative therapies covered by insurance are still limited by a lowered number of allowed visits per year. For example, Blue Cross California's PPO 40 Plan covers Physical and Occupational Therapy, chiropractic services, acupuncture and acupressure but each is limited to 12 visits per year. Most complementary therapies work as well as conventional therapies when it comes to non-emergency care and reducing the severity of chronic conditions. They often cost less and have fewer, if any, side effects. For example, acupuncture results in a reduction of arthritis pain with fewer side effects than medication, and St. John's Wort has been recently shown to effectively treat mild to moderate depression just as well as commonly prescribed antidepressant medication, while causing fewer side effects *[from: kaiserpermanente.org]*.

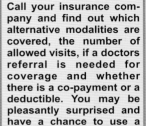

Call your insurance company and find out which alternative modalities are covered, the number of allowed visits, if a doctors referral is needed for coverage and whether there is a co-payment or a deductible. You may be pleasantly surprised and have a chance to use a services that you did not know were covered!

Why has the outlook changed recently? Is it just a trend? Many professionals have already noticed the shortcomings of a one-sided approach. Ultimately, the goal of every healthcare practitioner, no matter what their background, is to offer the best possible care for their patients. If scientific explanations for certain modalities are still unavailable (due to the inability to accurately measure velocities such as the human energy field, or lifeforce) practitioners will continue choosing to provide the most effective result-oriented care, based on their observation of what works. If science has not yet been able to prove the effectiveness of certain CAM modalities but the patients are happy with their treatment and results, naturally they will keep treating people with what works! Science and research will eventually catch up.

Complementary and alternative medicine (CAM) is an umbrella term for Alternative and Complementary medicine including practices that incorporate spiritual, metaphysical, or religious underpinnings; non-U.S. medical traditions, or newly developed approaches to healing. There are about 500 such systems.

-

"Healer's Guide 2007"

What exactly are the criteria for a CAM technique to be scientifically validated and subsequently approved? If symptom suppression or the subsiding of symptoms still continues to be considered success or validation, then it is possible that researchers are looking in the wrong direction. If success is measured by complete healing - returning one's health to the state prior to the illness, often inaccurately called spontaneous remission, this may be a more appropriate reflection of the rate of success. Another factor is often overlooked by the mind-oriented desire to have measurable proof. If inner-healing occurs on the mental, emotional or spiritual level, how is it possible to quantify, other than by the patient's testimonial? Is it possible that a shift in consciousness provides inner peace and healing far beyond what scientific equipment is able to measure?

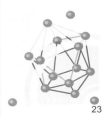

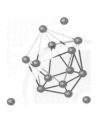

What appears to be practical or functional and what becomes mainstream practice often differs. There are two major objectives. First, there is the risk of under-treatment, by the sole use of CAM and second is the economical impact, yes, the money, and wisely so. The introduction of new services and solutions to take the place of or enhance the old services must move slowly, so as not to create economic chaos. At the same time, it is unfair to hang on to old systems for the sake of greed and profit. There have been mainstream medical discoveries within the past century, which have been proven to be effective and safe that were not accepted, and even banned as mainstream practice. New medical procedures costing a mere few hundred dollars, coupled with a measurable success rate and no side effects pose a threat to the complex, but well established medical system with advanced procedures costing tens of thousands of dollars. It always takes time to break a habit, especially one with an invested economy and a 100 year tradition. Complementary medicine, on the other hand, can be gradually integrated into the system, bringing great benefit and fitting into the economic structure.

In February of 2001, several medical professionals working in four small hospitals in Central Europe, discovered that by "choking" a malignant tumor inside a patient's body, they could trigger a unique immune system awakening. The malignant tumor, including its metastasis, were then quickly cleared up by the body's own intelligence. This relatively simple procedure

Research Details:

The first stage of clinical tests of the technique for the Devitalization of tumors (conducted at 4 hospitals in the Czech Republic, beginning February 2001) has fully confirmed two initial findings of Prague-born surgeon Dr. Karel Fortyn (1930-2001). According to the study:

Ligation of tumor, left in the body, but merely deprived of blood supply, results in no dangerous sepsis. Such tissues are not damaged, but "healthy" only "starving" to death the body being able to adjust to (and, therefore, cope with) gradually starving (which is to say, gradually dying tissues) and that it is essential to ligate both arteries and veins (leading to and from the tumor).

The primary discovery by Dr. Fortyn that the tumor, when dying of starvation, triggers an attack of the body's immune system against all cancer cells of the same type (resulting in their eventual eradication) could not be fully proved in this initial stage of clinical testing due to the fact(s) that:

(1) too short a period of time had passed to be able to objectively assess the final results, and (2) all of the participants in these initial tests were already by that time in the fourth stage of their cancers' development, and were already post-chemotherapy (which had seriously weakened their immune systems).

This effect had been proved on 20 of Dr. Fortyn's patients, and also on many others who had been (more or less "illegally") operated on by his colleagues and followers over the next 44 years, and also in animal cases in laboratory experiments and veterinary offices over the past thirty years.

" The ideal physician and surgeon is the man who is also a metaphysician; to the lack of this combination much of the present difficulty and confusion can be ascribed"

-

"Esoteric Healing 1998", D.K. by Alice A.

Based on results from the first stage of tests, the second stage of clinical testing is now being prepared for. The Czech Association of Patients has (as of October 14th, 2001) established a Scientific Council, the purpose of which is to cooperate with the Czech Ministry of Health on these preparations. New testings will more precisely follow the findings and recommendations of Dr. Fortyn (i.e., NO chemotherapy should be advised before devitalization, which should be performed earlier than in the fourth stage of cancer; ligature of the main tumor is to be preferred).
For more information visit: www.pacienti.cz/devitalization.htm

is one of several that have potential, and require further research and investigation; and may, in fact, leave patients cancer-free for an estimated cost of a few hundred dollars with enough support and recognition.

The above-mentioned research illustrates that for a long time it was believed and therefore taught in medical schools, that dying tissue inside the human body may be the cause of acute sepsis leading to the death of the patient. Now we know that this was not exactly correct. It was also believed that the Earth was a short cylinder with a flat, circular top. Anyone who did not support this idea was persecuted until Pythagoras (6th century BC) proved otherwise. Is it possible that alternative therapies just need more time to be confirmed by science?

Orthodox allopathy can be likened to a bundle of habits (methods of cure). Overall, these habits or techniques have an undoubtedly beneficial outcome and a proven record of success for improving one's health, but when these habits requires an upgrade or a more effective replacement, it must be processed by the machinery - including government, health departments and legal channels - before it is approved. This can be compared to feeding a pre-historic animal. You give it food on one end and expect it to come out on the other the next day, but to your surprise, there is a three week lag time. The current system is like a pre-historic animal, but slower. It doesn't matter if the outdated habit is no longer the best available, and logically should be replaced - by a new alternative or conventional method - it just takes too long.

Patient's requests for better medical care are primarily addressed to physicians or their administrative support who, under the load of responsibilities, may not have the time or energy to fight for these important changes. So, to create the necessary changes, the responsibility falls upon the shoulders of the patients (the consumer) who, by raising their voices, create a demand and speed up the process. The majority of health care professionals are already aware of the necessity of an integrative approach. Many pioneers have risked their medical licenses to start the battle, but their missing ally is the overwhelming force of the public (you included), openly requesting these changes.

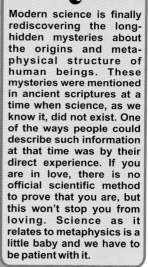

☯

Modern science is finally rediscovering the long-hidden mysteries about the origins and meta-physical structure of human beings. These mysteries were mentioned in ancient scriptures at a time when science, as we know it, did not exist. One of the ways people could describe such information at that time was by their direct experience. If you are in love, there is no official scientific method to prove that you are, but this won't stop you from loving. Science as it relates to metaphysics is a little baby and we have to be patient with it.

"Science will never be able to reduce the value of a sunset to arithmetic. Nor can it reduce friendship or statesmanship to a formula."

-

Louis M. Orr,
Head Coach at Seton Hall University,
2001-2006.

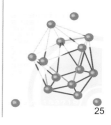

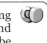

An Interview

with Emil Levin, M.D. on his view of alternative medicine professionals and orthodox allopathy today.

Dr. Levin, you are a medical doctor practicing holistically. You have studied homeopathy and naturopathy in Germany; have a medical degree in Russia and in the United States and many years of experience in the field. What is your opinion about the booming business with alternative health care modalities?

Competition is healthy and should be encouraged. The freedom of the patient should not be impeded in any way. Each patient must be allowed to choose the method of medical care appropriate for them. Narrow-minded healthcare standards by government agencies should not be enforced. Western Medical care only looks for the tip of the iceberg. It does not look for the marginal shifts in physiology which dramatically affect the patient's health.

Do you think that alternative and holistic care and the patients' shift in focus is a trend and that the excitement will cease?

No, I believe that the demand will increase tremendously. More and more people are looking for answers. They are seeking out holistic treatment because western medicine is not helping them to get well - it only treats their symptoms. The public will no longer tolerate the status quo established many years ago by the megagiants and pharmaceutical companies. One of my colleagues, a reputable western medical doctor who is a cardiologist, recently told me that some of his patients have questions about alternative medicine. One of the common questions they are asking is about his opinion on co-enzyme Q-10. This is not an unusual request. Patients are more knowledgeable today - they have access to a tremendous amount of information, which was previously unavailable to the public. Now, they are questioning their healthcare professionals and they expect their questions to be answered knowledgeably.

What do you think of the relationship today between orthodox medicine and alternative medicine?

Approximately twenty-five years ago, western doctors looked down on holistic doctors and called them quacks. But now, some of these western doctors are very interested in what holistic medicine has to offer. Western doctors who become holistic doctors are experiencing excellent results.

What do you think has motivated so many medical professional to change their mind and start accepting and incorporating holistic approach into their practice?

More and more, patients are spending their money on holistic care, even though most treatments and supplements are is not covered by insurance. They are spending money because they are getting results. Holistic doctors are needed today. The western doctors are going into this field because of the satisfaction in being able to help their patients. At the very least, alternative applications will influence, if not bring about a cure entirely. I have yet to find one disease that holistic medicine cannot favorably influence. The holistic doctors are experiencing tremendous results without chemicals or drugs.

There are two categories of western doctors. The first are those westerns medical doctors who are switching their services to a holistic practice. The result is that their patients are becoming well and benefitting from the treatment without any bad side-effects.

The second group are those who follow the western system exclusively. The classically trained medical doctors are told what to prescribe, how to treat and are given strict guidelines which they must follow. They come to depend on their high patent load and become very comfortable, financially. Therefore, they are not looking to learn and grow or to seek more holistic information on how they can help their patients.

What is your opinion of energy healers and other alternative or holistic care providers and their ability to influence the health of their clients?

Excellent. It happens in my office every day. I practice holistically and medically. My patients respond very well to those alternative treatments. If my patients require medical treatments or prescription drugs, I am able to do so, as well. If services are required beyond my medical training, then I will refer them to a specialist.

Would you recommend an alternative healing approach to your patients and if so what do you think their reaction would be, in general?

Most of our patients are already holistically-oriented. They live a holistic lifestyle, come in for regular, preventative treatment and take very good care of their health. They are knowledgeable in this field. They understand and appreciate the framework of my practice and the care I am able to offer.

Would you be willing to work with an experienced healer side-by-side and what difference do you think it would make to your patients?

Yes, it would definitely benefit our patients tremendously.

Do you think that it is realistic for a western medical professional to be a great doctor as well as an experienced healer simultaneously?

Everything is possible. I believe that both western and holistic doctors in their own way want to help their patients, within the framework of their

practice. But due to the fact that western doctors are unable to step outside of that framework, their knowledge is limited and therefore, they can only offer prescription drugs which suppress symptoms and always have side-effects. This type of care does not go to the cause of the problem. On the other hand, the holistic approach does.

Is there anything you would like to say or recommend to our readers?

Yes, absolutely. It is not about homeopathy vs. antibiotics, or vitamins vs. pharmaceutical drugs. People have to start thinking in terms of changing their lifestyle. Not many people want to or care to do so. "The doctor will give me a pill and I'll be fine" is not the way of the future. Look around you. If you want physical change, then you must change your diet. Diet is the major thing. The regular food in the United States is contaminated with chemicals and preservatives. These chemicals do not belong in the human body. Toxins are a huge problem. Start eliminating foods such as pizza, diet soda and soft drinks. (Soft drinks have an enormous amount of sugar). Good health is like building a house. You must prepare the foundation first. The foundation is the diet. If you want to preserve your health, you must eat right.

In Europe, you do not find hormones and antibiotics in the food, as is the case in the United States. This alters the ecology. Good food is not a cheap commodity – if food is cheap, it is lacking nutrients and quality.

Let's look at symptoms for a moment. Say you have dandruff. Weeks later, the skin is dry and begins to crack. Then, the intestinal tract becomes inflamed. After some time there is blood in stool – colitis. These symptoms are different pages of the same book. At the first sign of dandruff, you might visit the dermatologist or the local drug store, to get a special shampoo to cover up the dandruff. Then years go by and all of a sudden, there is blood in the bowel. Dandruff is often an early sign of a gluten sensitivity or lack of fatty acids. You need fish oil, not shampoo. Patients can easily get lost in specialization. Dermatologists, ear-nose-throat specialists, gastrointerologists, etc., all treat symptoms. This is a horrific injustice. In this example, if you address the initial problem holistically – you quickly find the cause of the problem – lack of quality oils, and avoid having the bigger problem of blood in your bowel years later.

Let's discuss cholesterol. The heart consumes fatty acids for its metabolism – borage, fish oil. Muscles run on glucose. We have been given wrong information. Butter is not a cursed word; egg is not a cursed word; cholesterol is not a cursed word. Without cholesterol people become sexless jellyfish. We need good cholesterol. It is produced by our bodies. The important thing to discuss is - what is good cholesterol and what are triglycerides? Only 10% of cholesterol in human body is diet-related. No one looks for a certified fire department fire extinguisher when you have a fire in your house – you look for the quickest solution - the nearest source of water. If you do not have enough antioxidants in the body, the body looks for the easiest solution. It will start to produce cholesterol to put out the fire, which soon oxidizes and damages the inside of your arteries. The body's primary business is to sustain life. People should search for the right knowledge regarding their metabolism and learn how to take care of themselves properly. Then, they will know how to choose the right doctor for their needs.

Constipation is a common problem, leading to more severe conditions. A lack of fiber is detrimental. Take care of the diet and increase the fiber in order to eliminate regularly. When constipated, the colon becomes toxic to the body. Women only need two simple things to remain healthy, enough sleep and proper elimination. When they have a full time career and children to take care of, often they are lacking sleep and suffer from poor elimination. This leads to reproductive system

dysfunction, problems with the levels of hormones, followed by fibroids in the uterus and then, in many cases, western doctors will recommend removing the uterus. A holistic doctor would not make this recommendation. A holistic doctor will suggest that the patient cleanse the colon and liver, eat proper diet, juicing and in some cases homeopathy. This same treatment would be recommended to women with PMS, as this is often caused by having a toxic liver.

Pay attention to minor symptoms. We are biochemical beings. Take care of the body's chemistry through proper diet and nutrition and it will take care of you.

[Holistic Medical Center, Emil Levin, M.D., see page 27]

Holistic Medical Center
Emil Levin, M.D.

Emil Levin, M.D., has practiced Homeopathic and Holistic Medicine since 1969. He uses various European methods to build up the immune system to fight diseases.

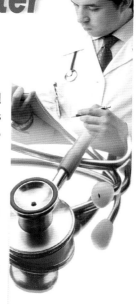

● Colon Hydrotherapy:
People can eliminate as much as 10 - 30lbs over a series of treatments by cleansing out their colon.

● Allergies:
Homeopathic method of desensitization to environmental & food allergies.

● Chelation Therapy:
Highly effective treatment for removal of metabolic and environmental toxins. Restoration of circulation for athero-sclerotic vascular disease. Reduces high blood pressure, controls blood sugar and prevents heart disease.

● Parasites:
21 million Americans are infected, leading to one of the major causes of chronic illness.

● Natural Weight Loss:
An Australian method, up to 5lbs. per week.

Specializing in:
- Viral Infections
- Arthritis
- Candidiasis
- Headache
- Asthma
- Hepatitis
- PMS
- Dermatitis
- Eczema
- Diabetes
- Constipation
- Colitis
- Cardiovascular Diseases

Emil Levin, M.D.
Holistic Medical Center
8264 Santa Monica Blvd.
Los Angeles, CA

(323) 650.9606

An interview

with Craig Alan Ravenscroft, D.C. on his view of alternative medicine professionals and orthodox allopathy today.

Dr. Ravenscroft, you are a Doctor of Chiropractic at the Health First Chiropractic & Wellness Center and you have 15 years experience in the field. What is your opinion of orthodox medicine?

I see more openness to alternative healing as MDs see more of their patients choosing alternative methods. I don't believe that they will accept alternatives on their own unless there is a attitude shift amongst people in general towards non-medicated, non-surgical methods of treatment. I think the medical associations are still trying to find ways to stifle alternatives, in the name of protecting the public.

What do you think drives your clients to visit your office instead of a conventional medical clinic?

They don't want to take drugs. They aren't getting better at their regular medical clinic.

Do you think alternative modalities could, in some cases, be more powerful than an allopathic approach and do you have an example of that?

Emphatically yes. I had a case recently where the patient came in with sciatica, was very guarded in his movements, and after the first treatment, he walked out normally with no sciatica.

What do you think the position of alternative medicine is in relation to allopathic medical care today?

Unfortunately, we are still subservient to the medical/insurance establishment.

What do you think has motivated so many medical professionals to change their approach and to start accepting and incorporating holistic elements into their practice?

For the most part, it is because they see their patients going to alternatives in larger numbers. Also, if alternative healers can develop a good relationship with MDs, then the MDs can personally see the effectiveness of alternative healing.

What is your feeling about the competence of CAM providers and the ability of CAM providers to influence the health conditions of their clients?

I think the abilities and competence of alternatives are all over the spectrum. Some are very talented. Some have a good heart, but not much skill. Some people are just in it for money. It is like any field anywhere.

Would you recommend an allopathic approach to your clients and if so what do you think their reaction would be in general?

Yes, and most people understand that at certain times they need stronger healing methods.

Would you be willing to work with side-by-side with an experienced medical doctor? What difference do you think it would make to your clients?

Yes, I think that most people who see me would think positively about that and I feel that for the patients, a variety of views and experience on healing can only be beneficial. No one way works for all people.

Do you think that it is realistic for a medical professional to be a great doctor as well as an experienced holistic healer, simultaneously?

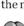

How can you be one without the other?

Is there anything you would like to say or recommend to our readers?

In order to understand health it is necessary to get an understanding of disease and the process to achieve health. All living beings are animated with a vital force or energy which the ancient Chinese gave the name "chi." It is this force which produces and maintains health in living beings. Unfortunately, in our life, we are subject to many external and internal processes that create blockages in the flow of chi throughout our body. Some of these negative influences are strong emotions, strong weather changes, improper diet, physical trauma, and infectious elements such as virus and bacteria. All have immediate and long lasting effects on our health. For example, the chicken pox that you had as a child does not completely leave your body. The virus remains latent in your nervous system and years later, when your immune system is weak, often with old age, you can develop a very painful condition called shingles which is a reactivation of the chicken pox virus.

Now, the job of all doctors, even though they may not know it, is to provide treatment to eliminate these blockages to the proper flow of chi. It can be in the form of chemical medicines, herbal medicine, acupuncture needles, acupressure, chiropractic adjustment, massage, exercise, and nutrition.

All of these methods work to restore your body's healing energy to function as it normally should. The art involved in using these various methods is to understand the strength of the disease versus the strength of the treatment and using that which is most appropriate. For example, when you use chemical medicines you are declaring full scale war on the disease. So you go in with the heavy artillery resulting in heavy collateral damage. Now, it is acceptable to have heavy collateral damage, *i.e.* side effects, when you are fighting an aggressive cancer, but why drop an atomic bomb when you

have a lone terrorist with a pistol, such as a cold.

The second job of the doctor, after providing treatments and therapies, is to educate the patient in methods to help eliminate the blockages and improve the strength and quality of chi flow. The doctor takes a less active role in this stage as the patient learns to understand how to live a balanced, harmonious lifestyle. Here, the patient must do the majority of the work, as experience is the only way to learn. The doctor can only stand on the sidelines and point the direction to go. At this point, the patient begins to take responsibility for doing the work, for deciding how to follow the doctors' advice, and for developing a knowledge of their personal physical limits, as well as accepting that they may have overdone an exercise resulting in pain afterwards. This is all part of the learning process that every one of us must undergo in our journey to full health. Ultimately, we have to accept that what happens in our life is our creation, positively or negatively.

Therapy and treatment will be more intensive in the beginning to remove the major blockages and to teach you how to eliminate, through exercise, meditation and nutrition, the minor blockages that remain. After several months to a year, treatments reduce to a maintenance level so that any developing blocks are handled before they cause major problems. With or without a doctor's care, the patient will continue to use the exercise and nutrition advice throughout the rest of their life.

[Health First Chiropractic, Dr. Craig Alan Ravenscroft - Frazier Park, CA]

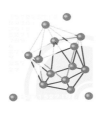

If you read carefully through the interviews, the viewpoint of holistic healthcare professionals is self-explanatory. The road to successful healing is the holistic approach where it is important to listen to the advice of both medical doctors and healers. This eliminates any confusion with regards to differences in treatment and it also ensures the safety of the healing process.

So how exactly does this new medical paradigm function? The emphasis is on the patient's individual effort to heal. This is to avoid the usual scenario: *"I went to my doctor. He prescribed some pills and told me to come back three weeks later for a check-up"* and to replacing it with: *"I went to my doctor and asked for holistic, integrative care. He gave me a diagnosis, prescribed medication and referred me to an alternative practitioner, who provided the additional treatment my physician was unable to offer."* This is the first and most important step. Patients must ask for the holistic approach.

The second step - and necessary part of the equation - is the ability of physicians to maintain critical open-mindedness and cooperate with alternative specialists. This has already begun! Statistics show that integrative care is emerging and holds a promising future. Kudos to all practitioners who are already there! While some medical clinics and smaller private practices are referring their

Many major hospitals have a Wellness Center or in-house program to provide CAM care. Physicians regard the Wellness Center as a valuable resource for the prevention of heart and lung disease, and might recommend programs for "borderline" patients as well as individuals with diabetes, cholesterol problems or who are overweight.

"The competent physician, before he attempts to give medicine to the patient, makes himself acquainted not only with the disease, but also with the habits and constitution of the sick man."

-
Marcus Tullius Cicero, philosopher of Ancient Rome (106 BC - 43 BC)

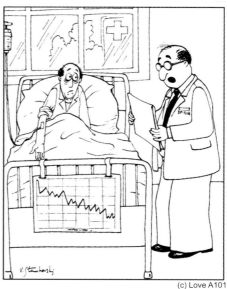

(c) Love A101

"Well Bob, I'm afraid we've exhausted our medical options, but we do have a few spells we can try...."

patients to alternative practitioners, others are sharing an office with an alternative healer to provide a wholesome approach. Medical clinics and hospitals are encouraged to offer mandatory training to educate their staff about the benefits of CAM treatments and when to recommend them. CAM practitioners and healers play an integral role and it is our hope, that soon they will be an inseparable part of the medical staff at all facilities.

Here is a voice representing a major hospital. Even though not local, their statement is a vote and a step towards the acceptance and recognition of alternative care by hospitals. *"Medical doctors, by and large, classify alternative practitioners as "quacks," which is defined by Webster as fraudulent doctors. If a patient goes to an allopathic doctor for months or years and eventually is told, "there is no more medicine can do for you," and then that patient turns to an alternative practitioner who helps them and may even cure them - who is the quack?"* [Kurt W. Donsbach, D.C., N.D., Ph.D.]

The third step is an expression of interest by the public that further encourages the widespread acceptance of CAM by government institutions. Several hearings at the White House Commission on Complementary and Alternative Medicine Policy addressed a wider and more accessible use of alternative modalities and recently resulted in a no-win situation. The scientists called for more research to find out which modalities are proven to work. This information will provide the basis for the decisions regarding which of the CAM therapies and treatments would be officially incorporated with conventional medicine and which will be excluded. Support this research by participating in CAM studies. These are the building blocks for the successful legislative changes which will make alternative care part of mainstream medicine. You can take action right now. Below are the websites to find more information.

> **Clinical trials where volunteers are needed:**
> ❏ www.cancer.uchc.edu/clinical_trials/
> ❏ www.nccam.nih.gov/clinicaltrials/factsheet/index.htm
> ❏ www.cancer.gov/cam/clinicaltrials_intro.html

Hospitals are business entities with overhead, including loans and wages to pay and income to generate, the same as any other business. Their income is derived from MediCare, Medicaid, Blue Cross/Shield, Commercial Ins., HMOs/PPOs, self-pay, workers compensation and other reimbursements generated by patients. The more patients treated, the more revenue. If patients get well quickly, no further medical care is necessary and no further income can be generated.

☯ Your physician may know of holistic solutions that could benefit you, but may not offer them. When you request holistic care, it sends a message to your physician that alternative medicine is a safe area of discussion with you and that holistic suggestions will be well received.

" It will be wise, for a very long time to come, for the spiritual healer to work always in collaboration with a trained physician. The healer will provide the required occult knowledge"
-
Esoteric Healing, 1998,
D.K. by Alice A. Bailey

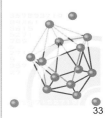

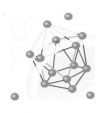

Could it happen that hospitals could lose income from the patients who get well by incorporating other healing modalities which are considerably cheaper than conventional care? It is estimated that a typical, insured American family of four, in one year, spent $13,382 in 2006 on medical care, with the family paying approximately 38% of this cost (approx. $5,050). It is also estimated that a family of four in California spends approximately $2,450 for alterative care. This is almost 50% of what is paid out-of-pocket towards conventional care. It is in everyone's interest that CAM therapies are included in the orthodox system - for the insured patient, the medical institutions, the insurance companies and those who stand behind the hospital funding counting their profits. Medical care is a consumer-driven business. If the consumer (patient) creates a sizable demand, the supply will change as well.

> Regular preventative holistic care such as massage therapy, energy healing, acupuncture, ayurveda, helps avoid financial devastation. Researchers at Harvard University surveyed 1,771 Americans in bankruptcy. About 50% answered that medical causes drove them to bankruptcy. Today it's easy to run up a $80,000 hospital bill. Even with 80% insurance coverage you would still have to pay $16,000 out of pocket.

The new form of medical care starts with the patient asking the following question when contacting the physician: "Doctor, would you be willing to consider my case from the holistic perspective and recommend other therapies I can integrate for the best results?" When visiting a CAM practitioner always ask: "Do you know of a conventional treatment that I should ask my medical doctor about in this case?" When implementing an integrative approach in your care program, the physical, emotional, mental, environmental and spiritual aspects are addressed. This represents a partial list of CAM professionals who are ready to assist:

● Chiropractor, Massage Therapist, Rolfer - to align the spine, improve nerve signals to the organs and brain, bring blood supply and nutrients to the tissues, remove waste products from tissues and lymph and improve the efficiency of the lymphatic system.

● Psychologist, Hypnotherapist - for the mental and emotional aspects related to the illness. To uncover old traumas locked in the subconscious mind which affect the overall health and often are the root of the illness.

● Neurofeedback - for imbalances or improper functioning of the brain, learning disabilities.

● Herbalist, Nutritionist - to provide the body a proper individualized nutrition plan, glandular support, etc.

● Energy Healer - to remove unsupportive energies or balance energetically congested, depleted or blocked areas, including blocks caused by old traumas, improve or increase energy flow where needed, restore proper function to the energetic

"I got the bill for my surgery. Now I know what those doctors were wearing masks for."
-
Dr. James H. Boren, internationally acclaimed humorist

centers (chakras), thereby influencing the health and condition of the endocrine system and entire body.

- Spiritual Counselors - help understand illness from a spiritual perspective. To receive guidance and help to implement a corresponding spiritual practice.

The true future of healthcare relies on a shift in the demand from the majority of the population and not solely on the physicians or CAM practitioners, who have already accepted the holistic ideal. When millions of people become aware of how effective the holistic approach is and raise their voices - out of sheer necessity - it may not be surprising to find that science will not be far behind and prove it to work. Take action now. Start asking the right questions!

> Your opinion helps health care practitioners to know exactly what the public wants and expects from their alternative or conventional medical care. Participate in our *Healer's Guide 2007* survey and help us to get practitioners on the same page.
>
> www.HealerGuide.com/survey2007

Cornerstones of the holistic philosophy:

❒ The best of the both worlds, conventional and CAM are combined.

❒ The human body, including the mental and emotional aspects, has an inborn ability to heal which is ultimately responsible for healing.

❒ Medical Diagnosis must always be accompanied by an attempt to understand the root cause of the illness.

❒ Treatments are designed to address the root cause of an illness, not just the symptoms.

❒ Treatment is result-oriented, meaning that restoring a patient's health is the priority and this can involve the use of "alternative" methods, as long as they are safe and helpful.

❒ Treatment is uniquely tailored to each patient based on their symptoms, personality, habits, background and the underlying cause of the illness. Practitoners refrain from a one-size-fits-all approach.

❒ Patients are perceived and respected as complex beings with physical, emotional, mental and spiritual aspects.

❒ The patient is ultimately responsible for the healing. The practitioners and their techniques or medications are only facilitators.

❒ The corresponding lifestyle management, education and prevention is always implemented with the treatment.

❒ Medication or surgery is an option, but utilized as a last resort.

❒ Death is a time of transition and spiritual help, prayer and healing must be administered at this time.

"The next major advance in the health of the American people will be determined by what the individual is willing to do for himself."

- John H. Knowles, M.D.

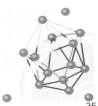

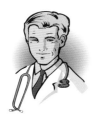

Respect & Discernment

Respect for Doctors and Healers Alike

Respect for medical professionals is quite common and has been in place for centuries. When visiting the doctor, patients switch to a submissive position, ready to receive and accept the verdict about their condition. Why question the diagnosis? The doctor knows best, no doubt.

After waiting from 30 minutes to one hour to see the doctor, patients anxiously look forward to having their symptoms assessed and their condition labeled, so they may quickly get back to their life routine with a prescription in hand to control their symptoms. Since most use a vacation or sick day for the doctor's visit and no one wants to spend the entire day at a medical clinic or resting in bed, the diagnosis and medication is quickly accepted without further question. Is this a delusion? Disease deserves one's full attention and it starts with an investigation and introspection as to the cause. Start asking questions. First of yourself, then of your care providers.

This will replace the "blind" respect for doctors with healthy respect and discernment. Taking time for a second opinion or a few days to think things through before deciding about a

> **Doctors and healers, both sacrificed years of their lives to learn their respective healing arts so that they may be in service to humanity. Although their training and techniques are a world apart, they are in essence two parts which complete each other to create a whole. They both deserve equal respect.**

"Patients - when they really have control over their lives and over their disease in some way I think are overall going to do better regardless of whether that comes from traditional treatments or a combination of western medicine plus other alternative approaches."

-
Bill Owen,
English actor
(1914 - 1999)

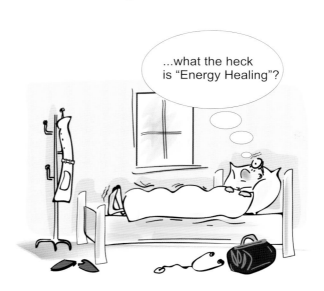

...what the heck is "Energy Healing"?

recommended procedure or taking prescription drugs is a good idea in a non-emergency situation.

Medical doctors studied for years to gain valuable knowledge. They literally sacrificed years of their lives to study and will spend the remainder helping others. This deserves healthy respect. If becoming a doctor was as easy as passing a driving test, we would be stuck in the traffic of doctors with no respect! They follow the guidelines and the system as they were taught, to the best of their knowledge, with the best intentions. But the system, like all man-made systems, has its flaws and human error, on occasion, is a part of life whether you are an accountant, construction worker, or a physician.

As children, we all have dreams about what profession we will choose. Many are told by their parents which occupation to choose - doctor, lawyer, politician. As we get older, we come to understand that one job is not superior over another. What truly matters is if we love our job. Respect belongs to those who work with love and integrity, regardless of their occupation. With this attitude, all jobs are equal; we all serve humanity.

There is a second group of caring souls who also felt called to help in the field of health care, but knew that in order to truly heal, the physical, emotional, mental, and spiritual aspects must be understood. Western medicine did not offer the broad scope of techniques and wisdom required to be an expert in this field, so they went on a quest for uncommon knowledge. Frequently prompted by personal health issues they traveled the world to find a cure. This led to the discovery of ancient healing techniques and spiritual studies with elders or masters, to uncover the roots of illness. Attending countless healing arts and self-improvement workshops they learned the secrets and mysteries of healing and spirituality. This journey resulted in an understanding of the psychological make-up of others as it relates to health; the ability to work with cosmic, natural laws and subtle energy to promote healing (described in detail in the *Body-Mind-Soul section, Part 2*); and an understanding of the importance of taking responsibility for one's personal well-being. Investigation of life's events and lessons brought a glimpse of the complexity of things and revealed the truths behind. They achieved balance, harmony and the know-how to discover and correct the underlying imbalances behind illness and its symptoms.

Through years of meditation, introspection and learning what is seldom taught, these seekers gained the Healer's Consciousness. This wisdom is distilled and translated into an invaluable service called a healing session. What is shown to clients in a few sessions would take a decade or more to learn. It is important to mention here that although healers utilize energy modalities and may apply a specific method, the kinds of techniques implemented in each healing session are as

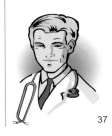

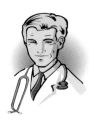

varied and unique as the individual seeking help. It may be an energy healing technique, it may be something as simple as a short conversation that shifts one's consciousness, or it may be nothing more than specific lifestyle instructions for the individual to follow that result in healing. It is virtually impossible to use the kinds of scientific tools currently available to measure soul wisdom and the profound healing effect it has on peoples lives.

Now, when we have an understanding and appreciation for the effort required to become a medical doctor or a healer and we have an equal and healthy respect for both, we must help build a friendly, professional bridge between them, encouraging healthy respect for each other. There are doctors and healers working in this capacity already. They are the pioneers of this virtue, providing an example for those who will follow in their footsteps.

You are responsible for your health, healing and wellbeing. Not your doctor, healer or other professional. They are there to advise, facilitate and assist. You must take control, use your guidance and decide wisely.

Medical doctors who respect and realize the value of CAM healers listen to their wisdom and suggestions. Healers, recognizing the success record of orthodox medical care, are able to work with a physician for the benefit of their patient.

Each time you visit a medical doctor promote this model relationship. Ask if they work holistically, or if they would be willing to research a holistic approach for your condition. Are they able to recommend a healer who is able to support healing on more than just a physical level? Ask your healer or practitioner if they are able to recommend an orthodox physician who will provide an accurate diagnosis and other forms of remedial treatment. Your questions will help to unite orthodox and alternative medicine.

Participate in the co-creation of the future of our new health care system. A system that integrates all aspects of the human being. A system where all things are inseparable. Purely physical, purely energetic or spiritual, they are merely different aspects of each human being.

Investigate, take responsibility and action. Interview healthcare professionals and use discernment when selecting your practitioner. Orthodox or alternative, help yourself to better health care. Health is not only the absence of disease, it is the highest level of wellbeing we can achieve.

Learn2heal
Getting to know us...

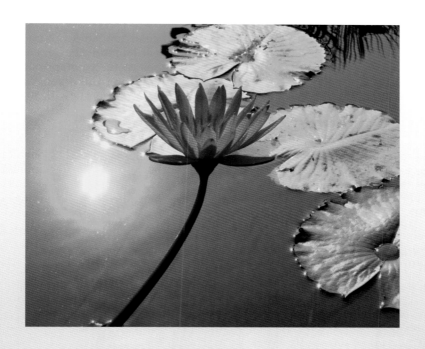

Professional Energy Healing Services and Quality Care
Healer and Therapist Training
Workshops and Spiritual Events

(310) 809 2237
www.Learn2heal.com

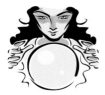

Selecting Your Practitioner

Things You Should Know

Before you start implementing your holistic healthcare goals, decide which modality or modalities are most appropriate. Learn which one or ones are the right match for your health concerns. Refer to the *Modalities* section in *Healer's Guide* for a list and their applications first.

Diabetes will have particular modalities more suitable for its care, as cancer will demand other choices. Next, discuss the modalities with your primary care physician, followed by asking those you know and trust if they have had any experiences with alternative health care. Your friends may be able to recommend qualified professionals they know. Ask what experiences they have had with the healing techniques and therapies you are considering. Chances are they will be able to offer a few pointers.

The following are helpful tips for finding your practitioner:

• Ask your doctor or other health professionals for a referral.

> Some people self-diagnose and then present their findings to their physician. The key to finding the right practitioner and the cure is to first find out what your health goal is and then look for someone to provide assistance. Some may say, "I have an upset stomach," when they could be asking, "How can I improve my digestion?"
>
> Self-diagnosing is the fastest way to medication, while setting the health goal brings the cure.

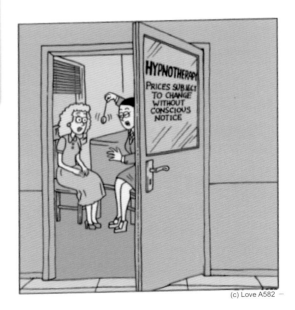

(c) Love A582

- Ask someone you know who has used alternative therapies for a recommendation.

- Contact your local medical center to find out if they staff alternative practitioners.

- Search the *Healer's Guide* for someone in your neighborhood.

- Contact the professional organization representing the modality you require. See the resource box below for a list of organizations. Organizations often provide referrals to practitioners in your area. If you are not sure whether a particular therapy or treatment is appropriate, they will offer guidelines as to the standards of practice as well as any recommended reference materials or literature explaining the modality. They will also let you know whether it is mandatory for practitioners to be licensed or certified and may verify that the practitioner you are considering has in fact, been trained according to industry standards and is able to provide quality service.

Selecting your conventional or CAM professional is like shopping for a car. Be prepared to invest some time and take several test drives before you find the right fit. After all, your health is worth more than a car! 150 years ago people were limited to having only one healthcare professional. Today we can choose. Shop for the best one; take your time to find the right match. Be prepared to try more than one!

Resources and guidelines on how to choose and locate health care practitioners:

❑ **American Academy of Family Physicians, (AAFP)** - Choose a Family Doctor (Smart Patient Guide) - www.familydoctor.org

❑ **American Holistic Medical Association, (AHMA) -** Direction for choosing a Holistic Practitioner www.holisticmedicine.org/public/pub_selecting.shtml

❑ **Holistic Health Network -** Find a Holistic Practitioner www.holisticnetwork.org

❑ **Spine-Health.com** - How to select the best chiropractor www.spine-health.com

❑ **National Center for Complementary and Alternative Medicine (NCCAM) -** Selecting a CAM Practitioner www.nccam.nih.gov/health/practitioner/index.htm

❑ **Alternative Medicine Foundation Inc. (AMFI)** - Choosing an Alternative or Complementary Medicine Practitioner www.amfoundation.org/practitioner.htm

❑ **The Richard & Hinda Rosenthal Center for Complementary & Alternative Medicine** - CAM Resources for Patients and Consumers www.rosenthal.hs.columbia.edu

Here are some helpful questions to ask the practitioner you have found:

- What is their education, licensing or certification?

- If you are not sure what level of schooling or training is required, check to see if the practitioner's qualifications meet the educational and training standards for that modality.

- Do they offer a consultation in person or by phone? This will give you the chance to ask any questions before scheduling an

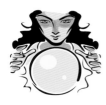

appointment. Keep in mind that some practitioners have a consultation fee.

● Do they specialize or have experience with your particular illness or problem?

● What is their general approach to treating or healing? You may also ask how effective and successful their approach has been with your particular illness. Some modalities will have scientific research or information relating to studies and if so, the practitioner will most likely direct you to or offer that information.

● How many patients does the practitioner typically see in a day, how long is each session and how much advance notice is required to schedule an appointment?

● Is there written material available so you may research further?

● What is the cancellation policy? How much advance notice must you give?

● Ask about charges and payment options. How much is the first visit or session and subsequent visits?

● Ask what happens during the first visit so you can be prepared.

● Does insurance cover this form of treatment and does the practitioner accept insurance? Do they bill the insurance company or give you a bill for future reimbursement?

● If you have physical difficulties and need an elevator or wheelchair access, ask.

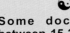

Some doctors see between 15-20 patients per day. There is a good reason why airlines do not schedule overworked pilots to fly planes and there also is a good reason why an overworked doctor should not be chosen to steer your health.

Above all, use your intuition, guidance and discernment. You will probably know right away if this is the right practitioner for you. See how your interaction goes and if you feel comfortable. Have you found someone you can communicate comfortably with and who listens to you? Here are a few guidelines for the initial interview (in-person or over the phone). The purpose of this conversation is not to treat or diagnose. Therefore be as direct and straight to the point without elaborating extensively about pains and symptoms. Do not ask or expect to be given the answers or solutions to your health problems in the consultation or over the phone. You are interviewing them to see if they are the right fit, not asking for advice or treatment yet.

If you are not sure about the practitioner, call another. Then assess the information given by both, to make an educated decision. Select the individual you feel will best serve your needs and whose image reflects what they practice. One who walks the talk. You won't choose a sick healer, an overweight person to help you loose weight, a broke person to give you financial advice or a psychologist who seems nuts!

Are We People or Are We Sheeple?
by: Michele Cohen, D.C.

Wouldn't it be great if our healthcare system really was about caring for the health of people? And wouldn't it be great if health insurance was really about insuring that people are, in fact, healthy? Well, unfortunately this is not the case.

While America is truly one of the best places to call home, our capitalistic ways have led us astray. There is no money in teaching people how to take care of themselves! Instead, we have created a disease care system that has cost everyone a lot of money, and that has made the pharmaceutical industry very rich and very powerful.

If our bodies were designed to fail, would we still be here? Absolutely not! Not even the best drugs in the world could keep us alive if we didn't have an innate perfection built into our systems. So how do we recapture the perfection that was created in all of us? We must take health into our own hands by learning about the REAL tenets of proper health. That means pursuing our health even if our insurance companies won't pay for it.

It is time to change our paradigm of thinking about the concept of "health" insurance. While the insurance industry has made forward strides by covering some forms of alternative healing, we are all still missing the boat about insurance. Health insurance must be treated the same way as auto insurance: get high coverage, with a higher deductible to keep the costs down, and pray that you never have to use it! Auto insurance doesn't pay for the regular upkeep of your car, does it? It's time to look at health insurance and preventative health care in the same light.

So many people are dissuaded from pursuing different avenues of well-being because their insurance doesn't cover that type of treatment. The truth is that health insurance is really for those major events requiring surgery and/or a hospital stay that would cost tens of thousands of dollars. In those cases, thank goodness for insurance! While there are some events that occur in spite of our efforts to be healthy, a large percentage of the reasons for which people undergo major medical procedures could have been avoided through basic knowledge and proper preventative care, not to mention an awareness towards physical, biochemical and emotional well-being.

The average American knows more about how their car functions than about how their bodies function and, they therefore take better care of their cars! Western medicine makes so many references to the fact that we are so much more advanced today in medicine, yet people are more sick today than they have ever been! In spite of the billions, perhaps trillions of dollars that have been spent on cancer research, more people have cancer than ever before! Does this not alarm you? What has changed? The focus on health has become a business; it has become so compartmentalized that people are viewed as parts rather than as a whole. This is what we have been blindly following and calling acceptable healthcare!

We must go back to believing in the power our bodies have to heal. Our bodies are dynamic self-healing, self-regulating life forms, but more importantly, no two bodies are the same and should, therefore, not be treated in a cookbook fashion. It is time to empower ourselves with knowledge and understanding. And we must not allow ourselves to be led, but rather we must lead ourselves into the arms of our own inborn perfection - our own perfect health!

[Dr. Michele Cohen, Illumina Healing Center - see page 44]

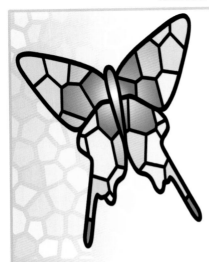

The Second Opinion

Know Your Options

Doubts and fears may arise when it comes to asking for a second opinion. A second opinion is the process of seeking an evaluation from another doctor or surgeon to confirm the diagnosis and treatment plan of a primary physician; or to offer an alternative diagnosis and/or treatment approach.

> Due to an increase in medical knowledge and available treatments, alternatives included, it is difficult for any one physician to be aware of all of the options. When patients seek a second opinion, it offers another chance to find a better approach. When patients share the efforts to find the best treatment, everyone benefits.

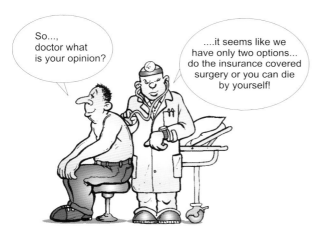

So..., doctor what is your opinion?

....it seems like we have only two options... do the insurance covered surgery or you can die by yourself!

Patients usually ask for a second opinion when a health problem involves more than a simple treatment. Second opinions are usually sought in cases of elective surgery, in which the patient has more time to consider their options. They are not as common in the case of emergencies because time is limited. Patients should let their doctors know they are seeking a second opinion and remember that it is their right. Embarrassment or fear of disapproval from their primary care provider is not a valid excuse and should not be an obstacle. A competent physician anticipates that their patients will be proactive and will not consider this action as an insult to their judgment or abilities. They may even suggest another doctor. In some cases, they may advise it, particularly when the advice from another surgeon with advanced training and expertise could provide more insight.

Without extensive research it's difficult to know whether your current physician is recommending the most up-to-date

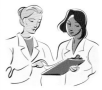

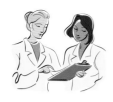

methods of treatment. The education, personal views and experiences of physicians may influence diagnosis and more frequently their recommendations. A second doctor may shed new light and recommend a completely different or more promising option. No doctor can know everything or make the right decision all the time. Different doctors, different viewpoints. One may prefer surgery, while another, a less invasive approach. Some will prefer to try other treatment options before recommending surgery and others may perform surgery to avoid further complications.

Getting a second opinion offers another perspective. It allows you to be well informed in order to make proper decisions and also enables you to confidently give your consent for procedures. From an emotional standpoint it provides peace of mind and reassurance, while reducing anxiety and uncertainty. From a financial standpoint, second opinions save insurance providers money by verifying the need for certain surgeries or procedures.

It is a good idea to get a second opinion if:

● You doubt the first one

● You would rather err on the side of caution

● You are dissatisfied with the information given or communication was unclear with your doctor. A 2002 Northwestern University study found that only 46% of patients coming into a breast cancer treatment center for a second opinion had been offered a complete discussion of treatment options during their initial consultation.

● You have been given a terminal diagnosis and there appears to be no hope, there is nothing to lose, and potentially, a lot to be gained.

● If your insurance provider is an HMO. HMOs do not refer outside their network, limiting available options. Certain HMOs omit their doctors from recommending certain procedures due to cost and you may not have access to the best procedure. You may wish to visit a doctor outside your HMO.

● Your doctor recommends a clinical trial. It's a good idea to get a second opinion before signing up. Research all options with other clinical trials before accepting.

● Your illness is rare. Find a physician who specializes in your particular illness. There may only be a few specialists if the illness is truly rare. If the expert is not in your city, have your doctor work with them by phone.

● Cancer: Obtain a copy of the pathology report. Pathology reports of the biopsy or surgical specimen are subject to

A "health panel" is comprised of professionals from different healthcare backgrounds who express their opinions on a given health condition. This idea is not revolutionary, yet the fact that it is being offered today, publicly, in a accessible format is.

Pathways to Healing is a panel event, presented by The Conscious Life Expo.

www.consciouslifeexpo.com

interpretation and human error. A study published in *The Annals of Surgical Oncology* in 2002 found that a pathological second opinion of breast cancers changed the initial diagnosis, prognosis, or treatment approach in 80% of the 340 study subjects. A different diagnosis can dramatically change the treatment and prognosis. Most hospitals have a tumor board. This is a regular meeting of specialists from departments such as surgery, radiation and oncology who will consider the best treatment for specific cases. If you or your doctor is uncertain about the diagnosis, ask if he would present your case to the board.

• Your illness requires a specialist. A reputation as a good doctor or surgeon is sometimes not enough. Find someone who specializes in the field you require. Each surgeon has their own area of specialization.

• Every time you are getting a non-holistic diagnosis and opinion of additional experts is needed.

Before visiting your doctor or alternative medicine practitioner, research and prepare a list of questions. This will prevent problems and misunderstandings. You do not have to be an M.D. or a healer to interview your healthcare professional. If they are caring, educated people, the conversation will take care of itself. Good doctors and healers are trained and know how to answer your questions. Remember, they may try to lead the conversation to maintain a professional look and keep on track with their busy schedule.

Conventional medical applications can be considered "last resort medicine"(except in emergency cases) and seeking holistic, natural health care, must be the first step to recovery. Obtaining a second or third opinion from a holistic M.D. or CAM professional is a priceless investment which can save your health and money in the long run.

Give your healthcare professional as much information as you are able. If the second opinion matches the first one, there is a good chance it is correct. If it contradicts the first, you can always get a third. Some insurance companies will pay for the third opinion if the previous two opinions do not significantly match. After receiving a diagnosis from a medical doctor who does not work with a healer or other alternative health care professional, consider the following:

"If you trust Google more than your doctor then maybe it's time to switch doctors."
-
Chasing Windmills, 2006,
Jadelr and Cristina Cordova

• Setting up an appointment with a healer to ask about a holistic approach for your health problem and to ask their advice and recommendations.

• Ask your doctor if he/she will consult and work with a healer of your choice. This means communicating and making the time to discuss the case with the alternative practitioner. You have nothing to lose by asking.

Be aware that alternative professionals may have quite a different approach than your medical doctor. It is all right, as long as they do not go against your medical doctor, but instead

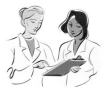

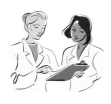

find ways to enhance or complement the medical care. When a disease is considered severe, it is preferable to work with both, simultaneously, or find a medical wellness center with doctors and CAM practitioners under one roof. Patients sometimes choose an alternative approach only, which may be enough in certain circumstances. It is always wise to include a visit to your physician and to have necessary clinical tests done for proper diagnosis. For effective and lasting recovery and healing, the expertise of both is recommended.

When requesting transfer of your medical records to a new physician, it my not be possible to recover documents dated 7 years or prior. CA Code Regs. Title 22, Chap 3, § 72543 states that "all medical records of persons aged 18 years or older and of emancipated minors shall be retained for seven 7 years from date of service.

The California Patient's Guide provides information on patients rights.

www.calpatientguide.org

Let's say that the nature of your condition, the results of the interview with your doctor, and your experience under his care indicates that it would be wise to make a change and find a new doctor, don't panic. After finding a new professional, simply inform the office of your previous doctor of your decision. Most of the time you will be dealing with their staff rather than with him directly. No business likes to see their clients leave. If questions arise, be as polite as possible. Remember, it is your right to change your health professional. Ask for your medical or health records to be transferred to your new healthcare professional. You also have the right to ask for a copy of those records for yourself (in most US states) and if some small copying fee applies, it is always worth the price.

Once you have located a qualified source, ask about the doctor's credentials, such as board certification, training, and experience. Bring all relevant medical records to your appointment, including test results, x-rays, and related materials. Often, the doctor will have requested the results of tests or procedures already performed. Bring a written list of questions, and paper and pen to take notes.

Second Opinion: Is a medical opinion provided by a second physician or medical expert, when one physician has provided a diagnosis or recommends surgery. Individuals are encouraged to obtain second opinions whenever a physician recommends surgery or presents an individual with a serious medical diagnosis.
-
Glossary for Health Consumers - 2006, www.healthinsurance.org

The following are a list of important questions for your western medical care professionals:

● Is surgery necessary? Are there any other less invasive possibilities that are equally effective?

● How soon should the surgery be done and what is the recovery time following the surgery? Is there postoperative pain? What is the success rate?

● What complications are associated with the surgery?

● What are all the treatment options? How are they performed?

● Are these options long term, permanent solutions and is any subsequent medication, additional treatment or follow-up required?

● What is the success rate of each option?

● What are the side effects of each treatment and how may they impact the quality of life? How long does each side effect endure?

● Outline the costs of all procedures including follow-up care.

Also visit both an energy healer and one other CAM practitioner to receive a second opinion from the Alternative Medicine point of view. This will get you started on a program of the correct alternative care and treatment for your illness. The alternative opinion does not represent, take the place of, or use the terminology of classical western medicine. A western medical diagnosis may only be given by a physician or a chiropractor. The alternative analysis, however, will explain your illness in the language of the particular modality. Certain treatments, therapies or supplements may be suggested which could save you from the possibly unnecessary and often drastic solutions associated with the orthodox approach.

If you find yourself in a situation where a suggestion seems too strange (drinking dragontails extracts or mosquito juice) or you feel uncomfortable, consider a second opinion from a different care provider of the same modality.

Some CAM professionals will provide a free evaluation or consultation. This is a great service especially in a case where insurance coverage or finances are an issue. Asking a CAM practitioner for their free opinion is a good introduction to a natural perspectives and holistic care.

After receiving a second opinion from both an orthodox and alternative practitioner, weigh all of your options. Surgery should be regarded as a last resort, after trying other conventional and alternative options. Before you admit yourself to hospital, consider that over 27% of deaths in hospitals are caused by secondary infections. In other words, by prolonging your stay in the hospital, you expose yourself to an extremely unhealthy environment, due to airborne bacteria and other influences, which may cause additional health

Second opinion medical resources:

❐ **University Library, Karolinska Institutet -** Resources on Internet for the general public and health care professionals.
www.mic.ki.se/Diseases/index.html

❐ **Second Opinions**: *Why, When, and Who Cancer Guide*, Steve Dunn
www.cancerguide.org/second_opinion.html

❐ **Robert S. Pashman, M.D.**, 444 S. San Vicente Blvd., # 800, Los Angeles, CA 90048, (310) 423-9983, (866) 567-7563 - www.espine.com

❐ **National Consumers League -** NCL helps consumers avoid alternative therapy pitfalls - www.nclnet.org/alterpr.htm

❐ **Health Grades, Inc.-** Research, compare and find new physicians
www.healthgrades.com

❐ **National Women's Health Information Center (NWHIC)**, Office on Women's Health (OWH), US Department of Health and Human Services (HHS) (800) 994-9662
www.4woman.gov/Tools/SecondOpinion.pdf

"Every patient carries her or his own doctor inside."

Albert Schweitzer, M.D.
(1875 - 1965)

problems or worsen your condition. If surgery is unavoidable and at-home care is an option available to you following surgery, and your physicians consent, this is a wise decision.

Minor surgeries are often unnecessarily recommended. Many minor surgeries can easily be avoided by the proper application

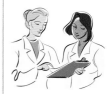

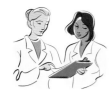

of effective alternative treatments, therapies or remedies. For example, rather than removing a gallbladder, there is a simple cleanse which opens the bile ducts and flushes out gallstones overnight. This is an effective solution recommended by alternative practitioners all over the world because there are no side effects. It is important to mention that this cleanse is preferably recommended before acute stages of gallbladder attacks. If gallstones are really large or physically fused to the gallbladder, then surgery may indeed be necessary.

There are two kinds of second opinions:

• **A second opinion can be done to confirm/disprove the nature or severity of the disease, possibly preventing unnecessary medical procedures.**

• **A second opinion can be done which sheds light on new or less invasive treatments.**

Typically, both are covered by most insurance companies and HMOs, but do not forget to ask if you are required to select from a specific group of affiliated doctors.

Navigating the insurance company rules regarding coverage of second opinions can be tricky. Here is some helpful advice: Call your insurance company and find out if second opinions are covered. Some insurance companies request one before major elective surgery. Some reserve the right to designate a physician in order to provide coverage. Most insurance companies will pay for a second opinion and frequently will not reimburse the cost of surgery if you do not have one. Obtaining a second opinion is an easy process. Keep the following in mind:

• The insurance company may not cover the second opinion doctors visit unless a diagnosis is given.

• You may have to make a worthwhile out of pocket investment, it may save your health and other unnecessary expenses.

• Insurance companies will not usually cover tests which are repeated for the second opinion.

As of mid-2003, Medicare Part B covered 80% of costs for surgical second opinions after deductible, and 80% for a third opinion if the first two opinions were contradictory."

It is not advisable to change your current healthcare professional on the basis of recommendations or advice found doing internet research. Be careful. The internet is often the king of misinformation with its pages of bold lies. The internet is easy and convenient to believe because the information feels so accessible. There may be many sites and pages related to your particular issue with false or misleading medical research, published side by side with products, money back guarantees, 100s of satisfied client testimonials and who knows what else, in order to sell you a supplement or other product.

Beware of any medical or health suggestions presented by a third party. You are looking for quality professional information or advice, presented by a legitimate healer or medical doctor. Not a supplement seller.

Be careful of certain online companies offering second opinion and evaluation services. Their intent is to file a lawsuit against your current health provider if it is found that you were misdiagnosed. This adds more gasoline to an already raging fire in the relationship between the medical establishment and patient trust. The wise thing to do is to address the error if possible, and move towards the promising direction of better care. Of course, proper legal action is necessary if major harm was caused due to medical fraud.

Making health-related decisions safely is like crossing the street. Look in all directions before making a move. The second opinion is one of the most important directions in which to look.

Common diseases frequently misdiagnosed:

- Breast Cancer
- Tuberculosis
- Lung Cancer
- Diabetes
- Prostate Cancer
- Cervical Cancer
- Ovarian Cancer
- Testicular Cancer
- Acute Myocardial Infarction (Heart Attack)
- Stroke
- Pulmonary Embolism
- Bacterial Meningitis
- Appendicitis

An online survey, conducted by U.K. marketing firm YouGov, asked people in the United States whether they or someone they knew had experienced a medical mistake in the last five years. About 35% of the 2,2001 patients who answered the survey said yes, while 58% said no. 50% of those who had experienced a medical error said the mistake was related to a misdiagnosis or a delay in diagnosis. Another 24% said they or someone they knew had experienced a medication error, while 18% said the errors were made during an operation or procedure.

Additional resources for a second opinion are listed below. Most of the resources listed in this chapter discuss the necessity for a correct conventional medical diagnosis. For a complementary opinion, in addition to a conventional approach, please refer to the *Healer's Guide, Part 3*.
You can also e-mail us at <u>alternativeopinion@healerguide.com</u> for local referrals.

Additional resources for a second opinion:

◻ The Armed Forces Institute of Pathology (AFIP) - this arm of the Department of Defense specializes in pathology consultation, education and research. www.afip.org

◻ FindCancerExperts - refers patients to nationally recognized doctors for expert second opinions. These pathologists specialize in all types of cancer diagnosis - www.findcancerexperts.com

◻ R.A. Bloch Cancer Foundation - offers a list of multi-disciplinary Second Opinion Institutions. These institutions when asked, work much like a tumor board, but the patient is actually present when their case is discussed - www.blochcancer.org

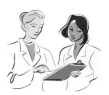

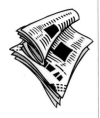

How Informed Are You?

The Message of Symptoms

To find a cure you must first find good, reliable information. As you research, trust yourself to know the truth of your health situation. Truth comes from within and everyone must find it on their own in order for it to be accepted. Such is the case with healing, Truth presented from the outside is just another opinion, nothing more and nothing less.

Symptoms, simply put, are red warning lights on the dashboard of life notifying us that something is wrong. The flashing light/symptom, is not the actual problem, it signals something deeper! Eliminating the symptom covers the flashing light with black tape and creates a false feeling about the state of your health. When you see an orange light in your car signaling that you are running out of gas, would it solve the problem to take out the fuse so it does not light up again? There are an army of "specialists" recommending and endorsing medications, supplements and surgical procedures to cover up your flashing light/symptoms.

Not only the media, but many other entities and authorities are ready to supply "the only proven medication" for any symptom we've got. Having skin problems? Buy this miraculous cream! Suffering from migraine headaches? Buy these doctor-recommended pills! Difficulty losing weight? Eat this food and you will loose 20lb in two weeks! Do you have sweaty palms? Here is the surgery! Having financial difficulties? Buy this proven method to get rich! The general label for such statements is B.S.

This barely scratches the surface of the terrible fraud we are programmed to accept. Some will argue that there are so many things to do: Go to work, solve problems, take care of the family, pay bills, feed the cat, the car needs an oil change and any of the 100 other things that are mistakenly made a priority before one's health; relationships and spiritual wellbeing, included. As a result, when it comes to self-care, the only energy most of us have left is used to visit isle four of the local grocery store to pick up headache medication. Why not? That is exactly what the TV commercial suggested, and what everyone else does.

Ignoring symptoms is dangerous. Doctors would rather see their patients more often and reassure them that nothing is wrong, than deal with full blown disease later. Have your symptoms evaluated from two basic standpoints:

• what disease is the symptom associated with?

• what is your body trying to tell you?

The answers are the two inseparable coordinates which lead you in the right direction.

"Pain (any pain-- emotional, physical, mental) has a message. The information it has about our life can be remarkably specific, but it usually falls into one of two categories: "We would be more alive if we did more of this," and, "Life would be more lovely if we did less of that." Once we get the pain's message, and follow its advice, the pain goes away."

Peter McWilliams, Author, *Life 101*

List of side effects of some common headache medications:

- an allergic reaction (difficulty breathing; closing of the throat; swelling of the lips, tongue, or face; or hives)

- chest pain, tightness, pressure, and/or heaviness

- neck, throat, or jaw pain, tightness, or pressure

- an irregular heartbeat

Other, less serious side effects may be more likely to occur. Talk to your doctor if you experience:

- nausea or vomiting

- drowsiness or dizziness

- numbness, tingling, flushing, warmth, redness, or heaviness in a body part

It appears that a somewhat dishonest reverse approach is used for advertising prescription drugs. Instead of starting with "If you experience migraine headaches take this clinically proven medication for fast relief," it would be more accurate to say "this chemical substance may or perhaps will cause at least one or more of the above mentioned symptoms and also may or may not help you with your headaches," but this would not sell!

Congratulations, you have just contributed to the fast growing wealth of one of the hundreds of drug companies and simultaneously missed a precious opportunity to discover what the true problem in your life. When you are 80, if you are lucky enough, and sitting on your bed with only a little time to live, you may regret the priority placed on all of life's little routines in which you were so conveniently buried, during the productive years. All the things which you considered important. It may dawn on you that you probably missed the chance, an opportunity to experience a much more vibrant life, a chance to grow, and a significantly happier old age. Sometimes the migraine headache or ulcer is a sign or "flashing light" that a job or relationship or other life situation change, may be long overdue. If the sign is heeded, one may find themselves in a much better and more supportive place. Not paying attention results in being stuck in the same situation, with the headache medication, temporary relief and an ugly medical future.

There is an intelligence that created the human body. If it was smart enough to create the brain, it could certainly foresee the body's diseases and symptoms as a language. With every symptom, the question arises "What does it mean?" Each question has an answer. This is how the body communicates. When symptoms appear, if the first question is "What medication can I take?" you're in trouble!

Find out more about your medication's side-effects:

❏ **Yahoo directory** - extensive information on virtually every prescription medication - http://health.yahoo.com/drug/

❏ **Drugs.com** - prescription drug and over the counter medicine information for consumers and professionals - www.drugs.com

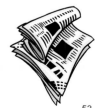

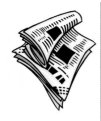

When irritating symptoms come, and they will, take a moment and put yourself first. Asking the right questions is a good start and if the answers don't come at first, keep asking because the answers will, eventually come. Why does this headache, ulcer, stomach pain, bladder infection, sinusitis keep coming back? What is the message? What is your body trying to tell you? Could it be the stress you're under? Do you work too hard without enough time for yourself? Could your fatigue be the result of a food allergy or is it the result of dealing with an unhealthy living situation?

The purpose of being grateful for our symptoms and investigating them instead of suppressing them is to cut to the chase while there is still time. Implementing this technique results in the enjoyment of better health on all levels. *(i.e.:* more vitality, peace, joy and passion; being able to fully experience your children; increased success and happiness which results in a better life.) Life is constant change, evolution. Disease or discomfort is a reminder that we are getting stuck or that we forgot to go with the flow of natural laws - simply a resistance to change.

If you must take medication, do so. Be thankful for it, but move past it when medically possible. It is a poor choice to join millions of others, with growing dependencies and fall into the trap of believing that medication creates health or takes troubles away. Getting off medication is as important as it was to get on it in the first place.

This primarily refers to the myriad of minor symptoms which at times can be overwhelming. Take insomnia for example. If you are not able to get a good sleep for many nights, it is, of course, difficult to function effectively at work or with your family. Chances are, symptoms include irritability and inability to concentrate. If the insomnia continues it could result in loss of employment. In this case, sleeping medication may be quite a blessing as an interim solution. But staying on it for a long time, may interrupt your chemical balance and the biorhythms of your body to such a degree that it may take years to fix.

When man-made medication is necessary - prescription or over-the-counter - and one accepts the possible side effects, one usually overlooks the secondary effects that may occur when the medication is no longer needed. Some drugs, when discontinued, may cause severe changes in one's wellbeing. This information may not be described in the list of side effects, as required by law.

"The more severe the pain or illness, the more severe will be the necessary changes. These may involve breaking bad habits, or acquiring some new and better ones."
-
Peter McWilliams, writer, *Life 101*

References for alternative treatments:

☐ **Alternative Medicine: The Definitive Guide** (2nd Edition) by Burton Goldberg, John W. Anderson, Larry Trivieri. "In the face of an increasingly inadequate system of conventional medicine, a growing number of people are turning to alternative medicine to address their needs..." - www.amazon.com - (Amazon ID: 1587611414)

Taking one medication often results in the subsequent recommendation of yet a second prescription drug to remedy the side effects caused by the first one, and so on. Be wise and be careful. Choose to take medication to gain back strength in the moment, but when you are strong again and in a calm and positive frame of mind, implement the question asking technique. Experiment with other choices, such as meditation or relaxation cds, yoga, exercise and diet. These natural choices require a little bit more effort than simply popping a pill, but will quickly and effectively   bring the body into balance and harmony. Not only that, but when time is made to honor yourself - body, mind and spirit - self love and self respect is the result. This personal gain is priceless and there are no negative side effects.

It may not appear that severe or chronic diseases would benefit by this approach, but they do. There are many conditions requiring the administration of prescription medication. Without medication, the quality of life would be so poor, or the pain so great, that the individual would not be able to lead a normal life, or would simply die from the disease. Although medication is required to manage, the proper effective holistic approach must be implemented simultaneously. The individual continues their treatment as prescribed by their physician, while seeking the support of holistic care. This may result in a cure or at the very least, a reduction in the prescribed medications. The types of diseases and the degree to which they afflict individuals are so varied, that one-size-fits-all recommendations cannot be made. Therefore, it is important that each case is handled individually, by the proper professionals, working together in an integrative fashion. One always has to look beyond the symptoms.

When one's symptoms are treated with medication, under the care of a non-holistic physician, and the symptoms subside, people often forget to address their imbalance from a holistic perspective. This can be compared to a person watching TV, while their house is on fire. They extinguish the fire in the living room, but leave the fire to rage on in the other rooms, where it doesn't bother them. For the moment.

"The first step toward a cure is to know what the disease is."
-
Latin proverb

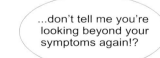

...don't tell me you're looking beyond your symptoms again!?

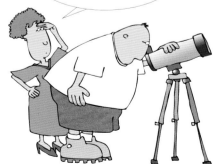

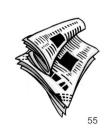

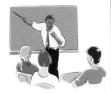

Education

Empower Yourself Through Knowledge

This chapter discusses holistic education. By definition it is learning and study based on the principle of interconnectedness or wholeness. Wholeness relates to the human body, education, civilization, social structures and ecosystems alike. Holistic education is based on the premise that each person finds their own identity, meaning and purpose in life through self-awareness, personal growth, supportive relationships and through a deepening practice and understanding of spiritual values such as love, forgiveness, compassion and peace.

> **☯**
>
> Education is one of the biggest influences determining important life choices such as selecting a place to live, food to eat, friends, or career. It has been said, "If someone gives you a fish it will feed you for a day. If you learn to fish, you will be fed for a lifetime." The quality of your life depends on the quality of your education.

The lifelong student obtains a well rounded education by paying attention to body, mind, emotions and spirit and through this process becomes self-empowered. Personal empowerment means that one accepts 100% responsibility for every life situation and eliminates the victim mentality in the process. Those supporting the movement towards holistic training maintain the belief that inadequate and insufficient education is the root of modern problems. This new education paradigm offers solutions and opportunities. When holistic education is introduced to orthodox medicine (where the long standing distinction or separation has been made between the body, mind and spirit), it is clear from witnessing the resistance, that the philosophy behind the allopathic medical approach does not consider, and is not willing to address all aspects of human nature. Health and self-healing reside within the body and the body's own innate healing ability makes healing possible at all. The degree of harmony and lack of resistance to one's environmental or external reality determines the quality of one's health and therein lies the secret to achieving wellness.

"Education's purpose is to replace an empty mind with an open one."

-
Malcolm Forbes,
Forbes Magazine,
(1919 - 1990)

The term holistic is often applied only to health, resulting in a narrow view of its' meaning. Holism (from "ὅλος" holos, a Greek word meaning all, entire) is the idea that all the properties of a given system - biological, chemical, social, economic, mental, linguistic, etc. - cannot be determined or explained by the sum of its component parts alone. Instead, the system as a whole determines, in an important way, how the parts behave. Holistic education is not limited to healthcare, but extends to every area of life. Teachers embodying holistic philosophy are found in, but not limited to, languages, arts, science, ethics, social, cultural and environmental education or religion. The principles of holistic care, and an understanding of it's reach can be grasped by acknowledging this wider perspective.

There is no single best way to study and there are many paths of learning. While few public schools are entirely committed to holistic principles, many teachers attempt to put holistic ideas into practice, albeit, despite the inherent resistance of the current school systems. Fostering collaboration rather than competition in classrooms creates community and ends isolation. This is one example which demonstrates its application. Throughout the 200-year history of public schooling, many forward thinking individuals have stated that educating human beings should involve much more than simply molding them into future workers or citizens. Education at any age should be an ongoing process that includes studies in moral, emotional, physical, psychological and spiritual dimensions as well as the development of practical life skills in the areas of health, finances, relationships, independent thinking and social skills, among others.

It takes several years to learn how to read and write in your native language. It may take only one weekend to learn how to improve your relationships with everyone in your life. Learning interpersonal skills belongs to the list of important knowledge. Besides the references in this chapter, refer to page 96 for additional resources.

It is possible to study and learn many practical healing tools, self-improvement skills and empowering techniques in as little as two weeks' time. When applied, they have the ability to make profound life changes. Introductory or basic workshops in the areas of energy healing, nutrition, meditation, yoga and hypnotherapy are just some of the options to choose from. Applicable knowledge is gained in a few short weekends.

"We don't receive wisdom; we must discover it for ourselves after a journey that no one can take for us or spare us."

-
Marcel Proust, French novelist
(1871 - 1922)

Take a minute and consider the most common, yet unsupportive routines. Perhaps your current eating habits consist primarily of cooked or processed food, with a couple of fast food drive-through meals weekly, because you are in a hurry or you are grabbing breakfast on the way to work. Vegetables are those annoying garnishes on the side of a plate. Then add a couple cups of coffee or soda and maybe a chocolate bar or a bag of chips every day. After coming home from work, there may be a microwavable dinner followed by one hour of television with two hours on internet (too tired to exercise) and a restless or only partially refreshing night's sleep. *[researchers from Stanford Institute for the Quantitative Study of Society found the average Internet user spends 3 hours per day online, study 2004]* If this has been going on for several years or decades, the result could be high cholesterol or blood pressure and pre-diabetes accompanied by fatigue, a doughy belly, digestive problems and headaches. Simultaneously, you may feel growing emotional turmoil and short temperdness. Relationships, if any, have more downs than ups. When casually observing friends or

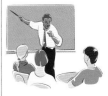

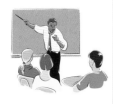

co-workers it appears most are on the same page and no one seems disturbed about it. Health problems seem to be a normal part of aging or life's natural progression. If this scenario sounds familiar, this chapter will provide much insight and encouragement for practical self-empowerment through knowledge and education. Presented here are suggestions, resources and opportunities to improve your quality of life. The lifestyle mentioned above and the resulting conditions are ABSOLUTELY NOT THE NORMAL PROGRESS OF LIFE!

Illness is the result of a chain reaction of poor habits and choices, which due to a prolonged period of negligence have overshadowed each other and led to the current condition. There have been many "red lights on the dashboard of life" along the way, signaling that which needed immediate attention. Ignored or suppressed symptoms are the pattern which eventually make life miserable beyond one's wildest nightmares. Of course, suppressing symptoms is much easier. This belief shared by the role models and many authorities of the orthodox health care system, is that the symptoms are the disease and that they must be treated. Medication is believed to be a cure. How funny, in a sad way.

"If you think you can make it, or if you think you can't, either way you are right."
Henry Ford
If scientists decide to prove or disprove something, enough supportive evidence can always be found, either way. Many health-related, scientific studies are only temporary statements, subject to change.

To understand why this sad approach is still followed, it is necessary to underline some faulty beliefs. One popular misconception and group belief is that illness is a natural by-product of aging. This belief comes from observing the common, unhealthy condition of the masses. It was never taught that chronic, self-inflicted conditions are not a normal state of health. The majority of the U.S. population has a condition or reason - usually unnecessarily prescribed, for taking medication. Blue pill, red pill, violet pill.

"Education is a progressive discovery of our own ignorance."
-
William James Durant, American philosopher, historian and writer (1885 - 1981)

So what is responsible for our nation's poor health? Is it the poor quality or selection of our food? Is it stress? The polluted environment? Is it the side effects from the drugs prescribed to alleviate the side effects of other drugs to "heal the symptoms?" Yes, all of the above are contributing factors for our lack of health, but that's not where the true responsibility lies. It starts with awareness followed by the action of each individual. As environmental and social influences are becoming stronger contributing factors to this condition, better lifestyle choices are necessary. The latest reports show that two-thirds of American's are overweight. Although obesity is commonly blamed on the improper diet or lifestyle of an individual, if one looks closely it becomes clear that this is not the originating cause. The root cause is the structure, beliefs and habits of our society itself.

The lack of knowledge, proper role models, life education - especially at an early age - ignorance, will power, and little communication with one's inner guidance or intuition are all symptoms of an unhealthy society. Of course the responsibility lies with each individual to develop a sound mind and judgement regarding what is right for them. How is it possible that unhealthy rhythms and habits are ingrained from an early age and override common sense and wisdom? Could it be inadequate education? The statistics do not lie. Refer to the statistics and research on page 60 which illustrate how many people in the United States succumb to common health conditions every year, as a direct or indirect result of their self-imposed unhealthy lifestyle.

Obesity, heart disease, cancer....the list goes on. In many cases diseases are expressions of wrong habits and stress and are completely preventable. Society must collectively shift its unhealthy patterns and belief structures. Preventative care, right lifestyle and the proper application of healing arts and sciences are the medicine of the future.

If you always find yourself working hard in order to achieve goals, it is a sign that you may not have enough knowledge or know-how to support your efforts. Fourteen days of study may save you fourteen years of hard work. If you have know-how, things go much easier, therefore it is a wise investment to obtain the right education, unless you enjoy hard work.

Our current health crisis is partially the result of a lack of information and education. If we were educated properly from an early age, teachings of wholesome living would imprint on the mind and soul of every child. Destructive habits would be less likely to develop. Public schools and colleges rarely teach this. Education for lifelong health should be mandatory. Extensive classes in nutrition, especially those encouraging the implementation of organic and raw food in the diet, as well as the consequences of unhealthy choices, must be taught. Healthy food must be served in the school's lunch rooms. It is everyone's responsibility not to become a victim of a poor social lifestyle due to a lack of proper education. It is easy to blame, but difficult to offer or implement a working solution. The tendency is to blame the media, the fast pace of life, genetics and others circumstances. Genetics are often a valid point but not in the case of more than 50% of adult Americans. Did you know that by maintaining positive thoughts, emotions and a clean lifestyle, there is a good chance that those "bad genes" will remain turned off? This will be Headline News from the scientific community in the years to come. Watch the movie *What the Bleep" Do We Know?* to learn about powerful scientific theories as they relate to human physiology.

"The aim of public education is not to spread enlightenment at all: it is simply to reduce as many individuals as possible to the same safe level, to breed a standard citizenry, to put down dissent and originality."

-

Henry Louis Mencken, journalist, satirist, social critic (1880-1956)

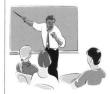

Consumer awareness is an important part of education and self-empowerment. Recently, there has been an influx of

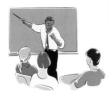

Statistics & Research:

A study *[by Mathew Reeves at Michigan State University]* **found that only 3% out of 153,000 respondents undertook four basic steps that define a healthy lifestyle – not smoking, keeping weight stable, eating right and exercising. "I was really quite surprised at how low that number was," said Reeves, an assistant professor of epidemiology. "These results illustrate the extraordinarily low prevalence of healthy lifestyles in the U.S. adult population."**

Less than 25% of Californian adults, about 5.5 million, walk on a regular basis, while about 6.8 million, barely walk at all. *[According to the UCLA Center for Health Policy Research]*

Chronic diseases are now the major cause of death and disability worldwide. Noncommunicable conditions, including cardiovascular diseases (CVD), diabetes, obesity, cancer and respiratory diseases, now account for 59% of the 57 million deaths annually and 46% of the global burden of disease. *[Facts related to chronic disease, www.who.int]*

Approximately 66.3% adults in the U.S., age 20 years and over, are overweight or obese and 32% are obese. *[National Health and Nutrition Examination Survey (NHANES) data on the Prevalence of Overweight and Obesity Among Adults - United States, 2003-2004, http://www.cdc.gov/nchs/fastats/overwt.htm]*

Obesity is a complex, multi-factored chronic disease involving environmental (social and cultural), genetic, physiologic, metabolic, behavioral and psychological components. It is the second leading cause of preventable death in the U.S and it helped kill 365,000 people in 2000.
[Jan. 19, 2005 – The Centers for Disease Control and Prevention]

- **80% of type II diabetes is related to obesity**

- **70% of Cardiovascular disease is related to obesity**

- **42% of breast & colon cancer is diagnosed among obese individuals**

- **30% of gallbladder surgery is related to obesity**

- **26% of obese people have high blood pressure**
 [References from the National Institute of Diabetes & Digestive & Kidney Diseases (NIDDK) and My.WebMD.com website. www.winltdusa.com]

 The American Obesity Association and Shape Up America!, Nonprofit organizations whose missions include combating obesity through

> "The great aim of education is not knowledge but action."
>
> -
> Herbert Spencer, English Philosopher (1820 - 1903)

products on the market that have not been approved by the FDA. The marketing and claims for these products and medications - isolated chemical compounds from natural or synthetic sources - are often untrue. These products claim to be backed by supportive research and are often labeled, "Doctor Approved." The research is usually financed by private corporations or pharmaceutical companies. If a company pays millions of dollars for a research team to find out if their product works or is safe, would they pick a team who will find that it doesn't?

Once in a while, products initially approved by the FDA are later proven to be harmful (for the complete list of recalled products or those with warnings visit: *http://www.fda.gov/cder/warn/ warn2006.htm*. This is not entirely the fault of the FDA. Private companies are anxious to flood the market with their products and too often present unfinished or misleading studies for the sake of rushing their product to market. Mandatory third party investigations and more independent research would put a stop to all of the pharmaceutical nightmares for the unsuspecting consumer.

The right education helps the consumer make wise decisions based on knowledge and a cautious approach, not on outer suggestions. In this case, the media is a huge unsupportive influence. Commercials of all kinds, forms and shapes, now even on little TVs attached to the cash registers at grocery stores are grossly misleading everyone. It is no surprise that the largest amount of money spent by consumers goes to the companies who heavily advertise their pharmaceutical products. This influence is indicative of a convenient, fast food society, but that does not mean everyone has to buy into it.

Listen to experts and study professional resources, instead of commercials where the nice looking actor, dressed as a doctor, ensures the safety and effectiveness of the new product. Advertising and commercials unfortunately cannot be trusted. The truth has to be found through holistic education.

Media, when used constructively is a powerful educational tool. Watching supportive, conscious media and reading quality educational materials is a good place to start *(see the chapter in Healer's Guide on Conscious Media)*. When watching television, it is recommended that you turn the sound off during the commercials. Turning off the TV a few nights a week is even better. Going to seminars or workshops instead and learning from people you can see, hear and touch is a positive change. It is essential to start learning something new today! Most local schools and colleges have community extension programs. A series of inexpensive public classes covering a broad range of topics including healthy diet, lifestyle, psychology, social skills, financial workshops, writing and more. Workshop fees range from $15 to $45. Less than the cost of dinner in a restaurant! The lessons and skills learned in the class stay forever. Provided is a list (on the next page) of community colleges. They post their schedule of classes on-line and will mail their up-to-date brochure upon request at no cost. Also, refer to the schools and other institutions featured at the end of this chapter.

Before you decide to make a profound shift in your life, meditate to find out what it is that you always wanted to be or to do. Then take action.
• **Review the resources in this chapter**
• **Follow your heart**
• **Pick up the phone**
• **Dial the right number**
• **Let a professional help you make the right course selection based on your interests and needs**
• **Sign up for the class**
• **Attend the class**

"Look at every path closely and deliberately. Try it as many times as you think necessary. Then ask yourself alone, one question. Does this path have a heart? If it does, the path is good; if it doesn't it is of no use."
-
Carlos Castaneda, author
(1925 - 1998)

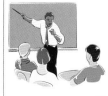

List of Community Colleges, Extension Programs:

- **Antelope Valley** - 3041 West Avenue K, Lancaster, CA 93536, (661) 722.6300 — avc.edu
- **Canyon Country** - 26455 N. Rockwell Canyon Rd., Santa Clarita, CA 91355, (661) 259.7800 — canyons.edu
- **Cerritos** - 11110 Alondra Boulevard, Norwalk, CA 90650, (562) 860.2451 — cerritos.edu
- **Compton** - 1111 East Artesia Boulevard, Compton, CA 90221, (310) 900.1600 — compton.edu
- **Costa Mesa** - 2701 Fairview Road, Costa Mesa, CA 92628, (714) 432.0202 orangecoastcollege.edu
- **Culver City** - 9000 Overland Avenue, Culver City, CA 90230, (310) 287.4200 — wlac.edu
- **Cypress** - 9200 Valley View Street, Cypress, CA 90630, (714) 484.7000 — cypresscollege.edu
- **East Los Angeles** - 1301 Ave. Cesar Chavez, Monterey Park, CA 91754, (323) 265.8650 — elac.edu
- **Fountain Valley** - 11460 Warner Avenue, Fountain Valley, CA 92708, (714) 546.7600 — coastline.edu
- **Fullerton** - 321 East Chapman Avenue, Fullerton, CA 92832, (714) 992.7000 — fullcoll.edu
- **Glendale** -1500 North Verdugo Road, Glendale, CA 91208, (818) 240.1000 — glendale.edu
- **Glendora** - 1000 West Foothill Boulevard, Glendora, CA 91741, (626) 963.0323 — citruscollege.edu
- **Huntington Beach** - 15744 Goldenwest St., Hunt. Beach, CA 92647, (714) 892.7711 — gwc.cccd.edu
- **Irvine** - 5500 Irvine Center Drive, Irvine, CA 92720, (949) 559.9300 — ivc.edu
- **Long Beach** - 4901 East Carson Street, Long Beach, CA 90808, (562) 938.4353 — lbcc.edu
- **Los Altos Hills** - 12345 El Monte Road, Los Altos Hills, CA 94022, (650) 949.7777 — foothill.edu
- **Los Angeles** - 855 North Vermont Ave., Los Angeles, CA 90029, (323) 953.4000 lacitycollege.edu
- **Los Angeles** - 1600 West Imperial Highway, Los Angeles, CA 90047, (323) 241.5225 — lasc.edu
- **Los Angeles** - 400 West Washington Boulevard, Los Angeles, CA 90015, (213) 763.7000 — lattc.edu
- **Mission Viejo** - 28000 Marguerite Pkwy, Mission Viejo, CA 92692, (949) 582.4500 — saddleback.edu
- **Moorpark** - 7075 Campus Road, Moorpark, CA 93201, (805) 378.1400 — moorparkcollege.edu
- **Orange** - 8045 E. Chapman Avenue, Orange, CA 92869, (714) 628.4900 — sccollege.edu
- **Oxnard** - 4000 South Rose Avenue, Oxnard CA 93033, (805) 986.5800 — oxnardcollege.edu
- **Pasadena** - 1570 E. Colorado Boulevard, Pasadena CA 91106, (626) 585.7123 — pasadena.edu
- **Rancho Cucamonga** - 5885 Haven Ave., Rancho Cucamonga, CA 91737, (909) 987.1737 chaffey.edu
- **Riverside** - 4800 Magnolia Avenue, Riverside, CA 92506, (915) 222.8000 — rcc.edu
- **San Bernardino** - 701 S. Mt. Vernon Ave., San Bernardino, CA 92410, (909) 384.4400 valleycollege.edu
- **San Jacinto** - 1499 North State Street, San Jacinto, CA 92583, (951) 487.6752 — msjc.edu
- **Santa Ana** - 1530 W. 17th Street, Santa Ana, CA 92706, (714) 564.6000 — sac.edu
- **Santa Monica** - 1900 Pico Boulevard, Santa Monica, CA 90405, (310) 434.4000 — smc.edu
- **Sylmar** - 13356 Eldridge Avenue, Sylmar, CA 91342, (818) 364.7600 — lamission.edu
- **Torrance** - 16007 Crenshaw Boulevard, Torrance, CA 90506, (310) 532.3670 — elcamino.edu
- **Van Nuys** - 5800 Fulton Avenue, Van Nuys, CA 91401, (818) 947.2600 — lavc.edu
- **Ventura** - 4667 Telegraph Road, Ventura, CA 93003, (805) 654.6400 — venturacollege.edu
- **Walnut** - 1100 North Grand Avenue, Walnut, CA 91789, (909) 594.5611 — mtsac.edu
- **Whittier** - 3600 Workman Mill Road, Whittier, CA 90601, (562) 692.0921 — riohondo.edu
- **Wilmington** - 1111 Figueroa Place, Wilmington, CA 90744, (310) 233.4000 — lahc.edu
- **Woodland Hills** - 6201 Winnetka Ave.,Woodland Hills, CA 91371, (818) 719.6401 — piercecollege.edu
- **Yucaipa** - 11711 Sand Canyon Road, Yucaipa, CA 92399, (909) 794.2161 — craftonhills.edu

There are a wide variety of professional, holistically-oriented workshops available through private institutions. They are generally on the alternative side and are relatively unknown to the mainstream community. They have years experience teaching valuable skills, and practical tools for self improvement in all areas - relationships, financial health, alternative healing, spiritual studies and more. Spending a mere $200 to $600 to gain valuable education may instantly change one's life. That's less than one car payment.

This knowledge will be retained for lifetime and sometimes beyond! Education is an excellent investment.

When attending live educational seminars or workshops, listen to your heart and intuition and feel if the information shared is helpful or right for you. With DVDs and television, the personal interaction is missing. It is not as easy to tune in and therefore, valuable insights, which would easily be seen in a live presentation may be missed.

It is time to start relying on our own ability and judgement to recognize what is right instead of solely depending on outer influences and suggestions. Listening to your inner voice and intuition aided by your education is an integral part of obtaining true guidance for your future.

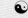

Find out, which courses are offered at your local community college. A list of schools is provided. Preview the current schedule of classes on the internet, or request a brochure by phone. Brochures are mailed free of charge and most schools send periodic updates.

Through personal development and self-discovery, countless individuals have found a passion for knowledge. They understand that self-education and personal growth ultimately enable them to be of service to others. With less than one year of study it is possible to become an expert in a field of your choice. It is a myth that one must study for 10 years to become a professional in a desired field. Times have changed. The learning methods and educational processes are quite different from those remembered from high school. Everything is evolving. When things are out of balance, educate yourself. Don't wait, start now! Your new-found knowledge will show you the way.

"Education is the power to think clearly, the power to act well in the world's work, and the power to appreciate life."

-
Brigham Young
LDS Church
President
(1801-1877)

Consider the possibility of a holistic health-oriented career. It is estimated that the number of visits to alternative medicine practitioners increased from 427 million in 1990 to 629 million in 1997. Approximately $27 billion were spent on alternative medicine therapies by 42% of American healthcare consumers. It is also estimated that more than 62% of those visiting health care professionals, in the United States used complementary or alternative therapies in 2006. The amount of money being spent on CAM care is growing exponentially each year. Countless geographical locations do not have enough qualified practitioners to serve the area. There are a variety of schools offering training and certification programs. It is also possible to study part-time or via distance learning programs. Refer to the list of recommended schools at the end of this chapter.

This may inspire you to be of assistance to others. Today's healthcare costs are overwhelming. Ideally, there would be one or two individuals within each extended family or group who has been trained in healing arts or therapy.

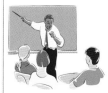

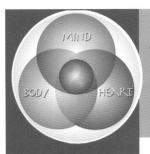

The chosen methods of study would depend on the family's needs. The family or community healer would monitor the health state and consciousness of the group and be available to provide in-home healing services when needed. Could that person be you?

When selecting a workshop or teacher, learn from the masters, from those who walk the talk. Unless one is guided by quality teachers, progress is limited. When in the presence of a Guru or teacher, not only is it possible to receive the most from the class, but it's easy to see if they "walk the talk," or if it is simply an ego trip on the way to becoming rich or famous. Judge the tree by its fruit. In the teachers' presence their abilities and competence are easily seen. Not necessarily from what they say, but from body language and other subtle hints. If you are not certain whether the teacher has enough experience to actually teach the subject matter, inquire about their accomplishments and experience. Don't be afraid to ask. What is the worst thing that can happen? If they really walk their talk, they will be happy to answer questions.

Each year thousands of people travel to Los Angeles to study courses unavailable in their country, especially those related to health or spirituality. Los Angeles is a Mecca for alternative education. To study here, others had to travel across the world. If you are here, why are you not taking advantage of this amazing opportunity?

One cannot give to others what they do not possess and that applies to those who teach. If you sign up for a seminar called "How to Heal Yourself" and your lecturer shows up smoking, find a different teacher. This applies to all other categories as well. If your "How to get Rich" seminar lecturer is driving 85' Toyota with bumper-stickers, it sends a strange message. It is difficult, if not impossible, to learn from someone who doesn't have it, even though they may be a brilliant speaker.

"Never trust the advice of a man in difficulties."

-
Aesop,
Greek fabulist
(620 BC - 560 BC)

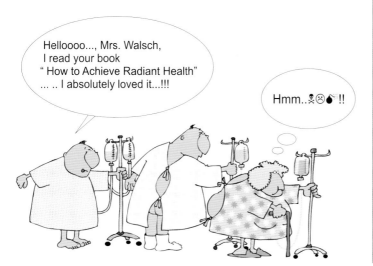

Helloooo..., Mrs. Walsch,
I read your book
" How to Achieve Radiant Health"
... .. I absolutely loved it...!!!

Hmm..♟☹☂☠ !!

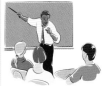

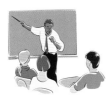

Make live interaction a priority. An important fact to remember; knowledge is not only transferred by what we hear, see or touch, but also by the radiatory field of the teacher which makes an imprint on our own field and works as a blueprint to set up a similar successful pattern in our lives.

Many years ago, I knew I wanted to study psychology. I applied with the hopes of being accepted to a prominent university offering a psychology program. That same year there were several thousand applications for that particular school and the limit was 400 students. During this time I was highly active in sports, so I decided to apply to a different university - The National University of Sports - which was coincidently offering the same psychology program. My plan was to get transferred during the first year of study, to the psychology program at the university which was my first choice (since there was a certain dropout of students in the first year, it was not usually a problem to be accepted via a transfer). What a perfect plan! I had started with sports at an early age and it was no problem to pass the exceptionally difficult entry tests - running, swimming, high jump, discus, gymnastics, etc. There was only one exercise on the bars, I was unable to do, no matter how hard I trained. I read books which explained step-by-step the proper way to perform it. I spoke with classmates and friends who claimed to know how, but every time I went to the gym and hung on the bars and tried to follow others' instructions, I failed. I was able to perform everything else except that one exercise and without it I could kiss my chances of being accepted good bye. One day I went to the gym with a friend. During the break, I asked if he knew how to do this exercise on the bars. He was in his 3rd year of architectural university and specialized in bridge building and was the last person I would expect to know. As absurd as it sounds, without a word, he jumped up on the bars and performed it perfectly. My jaw went down. I stood up, next to him and tried it myself. It didn't quite work the first time, but I began to have a feeling that I could actually do it. He showed me the exercise again and on my 5th or 6th attempt, I did it! Unbelievable! So many weeks of no luck, following books and the advice of others, and here, in the presence of someone who knew, I succeeded.

[M. Polak]

"90% of success begins with just showing up!"
-
Donald Trump

This story is nothing exceptional, but it clearly demonstrates how the presence of the teacher really works. By being in their field, which contains the actual experience and knowledge, it is far easier to learn something new, rather than figure it out by yourself. As someone cleverly said, sometimes things cannot be taught, they have to be caught!

On page 70 there is a reference list of recommended schools offering local or distance learning programs and courses focusing on alternative, integrative or spiritual areas of health care. When selecting a school, carefully examine the program. If the program or the information does not seem appropriate or interesting, continue searching until you find one which feels right to you. Either way, start today!

Our "Discovery" of Neurofeedback

by Siegfried Othmer, Ph.D., Chief
Scientist, The EEG Institute

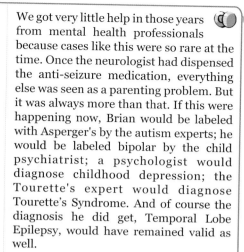

Our first child was born nearly forty years ago, while Sue and I were in graduate school at Cornell. There were some early signs that there was something odd about Brian, but this was before the terms Autism Spectrum or childhood bipolar disorder were commonly known.

Brian was in his own world in pre-school, but he was admitted to first grade despite his young age and relative immaturity. In first grade he was essentially a non-participant, but by second grade he was getting into trouble behaviorally. Eventually he was expelled from school. We were totally mystified by what was going on until his pediatrician suspected a neurological involvement and started him on anti-seizure medication. The violent episodes mercifully ceased, and we were grateful, although Brian remained a very troubled child.

Just as we did not understand his behavior, Brian was also a mystery to himself. At one point, when we came down on him for his awful behavior, he just collapsed into a whimper, "I guess I am just an evil person. I guess I am just going to go to prison when I grow up." We realized at that moment that he was struggling with something he had no control over. He could not have been more remorseful over his own behavior. His models were the well-behaved kids at school, and since he could not be like them, he felt that perhaps he was not even entitled to be alive. He was depressed to the point of being suicidal.

We got very little help in those years from mental health professionals because cases like this were so rare at the time. Once the neurologist had dispensed the anti-seizure medication, everything else was seen as a parenting problem. But it was always more than that. If this were happening now, Brian would be labeled with Asperger's by the autism experts; he would be labeled bipolar by the child psychiatrist; a psychologist would diagnose childhood depression; the Tourette's expert would diagnose Tourette's Syndrome. And of course the diagnosis he did get, Temporal Lobe Epilepsy, would have remained valid as well.

Fortunately we discovered neurofeedback when Brian was seventeen and a junior in High School. By that time, he had been on anti-seizure medication for some nine years, and life had been very difficult for both Brian and us throughout that time. We were only too happy to evaluate a new approach that seemed to make sense. As it happens, my wife, Sue Othmer, had received the relevant training in neurobiology at Cornell that allowed her to understand what was being proposed. The training was offered in Beverly Hills by a pioneering practitioner, Margaret Ayers, who had participated in the early research on the method at the Sepulveda Veterans Administration Hospital by Barry Sterman of the UCLA School of Medicine, now in emeritus status.

Ayers placed a few electrodes on Brian's head and turned on an instrument that showed him what his EEG was doing from moment to moment. Within weeks, Brian's behavior changed to the point where even casual acquaintances noticed. He started making eye contact. He started making friends and engaging in lengthy conversations. He became almost giddy at the realization that interactions with other people could be rewarding and positive.

He was also more academically successful, to the point where he was able to get himself into college. We enrolled him at Cal Lutheran, so he would be nearby in order to continue his neurofeedback training. After a couple of years he switched to Cal Poly in San Luis Obispo, where he ended up at the top of his class in computer science and was selected for the math honorary even though he was not even a math major.

Neurofeedback helped because Brian was dealing with a failure of brain regulation. The brain has the burden of controlling itself, of regulating bodily functions, and of organizing and supporting our higher functions at the conscious level. When the brain (or the central nervous system) is unable to regulate its affairs, the result may show up in a variety of ways. Brian had this problem more than most, and it was nearly his undoing. Now the remarkable finding was that with only this single technique of brain training, Brian improved functionally across the board. His sleep improved; his mood was more even; temper tantrums fell away; the paranoid episodes vanished; and he developed in so many positive directions.

How is it possible that one technique could accomplish all of that? The only explanation that makes sense here is that the technique caused the brain to reorder its affairs quite generally. One might think of this as a kind of brain exercise, by analogy to physical exercise. Physical exercise does not cure; but it does give us access to better function.

The neurofeedback was so compelling in our son's situation (and in many others that we got to witness along the way) that my wife and I decided to enter the field so that the training could be made available more widely. With Sue's background in neuroscience, and with my own background in physics, we were both on home turf. Both of these disciplines were relevant to the task at hand

when the issue was improving the function of our central control system, the brain.

This kind of work is now blossoming around the world. Margaret Ayers is still active in Beverly Hills, with a primary focus on traumatic brain injury and stroke. We began our own practice in Encino in the late eighties, and over the last few years have established the EEG Institute in Woodland Hills. Our task is to improve brain function using a variety of methods, with neurofeedback at the heart of it all. There are now thousands of practitioners around the country. We ourselves have trained over 4,000 since the early nineties. Many of these practitioners are listed at:

www.eegdirectory.com

As a direct extension of our early work with Brian, we are now helping children and adults with a variety of behavioral and emotional problems. The training avoids negative side effects because we are simply getting the brain to function as intended. The technique is complementary to medical management of these conditions.

[International Neurofeedback Organization, www.eeginfo.com see page 69]

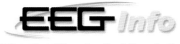

International Neurofeedback Organization

EEG Intro Courses

2007

January 25 - 28
Woodland Hills, CA

February 22 - 25
Miami, FL

April 12 - 15
Location TBA

May 3 - 6
Zurich, Switzerland

June 7 - 10
Woodland Hills, CA

August 9 - 12
Boston, MA

September 13 - 16
Woodland Hills, CA

October 18 - 21
Munich, Germany

December 6 - 9
Woodland Hills, CA

Learn **Neurofeedback**
from the *Experts*

Neurofeedback has been shown to enhance clinical outcomes in the management of attention, mood and behavior. Our comprehensive introduction to Neurofeedback will give you the foundation on which to build your practice.

Professional Clinical Course in Neurofeedback

Presented by Siegfried and Susan Othmer
32 CEs $1495

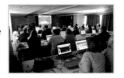

The Professional Clinical Course is a comprehensive introduction to the theory and clinical application of Neurofeedback including lecture, demonstration, discussion and hands-on practical experience. You will acquire the knowledge and experience to begin working with this exciting technique for improving self-regulation and enhancing brain function. Includes One-Day Introductory to Neurofeedback.

Introduction to Neurofeeback is available as a One-Day Course (qualifies for 8 CEs). Please call for more information.

Intro Course Now on DVD

$850

Instrumentation Supported:

NeuroAmp with BioExplorer

BrainMaster Technologies, Inc.

Thought Technology Ltd.

Siegfried Othmer, Ph.D., BCIAC
Susan Othmer, BCIAC

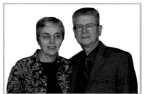

Neurofeedback pioneers Susan and Siegfried Othmer have been leaders in Neurofeedback training, research and development since 1985. A majority of today's practicing clinicians have participated in one or more of the Othmers' training courses.

The EEG Institute is approved by the American Psychological Association to sponsor continuing education for psychologists. The course meets the qualifications for 32 hours of continuing education credit for MFTs and/or LCSWs as required by the California Board of Behavioral Sciences; provider #3628. Provider approved by the California Board of Registered Nursing, provider #14536, for 27 contact hours.

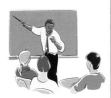

Recommended resources:

Acupuncture

● **Yo-San Acupuncture**
13315 Washington Blvd
Los Angeles, CA 90066
(310) 577-3000
www.yosan.edu

● **South Baylo University**
1126 North Brookhurst Street
Anaheim, CA 92801
(888) 642-2956
www.southbaylo.edu

● **Emperor's College**
1807 Wilshire Blvd.
Santa Monica, CA 90403
(310) 453-8300
www.emperors.edu

Ayurveda

● **Ayurveda Institute of America**
7466 Beverly Blvd.
Los Angeles, CA 90036
(800) 313-4372
www.ayurvedainstitute.com

● **American University of
Complementary Medicine**
11543 Olympic Blvd.
Los Angeles, CA 90064
(310) 914-4116
www.aucm.org

● **California College of Ayurveda**
(distance learning)
1117A E. Main St.
Grass Valley, CA 95945
(866) 541-6699
www.ayurvedacollege.com

Biofeedback

● **Bio-Medical Instruments**
(workshops in Los Angeles)
2387 East 8 Mile Rd.
Warren, MI 4809
(800) 521-4640
www.bio-medial.com

● **My Bio Body (Quantum)**
Sepulveda Blvd.
Los Angeles, CA 90064
(310) 202-0295
www.mybiobody.com
Additional information on page 246

Chiropractic

● **Cleveland Chiropractic**
590 N. Vermont
Los Angeles, CA 90004
(323) 660-6166
www.clevelandchiropractic.edu

● **Southern California University of
Health Sciences**
16200 E. Amber Valley Dr.
Whittier, CA 90604
(800) 221-5222
www.scuhs.edu

Colon Therapy/Hydrotherapy

● **Bryman College**
Los Angeles area
(888) 741-4270
www.bryman-college.com

Cranial Sacral Therapy

● **CalCopa**
18582 Beach Blvd, Suite 11
Huntington Beach, CA 92648
(714) 964-7744
www.calcopamassageschool.com

Crystal Healing

● **AIAS**
6251 Schaefer Ave. Unit C,
Chino, CA 91710
(888) 470-5656
www.pranichealing.com

Dietary Consultant

● **Eastern Michigan University**
(distance learning)
302 Everett L.
Ypsilanti, MI 48197
(734) 487-0918
www.ce.emich.edu

Energy Healing

● **Barbara Brennan School of Energy
Healing** - (distance learning)
500 NE Spanish River Blvd., Suite 108
Boca Raton, FL 33431
(800) 924-2564
www.barbarabrennan.com

● **AIAS, U.S. Pranic Healing Center**
Pranic Energy Healing Training,
6251 Schaefer Ave. Unit C,
Chino, CA 91710
(888) 470-5656
www.pranichealing.com

Feng Shui

● **American Feng Shui Institute**
111 N. Atlantic Blvd. #352
Monterey Park, CA 91754
(626) 571-2757
www.amfengshui.com

Herbal Medicine

● **Global College Of Natural Medicine**
250 Natural Bridges Drive
Santa Cruz, CA 95060
(800) 605-6520
www.gcnm.com

Homeopathy

● **The Homeopathic Academy**
2236 Rutherford Road
Carlsbad, CA 92008
(877) 800-4197
www.homeopathic-academy.com

"Everything you want
is out there waiting
for you to ask.
Everything you want
also wants you. But
you have to take
action to get it."
-
Jack Canfield,
motivational speaker,
trainer and author

● **American University of Complementary Medicine**
11543 Olympic Boulevard
Los Angeles, CA 90064
(310) 914-4116
www.aucm.org

Hypnotherapy

● **Hypnosis Motivational Institute**
18607 Ventura Blvd., # 310
Tarzana, CA 91356
(800) 479-9464
www.hypnosis.edu

Massage Therapy

● **Massage School of Santa Monica**
1453 Third Street Promenade #340
Santa Monica, CA 90401
(310) 393-7461
www.massageschoolsantamonica.com

● **Shiatsu-Anma Massage**
Shiatsu Massage School, 2309 Main Street Santa Monica, CA 90405
(310) 581-0097
www.shiatsumassageschool.org

● **Institute of Psycho-Structual Balancing (IPSB)**
5817 Uplander Way
Culver City, CA 90230
(310) 342-7130 - www.ipsb.com
Additional information on page 64

● **California Healing Arts College**
12217 Santa Monica Blvd. Suite 206
West Los Angeles, CA 90025
(310) 826-7622 - www.chac.edu

● **Touch Therapy**
15720 Ventura Blvd. # 101,
Encino CA 91436
(818) 788-1816
www.touchtherapyinstitute.com

Naturopathy

● **Southwest College of Naturopathic Medicine** (distance learning)
2140 E. Broadway Rd.
Tempe, AZ 85282
(480)858-9100
www.scnm.edu

Neurofeedback

● **EEG Institute**
22020 Clarendon St. # 305
Woodland Hills, CA 91367
(818) 373-1334 - www.eeginfo.com
Additional information o page 69

Neuro Linguistic Programming

● **Designed Thinking Seminars**
Encino, CA 91316
(866) 718-9995
www.designedthinking.net

● **The Christopher Howard Comp.**
1601 North Sepulveda Blvd., Suite 395
Manhattan Beach, CA 90266
(888) 877-8550 - www.chrishoward.com

Reiki Healing

● **The Reiki Center of Los Angeles**
16161 Ventura Blvd. # 802
Encino, CA 91436
(818) 881-5959 - www.reiki-center.org

● **American Reiki Academy**
Los Angeles, CA
(310) 397-2405 - www.reikiacademy.org

Rolfing

● **Integrated Manual Therapies**
1460 7th St.,
Santa Monica, CA 90405
(310) 395-3555
www.advancedrolfing.com

Spiritual Psychology

● **Barron University**
Los Angeles, CA
(866) 677-9465 - www.gobu.org

● **Transformations Incorporated**
(distance learning)
4200 West Good Hope Rd.
Milwaukee, Wisconsin 53209
(414) 351-5770
www.transformationsusa.com

Nutritional Counseling

● **Clayton College of Natural Health**
(distance learning programs)
(800) 659-8274 - www.ccnh.edu

Oriental Medicine

● **Samra University of O.M.**
3000 South Robertson Blvd.
Los Angeles, CA 90034
(310) 202-6444 - www.samra.edu

● **Emperor's College**
1807 Wilshire Blvd.
Santa Monica, CA 90403
(310) 453-8300 - www.emperors.edu

Polarity Therapy

● **Polarity Therapy Training**
19600 Cave Way
Topanga, CA, 90290
(310) 455-7873
www.polarityhealingarts.com

Pranic Healing

● **Learn2heal**
P.O.Box 6717
Pine Mountain Club, CA 93222
(310) 809-2237 - www.learn2heal.com
Additional information on page 39

● **AIAS, U.S. Pranic Healing Center**
6251 Schaefer Ave. Unit C,
Chino, CA 91710
(888) 470-5656
www.pranichealing.com

"I just wish people would realize that anything's possible, if you try; dreams are made, if people try."

Terry Fox,
Canadian humanitarian,
athlete, and cancer treatment activist
(1958 - 1981)

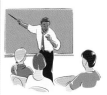

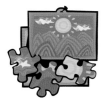

Treatment, Therapy or Healing?

A Personal Story of Growth & Understanding

These three terms are used so often and so little thought is given to their correct application. For instance, the definition of the word treatment is "Administration or application of remedies to a patient or for a disease or an injury; medicinal or surgical management; therapy." Any application of a practical remedy whether it be orthodox, complementary or alternative is a treatment. The word therapy comes from the Greek "therapeia" meaning "a service, an attendance," which, in turn, is related to the Greek verb "therapeuo" meaning "I wait upon." Therapy was, and is, a service done for the sick. Note the difference in the meaning of the word healing:

- To restore to health or soundness; cure.
- To become well; return to sound health.

The term healing is applied when the health of the individual is restored. The goal of all who treat, administer therapies, and heal should always be to restore health. Oftentimes, and unfortunately, applying a treatment is the only thing that happens. It is unfortunate that a treatment is incorrectly considered successful when the symptoms are covered up. This is often as far as some busy, overworked and over-booked conventional, healthcare professionals get. This is where the holistic practitioner comes in. They spend time, one-on-one for a full hour or more and can continue the healing work on other levels and in more depth where the medical doctor has left off.

To further clarify, treating or applying a therapy to ease symptoms and to promote wellness, is not a healing but may and often does bring about healing indirectly. Holistic treatments and therapies frequently bring about a variety of physiological, emotional and mental changes creating chemical balance and harmonizing the patient's system. This results in the free flow of an individual's energy. This healthy energy flow is what allows the body to heal. Healing occurs when the root of the illness is addressed and the client's main issue is substantially improved or completely cured. Here is another personal story shared with *Healer's Guide* that demonstrates the difference between treatment, therapy and healing:

> Every disease brings us a valuable lesson. Symptoms are the catalyst to awakening which leads us to the experience of treatment and therapy. This is the school in which one figures out what is wrong. This process offers us an opportunity to learn and self-educate. The healing is the reward for studying and doing our homework. Healing is the graduation from the life lesson.

> "Whoever survives a test, whatever it may be, must tell the story. That is his duty."
> -
> Elie Wiesel
> novelist, philosopher

A Personal Story

by Elissa Michaud, Hollywood, 1999

When I was in my early 20's I knew something wasn't right. I was tired all the time, I fell asleep on breaks and at lunch during work, sometimes even at my desk - at 10 in the morning. I justified it and told myself, I was simply overworked. I had two jobs, one full and one part-time. It would get better when things quieted down. Although there was some truth in that, there was much more than met the eye. In hindsight, I remember I had enough energy and enthusiasm for my evening job, which was much more interesting than my day job. I tried everything from special diets to fasting, studied as much as I could about herbs and tried them all.

Massage therapy and chiropractic treatments were a welcome relief from the aches and pains which I assumed were a result of the fatigue. They also helped with spinal alignment and organ function. However, what was going on as a whole seemed of no importance to either the massage therapist or the chiropractor. Massage therapists are not trained in medical intervention, nor is it a part of their service. At that time, neither were chiropractors. Nowadays, many modern holistic chiropractors incorporate an entire wellness service into their practice.

During this time, the best holistic treatment I received was from an naturopath. He had me answer a very thorough lifestyle and symptom questionnaire and carefully evaluated the answers. He then explained what he perceived were the areas of weakness (at 22 years of age!) and prescribed a treatment of psyllium husks to cleanse my intestinal tract, acidophilus to re-introduce healthy flora and build the natural balance of the intestines, chlorophyll to cleanse the blood, and cascara sagrada to move waste from the colon efficiently and in a timely matter. By following the treatment program I felt better after one month than in years! My energy level returned almost to full capacity - not amazing, but pretty good.

This newfound energy gave me the strength for a very positive career change. I had the mental energy and clarity to identify that the boredom of my day job and growing dissatisfaction with my second job, might not be the most supportive thing for me. I decided to start my own business. It was fun, I was enthusiastic and loved it! After a short time, the fatigue came again but this time it was much worse. Losing enthusiasm, because of my low energy and not being able to maintain a proper work schedule, caused the business to suffer. I took a few odd jobs to get by, nothing too strenuous, and figured that life must be leading me in a new direction. I looked for something fun and interesting to do, thinking that by doing something enjoyable, my health and energy would naturally pick up.

Next came an exciting move and the beginning of my next adventure. Much to my surprise, the big move from a small town to Los Angeles came with big challenges, financial difficulties and this time, severe and chronic illness and fatigue, which now included a host of infections from bladder to bronchial and of course, the flu. Now, only being able to work a couple of days a week, in a country without healthcare or support, caused me to suffer for many years. Falling back on what I knew worked best, gave welcome relief. Chiropractic treatments, massage and acupressure therapies, and the addition of acupuncture treatments and Chinese herbs helped, to a certain degree. The therapies and treatments relieved my aches and pains, increased my energy level and helped to boost my immune system. I was then able work full time again. Sometimes it would happen that a particular therapy or treatment didn't work or caused a problem. There was one time I tried several colonics and developed candida. The colon therapist failed to mention, that it was necessary to replenish my system with acidophilus after the sessions. This was followed by several months of trying to eradicate a systemic candida problem. After a particular visit, I would experience no relief at all, or sometimes feel worse. The important thing was that there was a marked improvement overall.

Throughout this time, I made occasional visits to medical doctors for antibiotics for flu-related lung infections or things of that nature. The orthodox physicians always ran the standard "look for white blood cell count," but really didn't seem to understand or be able to do anything for me when I explained my health history of the past 10 years. Most wanted to treat the immediate crisis and get me out the door, as fast as possible, with a prescription in hand. Was it worth it to try yet one more physician for the heck of it? I knew people my age didn't feel like this. There had to be something wrong. At one point, I felt physically like I was dying. At the same time, mentally I just didn't have the strength or will to live like this anymore. I sat in the next physician's office doing my best to explain what I had explained to many before her. As a 29 year old, I had been experiencing chronic fatigue, aches pains and most recently, short-term memory loss at the most profound level for the past 10 years (with a few good months here and there). I was on the verge of breaking down. Well, she must have had experience with this, because she proceeded to order a full-blood panel with the works. This one came back just as the others had in the past – perfectly normal, with my hormones a little low, but there was only one small detail on this test which had either been overlooked or not done on the others. Part of the test she ordered included checking the IGA, IGG, etc. levels in the blood, which typically indicate specific viral conditions. She discovered an imbalance in the IGG levels and explained that this, coupled with the symptoms indicated an Epstein-Barr viral infection. She explained that some people get the virus that causes mononucleosis and instead of it going away, it becomes chronic. Great! I was so excited! Someone finally was able to figure out what was wrong with me after all these years! I would have jumped up and down and hugged her if I had had enough energy! So how can you help me? What do we do now? I asked excitedly! "Nothing" she said, "there's nothing you can do for this. You will have good days and bad days. But, if you take care of your health and eat lots of good nutritious food like chicken noodle soup with lots of chicken fat you will feel better and be stronger." "Take care of my health?" I should be the healthiest person on the planet!" I eat right, exercise moderately and have spent thousands of dollars on health care plus another $400 right now and you're saying there is nothing you can do?" "Nothing, I'm sorry" was all she said. No alternative or holistic advise, just maintain a healthy lifestyle and eat chicken fat.

My parents would tell you that I never take no for an answer. I left there and knew there had to be a person with the answers. Someone who had been through this before or maybe, some healing practice which I hadn't heard of. This was the day my education really began. I began asking everyone I knew in the hopes of finding knowledgeable people. I told the producer of an independent movie, I was working on, and to my surprise, he knew just the person! A chiropractor, he said, "who did some really strange stuff." He didn't know how do explain what she did, but he said, " people just got better from

from illnesses that doctors didn't know how to cure." Several days later, I was in the presence of the "voodoo lady." It was $90 for every 15 minutes but I was happy to be there. She began with a very thorough written questionnaire, just like the first herbalist who was so helpful. She asked detailed questions about all aspects of my lifestyle and knew exactly what I was talking about. To her it seemed usual, just the kind of thing she saw on a day-to-day basis. She was confident in her approach and had the answers to many of my questions. She applied a form of energetic muscle testing, one step beyond standard kinesiology, which helped her determine which systems in my body were not functioning properly and which supplements would be most appropriate. She did a form of energetic medicine therapy designed to help jump-start the bodies' computer system, to make it function again. Her requests were simple – no caffeine, sugar or stimulants, no alcohol, no cell phones or cordless phones, a diet high in protein and the elimination of refined carbohydrates. Eat as much natural healthy foods as possible, rich in live minerals and enzymes. Reduce Stress. She explained exactly which systems in my body were affected and why. She recommended a building regimen comprised of a special immune system support product called *MGN3*, tried and tested through clinical studies. High dosages of glandular support nutritional therapy supplements containing vitamins and minerals for the endocrine system - the pituitary, adrenal and thyroid glands. It didn't matter which chronic virus was the problem, the most important thing was to strengthen my body's immune and endocrine systems and the body would throw off the virus and heal itself. Unlike voodoo, this was the most common sense I had heard so far. I followed the advise and recommendations exactly and took all the supplements, followed by one or two more office visits. The healing process was steady and consistent. I could feel the deep reserves and strength coming back as the weeks went by.

Now my interest was peaked with regards to energy work and the endocrine system. What the heck did she do anyways? How and where does one learn this?

I searched local holistic magazines for energy healing, and found that a donation-based energy healing clinic was taking place at a local spiritual bookstore. By this time, my finances were completely drained. I had spent tens of thousands of dollars on healthcare and was really happy to have this service available on a donation basis! I went to the clinic and awaited my turn. A nice middle-aged lady ushered me over to a chair and told me to just relax and close my eyes during the session – that was it! I peeked through my closed eyes to see her moving around me and moving her hands in the air around my body. Hmmm, that was strange. For the most part, it was very peaceful and relaxing, like a deep meditation might be. At one point different anxieties came up and I noticed a rapid heart beat for several minutes, then everything became peaceful again. After the session she explained that many times, the clients who have had chronic fatigue, have something in common. Most of them are very sensitive to subtle energy, but not aware of it and it has greatly affected their physical bodies.

Many with Chronic Fatigue were "sensitives" influenced by things that did not consciously affect most people and often, they naturally have great healing abilities. She stated that, generally, chronic fatigue clients were overly empathetic and quite intuitive and "took on" many things or too many responsibilities. I didn't feel all that different during the hours immediately following the session, only a feeling of lightness. In the days that followed, my energy improved dramatically. I felt "normal" – like a normal human being, having a normally healthy experience. I contemplated what she had said and kept asking myself "What was it the woman did?" After one week, my energy declined, but only a little. Only a few aches and pains crept back in. I desired more than anything to continue feeling "normal." So, I found a healer that practiced the same healing modality, Pranic Healing, and received four weeks of sessions. Since then I have been well.

When you receive energy work, you respond on an energetic level. The physical body follows the blueprint of the energy field and sometimes takes several weeks to adjust. These adjustments take place on all levels – emotional, mental and physical.

As a result of the healing, I began to be aware of certain patterns as they related to my use of my personal energy. I noticed that my energy level would remain strong and my body healthy until I came into the presence of people who were very negative, needy or draining. I found that I did not have strong boundaries or any boundaries with friends or strangers and unconsciously would be so empathetic as to allow others to "zap" my energy. I found that I said "yes" to others' requests because I wanted to please everyone on some level, again taking more of my life force. I had stayed in many unhappy or inappropriate situations in my life out of concern for the other person. I had ignored my own needs and worried about how others would feel as a result of my actions. I put everyone else ahead of me. As a result of working too much, there was not time to cultivate creativity or play. I realized that the place where I lived was inappropriate for me, due to the noise, amount of traffic and busy-ness . While some people may thrive in that excitement and fast pace, it's important to know what works for you. I discovered that through meditation and right lifestyle, I was able to generate enough vitality to not only live in an optimum state of health, but also to help others.

My interest had been peaked with regards to the nature of true healing based on my experience, especially as it related to healing with subtle energy. This prompted me to study many modalities, therapies and treatments. This was the catalyst that allowed me to make a monumental life change so that I may share this wisdom and insight with others, and hopefully, touch their lives with inspiration and hope. I believe that this gift of healing was the result of my desire to heal; willingness to do the work; in this case, really learning about myself; accepting complete responsibility and not buying into the common beliefs regarding chronic fatigue. It was also the result of finding the modalities which resonated with me. After speaking with others who have gone through similar journeys and come out victorious, I found they each had an experience with powerful modalities and lifestyle changes that worked for them. There are probably many other modalities which would have been effective and delivered the same gift, but these just happened to be the ones I found and that worked for me.

[Elissa Michaud]

This is an example of how powerful and helpful therapies and treatments are in not only helping to build the bodies' health and strength, but to understand ourselves at a deeper level. We all should take advantage of the wonderful holistic therapies and treatments appropriate for our health situation. It makes no sense to suffer unnecessarily, when there are so many helpful and kind souls, who are there to serve. Everyone has to go to work and pay the bills and in this modern day and age, we are not subject to the limitations of previous generations. Do what you can to get back on track as quickly as possible. Sometimes a therapy or treatment is all it takes to eliminate blockages, then the body is able to heal itself. You may also discover there are patterns and behaviors which underlie the problem causing a major or chronic health crisis. This is one example of a root cause. True and lasting healing does not usually occur until one comes to an understanding of the cause, and more importantly, learns how to heal by implementing the needed change in their behavior and their life.

Everyone who graduates from the school of conquering disease can be the motivation, inspiration and maybe even the healer for others. Don't keep the knowledge acquired through your healing process to yourself. Share your success to inspire others.

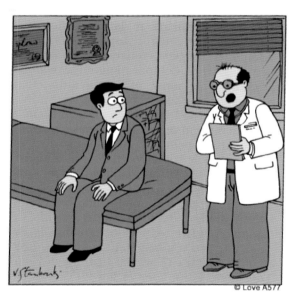

"We still don't have a diagnosis for your rash, so we're going to rub some more money on it and see what happens."

"As we advance in life it becomes more and more difficult, but in fighting the difficulties the inmost strength of the heart is developed."

Vincent Van Gogh, Dutch painter (1853 - 1890)

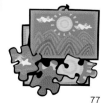

77

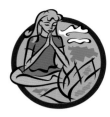

The Healer's Guide Structure

The Body-Mind Connection

I t is interesting to note the broad range of individual choices and beliefs when it comes to understanding one's own health. There are generally two extremes with a mixed bag of everything in between.

At one extreme there are those who identify solely with their physical body. Their reality is based only on what can be seen and touched. In this limited view, they address disease exclusively by the application of orthodox allopathy, without awareness or acceptance of alternatives. Is it possible, that by having a holistic attitude they would avoid recommended surgeries or medications a large percentage of the time? A one-sided approach brings harmful repercussions, especially when risky surgery or harsh drugs are prescribed. The results of unnecessary procedures include post-operative complications such as pain or motion restriction which are difficult to reverse. Orthodox medicine is lacking effective healing solutions for such complications, other than additional surgery, rehabilitation or more pre-scription drugs. Complications are an eye opener and present a window of opportunity to explore alternative methods, but this opportunity is often overlooked, and the route of additional surgical procedures and medication is chosen, resulting in a life filled with pain, without hope for relief. Examples of preventable surgeries (unless in the acute stage) include, spinal fusion, gallbladder removal, tonsil removal, hysterectomy and carpal tunnel release. Surgery for carpal tunnel syndrome is the second most common type of surgery, with well over 230,000 procedures performed annually. Surgery is generally recommended if symptoms last for six months or more (National Institute of Neurological Disorders). Some sources suggest that carpal tunnel surgery has a 57% failure rate and complications or similar symptoms begin anywhere from one day to six years following surgery. At least one of the following re-occur during this time: pain, numbness and tingling sensations. *(Source: Nancollas, et al, 1995. J. Hand Surgery)* If surgery is recommended after six months of painful symptoms, it is surprising that most make no serious attempts to search for healing alternatives during this

Body immunity is strongly influenced by thoughts and emotions. These subtle factors are mediated by the feedback between the nervous and endocrine systems, which form the powerful immunological mechanisms of PNI (psychoneuroimmunology). **The orthodox medical ap-proach tends to ignore the presence of innate human powers where mental fac-tors trigger the PNI system and employ the body's most effective and most powerful defense mech-anism. By cultivating this innate psychophysio-logical healing response with meditation, energy healing, and the power of positive thinking, individuals can learn how to cure and prevent dis-ease at home.** (inspired by: Daniel Reid, *The Tao of Health, Sex and Longevity*)
More information on PNI: www.cousinspni.org

time period. It is hard to believe that individuals in this group choose the option of a surgery with less than a 50% chance of success.

The second example of an extreme attitude is an individual who is solely oriented on alternative solutions and relates all problems to a "message from the soul" or something mystical in origin. Lacking proper perception and insight, they are easily influenced by outrageous claims from the black sheep of alternative healing and talked into undergoing trials of strange procedures which may result in direct harm to their physical organism, not to mention severe emotional and mental imbalances. Such individuals are often seen seeking advice from fortune tellers or "guides" they can communicate with through the special, "*zodiak pendant*" purchased online for $19.95. They become slowly detached from society and practical ways of living. For example: suffering from severe dermatitis, professional medical advice is not sought. An attempt to treat is undertaken by following a "guru -recommended" 10 day water fast found on the internet, accompanied by strong detoxification supplements and instructions to chant mantras repelling bad spirits. As if this isn't bad enough, following a sudden detox, the physical organs responsible for purifying the blood are overwhelmed, resulting in a different or more severe rash. Then, instead of consulting a physician, the sure diagnosis that this disease has its origin in a past life is given from the local fortune teller and the only way to have a healthy and happy life again is to listen what the "guides" are saying through the *zodiak pendant*. Then a mystical "bad karma removal" technique is applied for $300 a session. What results is a severely damaged person on all levels, possibly facing a financial breakdown and unable to return to a normal life just because of an allergy to a new detergent, which could have been discovered by a simple medical test and basic reasoning in the first place.

We are not suggesting, that all medical treatments, surgeries included, are risky or unnecessary, that all alternatives or gurus are fraudulent or dangerous, or that spiritual guides are nonsense. What we are suggesting is the middle path approach to obtain healthy professional opinions on any given subject. In this case, the subject is disease and the remedy is the selection of appropriate diagnostic methods and treatment.

How disappointing it is that little is done to create public awareness for health prevention and wellness. The popular slogan on cereal boxes stating that oatmeal will lower cholesterol is simply not enough. Dr. Michelle Cohen from

Uncovering health fraud is not easy. Especially when those selling it are 100% convinced that their services or supplements work. This makes them dealers of placebos, which incidently, may work, if one's faith is strong enough. Navigate by personal experience. Try once, if it works for you, stick with it. If it doesn't, remember the lesson.

"Psychoneuroimmunology (PNI) is a specialized field of research that studies the interactions between behavior, the brain, and the immune system of the body. The term was originally coined by Robert Ader and Nicholas Cohen at the University of Rochester in 1975. The *Placebo* effect and psychosomatic disease are part of this subject."
-
Wikipedia, The free Encyclopedia, www.wikipedia.org

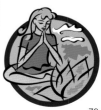

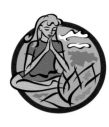

Illumina Healing Center summed it up with a simple statement: "People care more about their cars than they care about themselves. They regularly change the oil, brakes and tires to avoid further expensive repairs, but when it comes to their body, they are unwilling to invest the time, energy and a small amount of money into prevention. They behave as if the body unbreakable. The surprising thing is, few are willing to pay out-of-pocket for preventative healthcare and won't do so unless it is covered by insurance. But when it comes to their cars, preventative repairs and measures are done willingly and without hesitation, even if auto insurance does not cover these costs, because it is understood. It is the norm."

• If preventative healthcare was undertaken at regular intervals, just as preventative care is done for cars, 90% of all ailments would be eliminated.

• The technique used to bring about healing must adequately correspond to the disease in order to be efficient. "Do not use a sledgehammer to kill a mosquito or a BB gun to kill a dinosaur." (nothing against mosquitos or dinosaurs)

• A general education regarding all aspects of the human being - physical, etheric, emotional, mental and spiritual - must be understood before the right path of healing can be established.

• Extremes or excesses in any area are harmful.

• One opinion or diagnosis of a physical symptom is not enough. It is better for it to be complemented by an opinion addressing and assessing all aspects.

• The healing power is within the patient and does not come from the outside (doctor, healer, medication). These are merely tools that assist. The practitioner facilitates healing.

"It is well known that panic, despair, depression, hate, rage, exasperation, frustration all produce negative biochemical changes in the body."
-
Norman Cousins, prominent political journalist, author, professor
(1915 - 1990)

Success is the reward for those who try a remedy, carefully monitor their improvement, and try a different approach when the desired result is not achieved. Practical analysis, common sense, accurate perception, continuous education and being connected to inner guidance is necessary for the best results.

The chapters that follow, including the second section of the *Healer's Guide,* introduce the nature of all aspects of the whole human being. Every human being is made up of physical, etheric, emotional, mental and spiritual aspects. Holistic professionals describe these aspects as five separate "bodies." These bodies require care, nurturing and nourishment, attention and repair. Neglecting, abusing or using in excess any one of them leads to disharmony or disease. Think of the five bodies as five interconnected, dependent, fully functioning parts. These five parts communicate or share information. When there is trouble in one, the others are affected. Therefore, physical illness can not be treated solely by addressing the physical body without considering the corresponding aspects in the other subtle bodies. An emotional disease cannot be treated solely on an emotional level as it's counterpart exists in the mental body and other levels as well. To further illustrate this point, depression and irritability treated by a psychologist will not likely uncover a chemical or nutritional imbalance, easily diagnosed through blood and tissue analysis. Chemical or nutritional imbalances in the physical body are frequently responsible for causing depression or irritability. And vice versa, unresolved mental or emotional issues may cause chemical imbalances.

> The human body is the soul's vehicle and needs maintenance as every other vehicle. Every time you schedule your car for a new oil change, schedule yourself for a preventative healing session and medical checkup. Dental cleaning, energy healing, mammogram, routine blood work, pick one, but make it a habit.

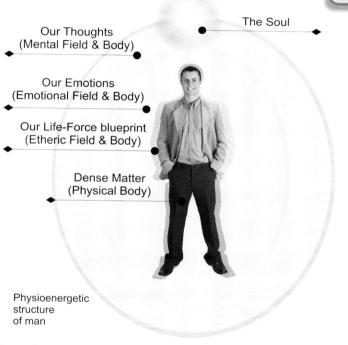

The Soul

Our Thoughts
(Mental Field & Body)

Our Emotions
(Emotional Field & Body)

Our Life-Force blueprint
(Etheric Field & Body)

Dense Matter
(Physical Body)

Physioenergetic
structure
of man

"In everything the middle course is best; all things in excess bring trouble."
-
Titus Maccius Plautus, playwright of Ancient Rome

By taking care of the whole system, rapid healing occurs. A tumor does not grow out of the blue. Something had to cause it. If illness is treated on the physical level only, for example, a tumor removed by surgery or radiation, it may grow back again and often it does. Maybe not in the same location, but as a different manifestation. Because the underlying root cause was not addressed, the tumor information remains in one or more subtle bodies and serves as a blueprint for the physical body to follow.

This explanation will assist you in understanding the structure of Part 2 of *Healer's Guide*. The chapters are broken down into the five body categories mentioned above. Each body category

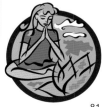

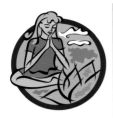

contains information pertaining to it's proper care, including effective healing modalities, techniques and suggestions for self-care. All the while, demonstrating their interconnectedness and interdependence. This is the easiest way to understand the complex nature of your human system. This allows for the discovery of choices that can be made with regards to one's unique healing plan. Part 2 also presents guidelines for achieving a personal experience of feeling, and possibly seeing, subtle energies (life-force). This may enhance one's insight. The way of "The Golden Middle Path," safely leads to a discovery of alternatives used to balance the whole person. This results in true healing and eliminating the dangers of unhealthy extremes. Whether suffering from chronic pain, physical illness or other manifestations of disease such as relationship problems, financial difficulties or spiritual delusion, *Healer's Guide* brings new hope for fast relief with its unique approach tailored to the Los Angeles environment.

> Every aspect of our being (spiritual, mental, emotional and physical) requires attention. The second part of the *Healer's Guide* provides essential information and how-tos on each of these aspects. Refer to *Healer's Guide* Section 2 anytime.

Part 3 includes a detailed explanation of many healing modalities, their applications and cautions, if any. This section also contains immediate referral resources for practitioners and healing centers offering the modalities.

The therapies one chooses are simply tools to assist in healing the body. They offer the opportunity to learn different life perspectives, wisdom and healing techniques from each practitioner. Utilize this process to your advantage and soon you will find yourself sharing the knowledge gained through personal experience with others. The soul has profound wisdom which leads us all through the journey of life's lessons and experiences. Honor this sacred process. The soul determines when the experience of illness has served its purpose. Lessons can be postponed, or altered in form, but never forfeited. The laws of the Universe are exact and push us constantly forward on the evolutionary path.

"It is well known that panic, despair, depression, hate, rage, exasperation, frustration all produce negative biochemical changes in the body."
-
Norman Cousins, prominent political journalist, author, professor
(1915 - 1990)

Hopefully this inspires everyone to read more, grasp the essentials of our human structure and take immediate action, first to realize your own responsibility and secondly to follow up by seeking appropriate professional help, if needed.

After weeks of severe back pain I sought a consultation with a medical doctor. A muscle relaxing medication was prescribed but did not work for long. A friend suggested to try chiropractic treatments. The chiropractor recommended 20 spine adjustment visits. After one week the pain disappeared but returned even more severely the week after. Waiting for my next adjustment, I met a woman who told me, that this type of pain is caused by toxicity in the body and recommended me to a person who specialized in detoxification and colon therapy. After 10 days of losing weight and with a colon cleaner than Christmas snow and no significant improvement, I went to church and prayed for help. A couple of days later the pain was so unbearable I ended up in the hospital emergency room. There I was ensured that my blood was fine, heartbeat, pressure and temperature was normal and there were no signs of STD's. I left with a $1600 bill, four painkillers in a paper bag and a recommendation to a local specialist. This was the last drop in the glass of my patience. A realization, that no one would help me unless I would consciously seek the truth for myself, prompted me to visit a holistic doctor whose reference I found in a local newspaper. He requested tests for my urine, blood and a hair analysis. I had to spend $310 out-of-pocket when I had just spent $1600 on the ER (my medical insurance had a $3000 deductible), plus at least $160 in related charges. When my results came back it was obvious that my body was dangerously low in minerals, depleted due to long-lasting work-related stress. The doctor explained that this could be responsible for my severe muscle pains. A highly absorbable mineral product from my local health food store took care of my debilitating condition within three days and I realized that, due to the detoxification and colon therapy, I had lost 15 lb. The daily headaches I had been self-treating with a grande latte until now and the reoccurring sciatica from the past disappeared thanks to the chiropractic sessions, and I sought a therapist who in a few visits dissolved my work-related stress. The positive side effect was that I could enjoy my family life again. When I was praying for help, the last thing I expected was to get worse, but ultimately that was the kick I needed to take responsibility into my own hands. I also realized that prayer soothed something very deep in my being and for the first time I experienced the feeling that I am actually not the mind but something much greater. One thing still bothers me, what lesson exactly did I learn by paying the $1600 to the emergency room?

Do you have a story which would inspire others and would like to be published? Does your story support or illustrate the complexity of illness as it relates to each aspect of human being?
Have your article published in Healer's Guide 2008! Email your story to article@healerguide.com before Sept. 16th, 2007.

"One cannot tell when he is going to be healed, so do not try to set an exact time limit. Faith, not time, will determine when the cure will be effected."

-
Paramahansa Yogananda,
Indian yogi and guru
(1893 - 1952)

[M. Polak]

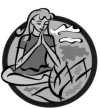

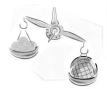

Additional Areas of Health

Finances & Relationships

The shape and condition of one's finances and relationships are an inseparable part of health. True health is not only measured by the absence of disease but by the quality and quantity of personal energy, abundance, social life, wellness and success. Financial and relationship difficulties are often indicative of underlying issues in need of healing and transformation.

Just as a person with a healthy body that suffers from depression is not in a state of true health, the person having physical and emotional health but suffering with relationships and finances is not experiencing true health, either. Of course, a financially poor person is capable of experiencing joy and good health, regardless of their financial situation.

A feeling of satisfaction is gained and a tremendous amount of good can be done with the money one earns. The pursuit of personal goals and spiritual development requires an effort of will, proper choices, and the necessary finances. Those who are less fortunate are greatly assisted by the generosity of others. What about all of those projects, missions and ideas which would be of great help, but are as yet unrealized because of a lack of money? Ideas and projects that have the potential to improve the quality of life and further the evolution of mankind? Even humanitarian efforts require money.

Everyone is familiar with the saying that "*money is the root of all evil.*" In actuality, money used for purely selfish purposes or earned at the expense of others, is the root of all evil. Money earned to invest in personal growth, education, spiritual development and to help others is the energy of love materialized.

Those who live in abundant countries such as the U.S., are gifted with the opportunity to materialize humanitarian projects quite easily. Because of our standard of living we have the freedom to help others in countless ways.

According to a study that examined a database of 34,000 patients with two or more psychiatric hospitalizations during 1994-2000, unemployment, poverty & housing un-affordability were correlated with a risk of mental illness. This finding was reported in the *American Journal of Orthopsychiatry*, published by the American Psychological Association (APA). "The poorer one's socioeconomic conditions are, the higher one's risk is for mental disability and psychiatric hospitalization," said author Christopher Hudson, Ph.D.

"Lack of money is the root of all evil."
-
George Bernard Shaw,
Irish playwright
(1856 - 1950)

There are two simple principles to follow to create abundance:

- Eliminate unsupportive belief structures or patterns surrounding money and replace them with correct perceptions and the right attitude.

- Put service goals fostering goodwill into action through a vocation or avocation. This will bring abundant rewards and help the personal evolution of yourself and others. Follow the basic law that says, "As you give, so shall you receive."

The important questions are: How can one shift unsupportive patterns and related conscious or sub-conscious beliefs? What are the necessary key steps?

- The first key has already been mentioned. Make the shift from service purely to self, to include service to others. What is the purpose of living one's life only for oneself? Eliminate self-centeredness. The activities chosen may be done as either a vocation or as part-time service.

- The second key involves taking the necessary steps to heal unsupportive conscious and subconscious beliefs as they pertain to your relationship with money. Read the following statements about money and see which ones sound familiar.

- You have to work hard to make money.
- It takes too much effort to earn money.
- You have to be born into a rich family to succeed.
- Money is dirty, or money is the root of all evil.
- I could become dependant on money.

$3 could be the whole daily food budget of a homeless person. The fastest way to gain wealth is to transform your daily "latte" into food for those in need. As you give, you shall receive. When you start giving, it sets a chain reaction in motion. The more you give, the more comes back, only you can stop it from returning to you by saying, "I do not want any more money." Experiment with it but don't use your creditcard.

"One of the reasons the rich get richer, the poor get poorer and the middle class struggles in debt is because the subject of money is taught at home, not at school."

Robert T. Kiyosaki, Author of "Rich Dad, Poor Dad"

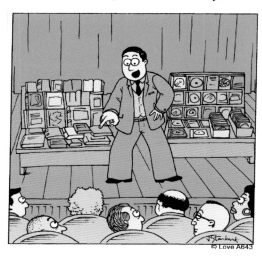

"So you say. 'Tom, how do I become filthy rich? Why. that's easy. By scamming others the way I am about to scam you"

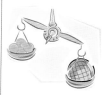

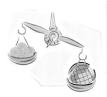

- People with money are greedy, dishonest and uncaring.
- I will attract the unwanted envy and jealousy of others.
- If I have money, I will loose my privacy.
- I am unworthy of having money.
- Money is not spiritual.
- I will never have enough money.
- We can't afford that.

Stress is difficult to define because it is so different for each of us. It is usually described as great mental or emotional over-strain. This over-strain has often been mistakenly related solely to the influence of negative inputs while the positive inputs are over-looked. A person who takes a vacation to Hawaii for the first time in his life and then gets sick, could be seen as succumbing to the effects of positive stress.

Hypnotherapy, psychotherapy, financial counseling and energy healing are very effective for addressing the root cause of your money problems. Hypnotherapy works on the subconscious. Psychotherapy and financial counseling on the conscious mind and energy healing on the bio-energetic field, which is the blueprint for the physical life, including finances. There are many mind-based scientific therapies such as Holosync Technology from Centerpointe Institute (page 174), a powerful tool, designed for subconscious brain re-patterning and raising the threshold levels of the positive and negative inputs one can handle. When people experience sudden success, they may become self-destructive and sabotage themselves due to the shift from their habitual comfort zone, which is predominantly defined by the subconscious mind. The subconscious mind of a person living in poverty for forty years will interpret an event of sudden financial success as a life-threatening change, resulting in self-sabotaging behavior

"A wise man should have money in his head, but not in his heart."

-
Jonathan Swift,
Irish cleric, satirist, essayist
(1667 - 1745)

Prosperity consciousness exercises:

Our energetic field (aura) is responsible for attracting us to situations which correspond to the character and quality of the energy in it. We are responsible for the energy field and therefore, fully responsible for what we attract. If our field is filled with the energy of abundance and prosperity, that is exactly what will be attracted to us, in the form of physical situations. To change the quality of our field from poor to rich is easy. For those who are prosperous already or grew up in a prosperous environment, it is easy to generate thoughts and feelings of prosperity since the surroundings already support this. The person who lives paycheck-to-paycheck won't have enough prosperity energy in their field. They must generate some before prosperous events can happen. The energy field is formed by our thoughts and emotions and our brain can easily be fooled for our benefit. There are several options. The old fashioned way was to go to fancy restaurants and golf clubs to socialize with rich people. This created feelings of wealth and sooner or later, attracted physical success. However, for a person who had thoughts of jealousy or envy (even subconsciously) it would not work, because their focus was on what they didn't have which changed their field to attract even bigger poverty. Another method of attracting success was to purchase items which were supposed to bring prosperity. This was very limiting for the person who actually didn't believe in it. No belief, no thoughts or feelings, resulted in no prosperity. Here are two very simple exercises which will generate amazing results. They are easy to do and don't cost a thing!

● **When you are reading a magazine or newspaper, focus on the pictures you like that represent prosperity or that which you would like to have in your life. Then silently affirm that this picture you are looking at is actually a real photograph of what you already have. See the nice car, affirm "Oh, yeah, this is my car I have it in the garage" or " Oh, yeah, this is my diamond necklace in my safety deposit box" etc. Practicing for 15 minutes each day will produce results. Would you like to make it even more powerful? Start collecting pictures that represent abundance & prosperity to you and create your own magazine with them. Simply glue the pictures in a notebook and as time goes by add more and more pictures of your choice. Then, take a moment three times a day to look through it with the above-mentioned affirmations. Allow yourself to be completely convinced that what you see is an actual reality in your life.**

(caution: no violence or items of violence, drinking, smoking, doing drugs, representation of racism, or acts against religion or spirituality can be used in your notebook!)

● **When you lie down in your bed, ready to fall asleep, repeat a short affirmation in the present tense i.e., "Money is coming to me right now, I am very prosperous" or "I am a millionaire." This should be repeated until you fall asleep. If you usually count sheep to help you sleep, this may be a more productive option.**

The first exercise is quite powerful and will generate enough prosperity energy in your field that you may be attracted to prosperous situations. The second exercise will partially influence your subconscious mind by carrying the affirmation through the opening in your mind barrier which happens at the moment of falling asleep.

When the prosperity flows in, follow these steps to ensure the continuation:

● 10% or more should be donated to a charity or to people in need

● 10% should be invested in your education and spiritual development

● 80% is at your disposal but can not be used to harm

The results will arrive much faster if you refrain from telling others about your practice. If you would like to share this with your loved ones or employees, give them a *Healer's Guide* as a gift.

"If your only goal is to become rich, you will never achieve it."
-
John Davison Rockefeller, Sr., American industrialist and philanthropist (1839 – 1937)

in an attempt to return to the "safe environment" of the past. Clearing the subconscious mind by brain re-patterning, raises thresholds and the ability to adjust to a new level of prosperity.

They third key is proper education. Workshops that teach financial skills, improving your relationship with money and learning how to invest wisely are a good start. Take a class or private coaching session from a professional and learn as much as you can about managing and manifesting wealth. Improve your work skills and abilities through specialized training and education. As an employee, you are an invaluable asset and most likely will be offered lucrative promotions and advancement opportunities. If you are self-employed, your business will improve as a result of implementing your new skills.

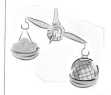

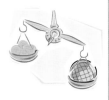

The fourth key is to create supportive surrounding influences. Surround yourself with successful people who have prosperous philosophies and approaches, as mentors, business associates and friends. It is not good enough to follow people who although rich, have undesirable motives and lack integrity. Don't overlook your home and work environment. A Feng Shui consultant can identify and neutralize destructive influences and help create an environment to boost health and wealth.

One of the most personally destructive habits is the overuse of credit cards, that take advantage of your cognitive and behavioral vulnerabilities. Marketing techniques used by credit card companies induce consumers to under-estimate their debt and promote snap decisions to spend what they do not have. Credit cards are a good safety net but that doesn't mean they should be ready and convenient in your wallet. Credit card debt is the second biggest cause of bankruptcies after hospital bills.

The fifth key is self-evaluation. Which destructive personal habits do you possess that do not support financial success? Here is a short list to review. Laziness, inability to complete things, misplaced priorities, clutter, difficulty being on time, a defeatist attitude, overall negativity, petty behavior, lack of emotional control, not believing in yourself. Make a personal list and put a check beside each one that stands in your way. These are obstacles which must be gradually healed through strong determination and will. If certain habits are difficult to overcome, have a professional practitioner help you. Try tackling one habit every month. Start small and build confidence.

Key number six: Investigate the personal habits of financially successful people, especially those you admire. Do they take the time to get to know others and are they kind? Are they always on time or five minutes early? Are they meticulous with their manner of dress? Is their car always spotless? What is their mind set? Core beliefs? Do they have a spiritual practice? Choose and implement one new habit (or more) every month.

You are work in progress. Just taking the first step on the path, does not guarantee immediate success. Keep focused on positive, steady progress. Although rapid results are possible by being proactive, this is usually not the case. Aim for steady results, but don't get discouraged and give up if progress seems slow. It took years of social conditioning, negative program-ming by family and peers, and years of bad habits to produce an environment of lack, so be patient.

"From borrowing one gets poorer and from work one gets richer."
-
Isaac Bashevis Singer, Author
(1902 – 1991)

Financial educational workshops:

☐ **Mastery University - Wealth Mastery,** Anthony Robbins Companies, shows you how to regain your financial footing and grow and sustain your wealth, as well as multiple ways to make and save money and defensive strategies to protect your portfolio, (800)898-8669 - www.anthonyrobbins.com

☐ **Financial Freedom Society, Inc.,** On-line & over the phone education, Financial Freedom Society, Inc. - eliminate financial problems by providing specialized education, professional services and tools for a low monthly fee. 9705 Sea Rider Way, Lutz, FL 33559, (813) 960-3131 www.ffsi.com

☐ **The One Minute Millionaire,** The Enlightened Way to Wealth, Robert G. Allen, workshops and books to help you create financial abundance - www.oneminutemillionaire.com

☐ **Peak Potentials Training,** Home of the world-famous 3-day Millionaire Mind Intensive, specializing in inner-world principles for real world success, helping identify and overcome the hidden obstacles that hold you back from reaching your full potential in terms of both success and happiness, (604) 983-3344 - www.peakpotentials.com

☐ **Art of Allowing Workshops,** Abraham-Hicks Publications, offered in over forty U.S. cities each year, helping you to create abundance (830) 755-2299 - www.abraham-teachings.com

☐ **The Leading Edge Training,** The Science of Manifesting, Steven S. Sadleir, offering tools, training and support for executives and entrepreneurs, 668 N Coast Hwy #417, Laguna Beach, CA 92651 (949) 497-9954 - www.theleadingedgecorp.net

☐ **GMCKS - Kriya$hakti,** Use thought power and the active generation of Good Karma to create material abundance. AIAS, (888) 234-9876 - www.pranichealing.com

☐ **Financial Healers, Inc.,** The intention is to clearly heal the negative emotions, thoughts and beliefs associated with your perception of money which keep you in financial bondage. The Healing Your Finance process will breakthrough illusions of lack, limitation and guide you back to your financial truth, (310) 364-3500 - www.financialhealersinc.com

"Prosperity belongs to those who learn new things the fastest."
-
Paul Zane Pilzer, an economist, entrepreneur, college professor, author

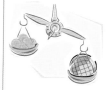

89

Financial Bondage
by Jeanette Perez, ALSP

The financial aspects of your life determine how you live and In most cases, tend to have dominion over all of your affairs. Thus, is it possible to create financial freedom in your life? How do we remove the shackles that keep us in financial bondage?

We live in a society where values have shifted and in changing these values, we have ultimately turned away from our purpose as individuals and society, as a whole. We are no longer living our truth; therefore, our purpose has little or no meaning at all. Now let us examine the significance of this dilemma: Profit and or gain appear to be the focus of today's society, which in turn affects the consciousness of the human race. The intensity placed on the end result, profit and/or gain, diminishes our personal values. Progress is evident in our society; however this progress is only in the material world. We have become masters in attaining material wealth. We are currently living in a world where many individuals are experiencing lack and limitation from a financial perspective. This is contrary to our natural birthright - abundance and prosperity. The need for change is evident and long overdue. While all else in our society has changed and is constantly changing, our money systems have not. We are using antiquated systems which have not evolved into the 21st Century. The biggest misconception is that there is never enough. The truth is, there is no such thing as lack. The use of this antiquated model has negatively impacted companies, families and individuals.

We are being called to redefine the financial aspect of our lives. If lack does not exist, why are so many individuals experiencing poverty? Poverty consciousness is the result of the belief in lack, which we call "not enoughness." Poverty conscious-ness is having its way with our society. It is also prevalent in individuals who continue to feel discontent with their material abundance. Wanting is the condensation of lack. The outpictur-ing of our lives mirrors our thoughts and

beliefs. Where do we begin? Teaching and empowering others to breakthrough old thoughts and beliefs, developing financial systems that support our renewed beliefs. We must bring money back to its original intention and service is an essential part of the equation. Money is a tool used to honor service. In honoring service, we are honoring each other. When in service, you are assisting something or someone and operating from your heart space. We are here to be of service to one another.

All industries/companies offer a service, however, more often than not, the focus is placed solely on profits. Operating from this perspective creates an avenue in which the value of service ceases. The energy created in this environment can be detrimental to the success of any given organization. In order to create a success-ful organization, true service must be part of the equation. True service provides personal fulfillment. In return, the energy birthed in this powerful truth produces positive results, including profits. Service qualifies the organization and all those who participate to attract experiences to support this positive energy.

From an individual perspective, the work needs to be done around debt. What emotions have you attached to debt? Fear? Shame? Fear of not having enough, shame for being in debt. These are considered low frequency emotions. If you are aligned with these emotions, you are in financial bondage. Debt is the word that describes the financial outflow of our lives. If we were to stop and examine the truth of debt, fear or shame would not exist. When you remove these emotions from debt, the truth is revealed. Your creditors have provided a service which has enhanced your life in one form or another. Therefore, they are not creditors, they are contri-butors. Shame and fear are replaced with gratitude. Allow gratitude to dictate your experience. Hence, you will attract experiences that will keep you anchored in gratitude. When you are paying your bills, you are gifting and honoring your contributors back. Become an observer of your thoughts and release the hidden beliefs which keep you in financial bondage. Live the life you were intended to live!

see page 91

Healing Your Finances

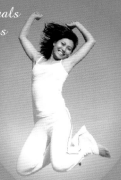

We live in an abundant universe, and yet many individuals are living in poverty consciousness. The human race has evolved on many levels, and still prosperity remains stagnant in many lives. Where do we begin? What is required to remove the misconceptions around money? The Healing Your Finances process will provide practical tools, which will empower you to manifest financial freedom.

Examine the origin of hidden beliefs & how they affect the out picturing of your life.

Breakthrough illusions of lack and limitation

Look at specific emotions, thoughts & beliefs which block the flow of money

Examine the language of the financial world which keeps you in financial bondage

How to create opportunities and options to increase your inflow/income

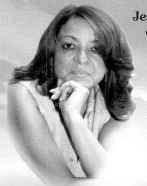

Jeanette Perez has worked in the financial arena for over twenty-five years. Her experience in the financial world has provided her with profound insights and revelations regarding society's perception of money. Jeanette, an avid student of New Thought/Ancient Wisdom, has combined these teachings with her career in the financial arena. This powerful combination birthed the Healing Your Finances Process. Jeanette is an Agape Licensed Spiritual Practitioner (Spiritual Counselor) who is committed in assisting others transform their lives

Unleash your earning power today!!!

For more information on Jeanette Perez and Financial Healers
310 364-3500
www.financialhealersinc.com

Relat—◆— Relationships —◆—

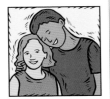

The subject of relationships is so complex, there could be an entire guide just for the topic. Presented here are the common themes, messages and energies at work which underlie all relationships as they pertain to overall health.

It is quite easy to recognize whether something works, and whether or not we have good, or not so good, relationships. Every relationship, be it intimate, family, friends or work, must be evaluated separately. There are different measures for each of them but the mutual aspects to be considered are:

- Is there, or is there not, a relationship?
- Is the relationship supportive or destructive or both?
- Is the relationship based on truth or lies?

Relationships cannot survive without healthy communication between the partners. Mastering the ability to communicate with your partner can easily resolve any issue your relationship may currently have.

Communication is the most important aspect of a successful relationship.

To figure out that there is something wrong with your physical body doesn't take much effort. To discover that your financial health is in need of healing, takes even less, but to determine if a relationship needs healing, takes quite a bit of work. Not because we lack the ability to see that there is something wrong, but because we have the ability to pretend that nothing is wrong and that everything will be all right. This is called *wishful thinking*!

Relationships are one of life's learning tools. They grow our spirit and force us to become better people. There are lessons to be learned and personal growth is gained from every relationship. Ideally, this growth enables us to move forward to a wiser and more harmonious place. Resisting this growth creates stagnation and disease. Relationships have a tendency to last when growth is continuous and encouraged between both parties in a healthy, harmonious way. Each party remains in the relationship based on their free will and choice. When growth opportunities are limited or unhealthy, relationships tend to dissolve.

"Assumptions are the termites of relationships."
-
Henry Franklin Winkler,
actor, director, producer

Subtle signs and hints, that let us know that a relationship is not a good fit for us, are usually present at the beginning. These signs are what enable us to decide if the new relationship will be good (growth) or will be harmful (stagnation). These are often overlooked for several reasons. For example, some want to have a relationship so much that anyone will do. They will ignore the signs or pretend they mean something else. Pain and suffering is the result when it comes time to deal with them later. Relationships based on physical appearance, money, and other material factors typically do not last.

The next logical question is, "what are the subtle signs that occur before entering a relationship" that have the ability to inform us whether it will be the right match and be helpful for our growth? These signs are part of your internal barometer. By listening to both your heart and mind, being aware and present, and following the flow or intuition, we will end up in a relationship that is the right match for our needs and evolution. By blinding ourselves with material reasons or physical appearance, a detour may lead us in a different direction for years before offering another opportunity to make a better choice.

We would be missing part of the picture if we believed that only happy, prosperous, faithful, joyous and other highly valued aspects of relationships are good and that those filled with pain, suffering, poverty, violence and ignorance are not. Relationships exist to help us evolve. Some appear to be very loving and harmonious, but offer no challenge. Not being able to stand up or not knowing how to protect yourself, physically, emotionally or mentally, may lead to the attraction of violent or abusive relationships. Of course, those who make the conscious decision to actively work on certain weaknesses, possibly working with a professional who can help them understand why they may be attracting these types of relationships, may no longer have to attract such unpleasant learning experiences. Rather, they may choose to participate in a seminar teaching assertiveness or communication skills. For the rest, who are too busy to consciously enter into the arena of personal growth, they leave the Universe no other choice than a relationship adventure and some hard knocks schooling.

Relationships reflect, as mirrors do, aspects which require learning and growth. Remember that a mirror's reflection is always reversed. For example a woman who is unorganized and messy in a relationship with an uptight clean freak has her mirror image. She is reminded daily to get organized, while he is reminded to loosen up and relax once in a while.

Taking deliberate action to work on our shortcomings before they are delivered in a more forceful manner by other life circumstances, liberates you from the endless cycles of same old patterns. Success in this area also depends, in part, on the ability of the partner, business, or coworker, to achieve the same willingness to grow. Deciding to break an agreement and end a relationship prematurely, without taking advantage of the opportunity to work on our issues, results in reoccurring patterns and similar situations. The next relationship will often repeat the same patterns and have identical issues.

The foundation of every successful, happy relationship is the strength of each partner's mental and emotional health. To find or maintain a healthy relationship is only possible when you are healthy. It is the responsibility of each partner to bring mental and emotional maturity, responsibility and stability to the table. An individual lacking emotionally stability cannot expect a healthy relationship.

"Lots of people want to ride with you in the limo, but what you want is someone who will take the bus with you when the limo breaks down."

Oprah Winfrey, talk show host

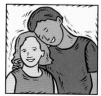

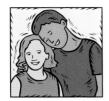

For those currently in dysfunctional relationships with family, friends or partners, who feel disillusioned by this information, do some introspection and try to analyze what the relationship may be teaching you about yourself and what may be the lesson for your counterpart. If they are open to it, have a conversation about those things and work on them together. Some relationship dynamics are too complex to apply the approach above. However, our personal growth is the underlying current behind all relationships. When there is enough strength and willingness to learn, coupled with conscious action and acceptance, a seemingly hopeless situation can be magically transformed. An unpleasant work situation can grow into a great business opportunity, maybe the company is suddenly sold and new management comes in, or a 20 year partnership with an abusive person ends and we realize how much happiness, freedom and new opportunities we have.

When both parties make conscious progress and the willingness to go forward is mutual, we shift into a whole new dimension. From the dysfunctional relationship, a compatible team or friendship is established. This is a much more secure place to start from, when difficulties or life lessons arise. In a team, personality imperfections can be pointed out and corrected without unnecessary suffering.

Improving a current relationship or increasing the possibility of establishing a new harmonious one, requires effort and determination to learn from previous mistakes. Increasing our reservoir of skills and knowledge in the area of inter-human communication leads to success. By listening to our hearts and re-evaluating decisions with sharpness of mind, stripped from the destructive patterns and programming of parents and society, the new, evolved relationship model is created.

> To listen to our partner is another essential aspect of a healthy relationship.
>
> "In order to truly listen it is necessary to be present, and the difficulty with being present is caused by unhealed emotional wounds. If we are not able to be emotionally honest with ourselves then it is impossible to be present and comfortable in our own skin in the moment. Obviously then, we are also incapable of being present with, and emotionally honest with, others. "
>
> [Robert Burney, author, www.joy2meu.com, www.Suite101.com]

"Love lasts when the relationship comes first."

-
Abraham Lincoln,
16th President of the
United States
(1809 - 1865)

The easiest way to recognize if a relationship is supportive is:

• By realizing if there is or there is not a relationship. This requires proper perception and acknowledging that a relationsip is truly an agreement of all parties. If only one party demands or attempts to establish a relationship with no obvious intention of the other party to participate, then there is no relationship and further self-convincing will bring disappointment.

• The relationship is supportive or destructive or a mixture of both. If the relationship is mostly supportive, great! If the relationship is destructive and continues in the same pattern, something must be addressed. The easiest and fastest way out of a destructive relationship is to identify the point of friction and learn as much as possible about it. This brings an opportunity to understand the issue much faster and eliminates the need to learn it painfully from the relationship. When the lesson is learned, we move on.

• The relationship is based on truth or lies. This requires self-honesty and introspection. Are we ourselves or playing a role? The latter deliberately creates an illusion, possibly helping our counterpart to grow at our expense, but most likely keeping them in a vacuum that will result in stagnation.

Remaining in one of these three situations creates a disconnect or separation between what we think, feel and actually do. This separation creates disturbances in the energy field (see Part 2). When this pattern is held for some time, it manifests as a blockage in the complex mechanism of the energetic anatomy, eventually resulting in physical disease. Following the physical symptoms provides an opportunity to discover and heal the more severe, underlying problems, often found in relationships, otherwise unconsciously ignored or overlooked and vise versa. Staying in a relationship that creates a constant charge of negative thoughts and emotions clogs up our bio-energy flow and results in physical disease.

The following signs of relationship difficulties are frequently suggested to be an indicator that it is time to end a relationship, but in fact they are only symptoms and may exist just to let you know that the relationship is in need of healing.

- A feeling of continuous frustration about the relationship.
- Finding reasons to spend time apart.
- One or both partners are physically or verbally abusive.
- Sex or other intimacies are demanded under pressure.
- One partner changes his or her core values, beliefs and goals to please the partner in hopes that relationship will become better.
- When appearance changes (*i.e.* cosmetic surgeries) are used to keep the other party interested.
- A growing feeling of emptiness.
- Close relationships with others (*i.e.* friends, family, coworkers) are discontinued to please the other party.
- When pretending to be someone else. Not being real.

Identifying unhealthy relationship symptoms that can be healed is the first successful step towards positive change, but this step should not be followed by running away. This is the time to realize what the lesson is and learn it at all costs.

As children, we looked up to our parents and learned about life by observing their actions. This is how we first learned about relationships. Dysfunctional family situations create underlying negative emotions in children and later serve as hidden magnets, attracting relationships which create similar negative emotions. The fastest way to improving relationships is to first resolve one's issues with one's parents.

"The objective of two lovers is almost always the same; to find meaning in their individual lives and in their life together."

-
Paul Pearsall Ph.D.
"Using the Power of an Intimate, Loving Relationship to Heal Your Body and Soul"

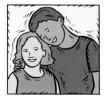

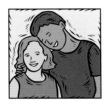

Learn in a weekend workshop, from a tape or book, from a friend, or on-line, but learn it. Then proceed with your fight or flight. At this point it may come as a surprise that the relationship will suddenly shift to a new level or will end gracefully without effort because you have graduated to a new level of wholeness.

By breaking off a relationship (intimate or professional) prematurely the opportunity of learning the lesson is lost. Don't do it yet. Implement a holistic approach before suppressing the symptoms and leaving the relationship. Try to investigate and understand what it represents for you. If violence is present it is a different circumstance. Violence can be one of the worst things to deal with. First make sure you are physically safe, and that proper legal actions have been taken for your protection. Then, attempt to understand the significance, so that it does not happen again. What attracted you to this person in the first place? Did you overlook important signs in the beginning of the relationship? Why would someone hit a person they respect? Even violent people rarely hit those they admire or respect. Perhaps there is an underlying issue with self-esteem or self-confidence that deserves attention. No one has any right to use violence towards anyone. Healing yourself always results in healing your relationships.

At the National Domestic Violence Hotline, help is available to callers 24 hours a day, 365 days a year. Hotline advocates are available for victims and anyone calling on their behalf.

1-800-799-7233

"People change and forget to tell each other."
-
Lillian Hellman, Author and playwright (1905 - 1984)

Relationship improvement workshops:

◻ **Mastery University -** Date With Destiny, Anthony Robbins Companies, (800)898-8669 - www.anthonyrobbins.com

◻ **Relationship Coaching Institute (RCI) -** relationship coaching training and support, P.O. Box 111783, Campbell, CA 95011 (888) 268-4074 - www.relationshipcoachinginstitute.com

◻ **The Bonding Weekend (TBW)** - Healing our relationships and feeling empowered in our lives, (805) 899-1970 - www.bondingweekend.com

◻ **Six Steps to Improve Every Relationship in Your Life -** 6161 El Cajon Boulevard #306 San Diego, CA 92115 - Southern CA Events, (619) 807-2473 - www.everyrelationship.com

◻ **SkillPath Seminars** - United States, PO Box 2768 · Mission, KS 66201, (800) 873-7545 - www.skillpath.com

◻ **Southern California Neighborhood Guide**, Classes & Seminars section - www.socal.com/events/

◻ **PAX Programs** - Understand how the most basic instincts of men and women pit us against each other in the world of dating and relationships, (80) 418-9924 - www.understandmen.com

◻ **Embody Tantra** - simple exercises to uncover the bliss of this moment and translate this presence in your relationships. Morning meditations, monthly classes, private sessions for women and couples, (323) 363-3135 - www.embodytantra.com

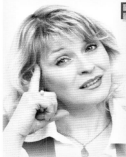

Psycho-Spiritual
Relationship Healing

...those with relationship
...those seeking relationship

Singles or Couples

No matter where you are in your relationships, this can take you to the next level. Attract a supportive nurturing relationship or evolve the current one.

◇ Clearing the build up of negative emotions stored as an energetic "charge" such as resentments from previous arguments and situations.

◇ Healing the energetic patterns which prevent you and your partner from having complete acceptance of each other.

◇ Removing energetic obstacles that prevent both partners from giving and receiving love and affection.

◇ Clearing others' jealousy, envy and wishes of failure towards your partnership.

◇ Re-establishing healthy energetic connections on the physical, mental, emotional and spiritual levels.

◇ Re-charging the relationship with blessings of love, peace, happiness, harmony, passion and understanding.

◇ Shielding the relationship from future harm and danger.

◇ Removing obstacles which prevent you from attracting and establishing a new supportive relationship.

◇ Heal energetic patterns or attitudes such as unhealthy ideas towards opposite sex. These may be based on conditioning or stored traumas from past experiences.

◇ Healing your fears and phobias surrounding romantic relationships.

◇ Clearing obstructive energies from parents or unsupportive patterns of their relationship which may have been passed to you.

◇ Tips and easy exercises to attract right partner.

◇ Clearing energetic patterns that prevent you from giving and receiving love and affection.

◇ Energetic psychotherapy to transmute and minimize trauma of abuse.

Healing includes spiritual healing and professional psychology session

Distance & In-Person Sessions are available.

www.relationshiphealing.us

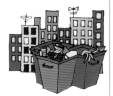

Environmental Health

The Influence of Your Environment

There are a multitude of environmental factors in our immediate surroundings that contribute to poor health or lack of vitality. Not to mention an endless list of chemicals, pollutants and additives. Even so, the human body is continuously evolving and adapting and mankind has survived the most destructive influences and will continue to do so. Before shedding light on several of the most influential environmental forces and their practical solutions, let us first look at the bigger picture.

Imagine yourself in the cockpit of an airplane with a see-through floor. Now look down on the Earth. There are areas of deep forests, broad deserts, oceans and lakes. Using intuition and logic, which areas appear to be best able to support life? Which would you consider a healthy place to live? Take a good look at the city of Los Angeles and if you were to rate it on a scale of one to ten, with ten being the most supportive, which number would you choose?

Major influences always supersede minor ones. Here is another example: let's say you are a fish living in an

"Progression of environmental illness tends to be a lot of allergies, and then people begin to develop multi-symptom disease that resists conventional treatment, such as PMS with colitis or spastic colon, heart arrhythmias, maybe asthma, or a combination of these things. Brain dysfunction is a common problem that we see - short-term memory loss, imbalance, dizziness, vertigo. Anybody who has an inflammatory disease of unknown cause can have environmental overload. These diseases can include lupus, scleroderma, vasculitis, non-specific colitis, general indigestion, and arthritis."

John R. Lee, M.D. interview with William J. Rea, M.D
www.ehcd.com

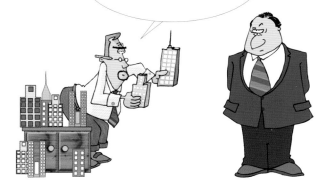

aquarium and the water happens to be dirty and disease-laden with bacteria. Even though you get adequate exercise by swimming, eat the healthiest fish food, meditate and pray every morning, chances are your energy, vitality and the quality of your life are less than perfect. The chances of getting sick are increased tremendously to the point that it is inevitable, because the environmental field or aquarium water is simply not supportive to life. Now, if you, as that same fish don't exercise, meditate or pray and eat fish junk food, but live in the waters of the Amazons, it is much less likely that ill health will manifest, due to the extremely life-supportive Amazonian field. Healthy environmental fields can override bad personal habits, to a certain extent.

Given the above scenario, the first question to ask is "Is my environment life-supportive?" If the answer is yes, then it's time to pay attention to the more minor details. If not, moving to a healthier environment is not such a bad idea. Following this advice does not necessarily mean moving out of town, unless of course, this choice appeals to you and is feasible. It may simply mean moving to a more environmentally supportive area of the city, maybe from downtown Los Angeles to Santa Monica, or from a house beside the freeway, to one close to a park or ocean.

When someone passes away, it is tradition for family members to place a headstone at their grave. In addition you may want to plant a tree in their memory. A tree is a meaningful way to express your sympathy and the memorial planting is a symbolic remembrance of the past and a renewal of life. This is a legacy that benefits the environment for years to come.

All living creatures, including humans, have an energy field, a bubble of life-force surrounding and permeating their bodies, called the aura. When we live in close proximity to each other, these fields mingle. If you could see these energy fields from a plane, you would see a huge mass of mingled fields in the big cities, creating a collective field. This collective field affects individual energy fields positively or negatively and influences the condition of one's health. The degree of influence depends on several factors. The following experiment further demonstrates this. When a calm, emotionally balanced person enters a room filled with ten anxious, upset or stressed out people, he or she will have a tendency to become stressed out as well, due to the group influence of the bio-energetic or radiatory field (auras) of the others. If you have never been exposed to or noticed your reaction to this common occurrence, try observing the shift in your thoughts, emotions and energy level while being stuck in rush hour traffic.

"You are a product of your environment. So choose the environment that will best develop you toward your objective. Analyze your life in terms of its environment. Are the things around you helping you toward success -- or are they holding you back?"
-
W. Clement Stone, philanthropist and self-help book author (1902 - 2002)

This influential ability of the collective energetic field affects but is not limited to health, relationships and finances. Observe the predominant characteristics of the field you live in or are surrounded by daily. If the environment is unhealthy or unsupportive, implement changes wherever and whenever possible. Even though it may seem like too big of a step to make

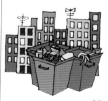

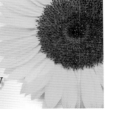

TRUE FENG SHUI®

The Ancient Art & Science of Environmental Mastery

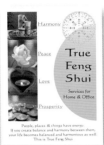

✓ Complete Feng Shui Assessment of your Home or Office

✓ Explanation of all seen/unseen factors and influences

✓ Detailed analysis of problem areas or situations (if any)

✓ Solutions to counterbalance these any problem areas

✓ Outline of the energetic blueprint of your place and how it affects you

✓ Assessment of the supportive and obstructive influences/energies

✓ Explanation of how to enhance or minimize these influences

✓ Detailed assessment of each room including furniture placement, color schemes, etc.

✓ Which energies, based on natural laws, are lacking in your environment and how to boost them

✓ Proper sleeping and working directions for each individual who uses the space

For Commercial Consultation we additionally offer:

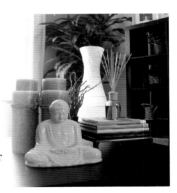

● Energetic Employee Evaluation (up to 10 employees)

● Business Forecast

● Business Relationship Evaluation

Consultation takes about 2 hours for residential locations and 3-4 hours for commercial locations.

● **Relationship**
● **Prosperity**
● **Success**
● **Health**
● **Spiritual Life**

$50 off your first Feng Shui services if you mention this ad

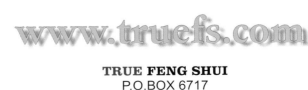

www.truefs.com

TRUE FENG SHUI
P.O.BOX 6717
Pine Mountain Club, CA 93222
Office Valencia: (661) 242 2477
Office Malibu: (310) 809 2237
Fax: (661) 242 2477

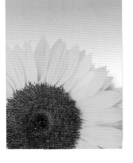

the payoff is an improved quality of life on many levels. If the fish in the above example decided to move from its polluted environment, it may not be easy to change aquariums - maybe the fish is accustomed to the tank and likes its water castle and plastic diver with bubbles. Over time, it became used to the diseased conditions to such an extent, that it seems impossible to change the habit of being in such an environment. What if the fish knew that by moving into cleaner water, not only would health problems diminish, but the change would open up new life and career opportunities? The fish would see the value of enduring a small amount of initial discomfort for the satisfying result of having a newer, even bigger, water castle, this time with a treasure chest. Isn't that a smart idea?

After taking care of the major influences it is time to start correcting the secondary influences (the minor ones). The sum of many negative minor influences may be as detrimental to one's health as living in a garbage dump. Many of these corrections are easy to do on your own. If your are unable to investigate whether your home or office environment is unsupportive or harmful, work with a Feng Shui practitioner. Feng Shui is the healing modality that investigates and corrects unsupportive environmental influences. Professional Feng Shui practitioners apply and utilize the laws of nature to balance the environment of a home or office, helping create balance and harmony by promoting the flow of positive energy and neutralizing, or minimizing, negative or destructive energy. Feng Shui is rapidly becoming a standard practice for creating an ideal and balanced environment in which to live and work. Following are some secondary influences to consider:

• **Neighbors:** If you live with or next to people who are negative, pessimistic, fighting, or always complaining about something, move. They could be neighbors, roommates, or family members. It is not advisable to live with toxic people. Make a list of the ten people you spend the most time with (friends, family, co-workers etc.) Assess their health, relationship, prosperity and success. It is typical that your own life situation is not far from the median of your group.

"Health consists of having the same diseases as one's neighbors. "
-
Quentin Crisp, English writer (1908 - 1999)

• **History and location of home or land:** Houses or apartments built in the proximity of what is or was a cemetery, hospital, slaughter house, police station or jail, military outpost, casino, etc., are not recommended. The energetic field of such sites is typically contaminated with destructive or unhealthy energies. Instead choose a supportive location instead close to a park, garden, ocean or lake. In a big city choose your surroundings carefully by investigating the neighborhood.

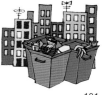

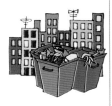

● **Air Inside of your house or apartment:** Air in the home is approximately 14 or more times polluted than the air outside, due to the evaporation of chemicals such as wall paint, carpet or wood impregnations, mold spores found in the space between walls, and chemical cleaning supplies, among others. These influences cause illness, especially respiratory problems, and make healing difficult as they burden the body with extra toxins. Make sure your home is well ventilated and buy an air cleaner or ionic air purifier to eliminate pollutants from indoor air or devices that pull air through and clean it. They are not the nice smelling chemical air fresheners or synthetic preparations, which actually create toxic air.

● **Clutter:** *The Law of Correspondence* has to do with the cause and effect of visible and invisible influences. The law states that what is on the outside is on the inside and vise versa. Your feelings are expressed by the way you create and maintain your environment, but conversely, your environment affects the way you feel about yourself and your life. Clutter falls under the category of producing both visible and invisible harmful influences, especially in relation to your psychological well being, productivity, relationships and finances. Tidy up and throw away or donate things which you do not like or will not use, even if they are gifts from your mother-in-law! A clean, uncluttered home or office offers peace and supports emotional and mental well-being.

Feng Shui states that what we carry inside of ourselves has a tendency to manifest correspondingly outside of us, and vice versa. A clean, organized and creative environment is indicative of a clean, organized and creative personality. Feng Shui improves one's surroundings, which helps to create the desired changes in one's personality.

● **Electromagnetic Frequencies (''EMFs''):**
Countless studies and research have been done and so little truth has actually been uncovered. It is impossible in this day and age to avoid EMFs unless you live in a Faraday cage. Electromagnetic fields are everywhere. Radiation from cell phone towers, television and radio transmitters, satellite broadcasts, military and emergency frequencies, all kinds of radars and who knows what else? You can't escape! Eliminating those in close proximity is the best defense. Never sleep closer than five feet to an electronic device such as alarm clock. When using cell phones, use an ear piece and try not to remain on a lengthy call with a cell phone attached to your head. Here is a simple experiment. Dial a number from your cell phone. While the phone is still dialing, cover the antenna with the tips of your fingers. You may experience a sharp pain or burning in your fingertips. For those who can feel it, think about the important part of your body that is being exposed to the cell phone antenna. Get an earpiece! Many "magical pendants" have recently flooded the market, with the promise of protecting you from all harmful EMFs. It is possible that certain devices, generating magnetic impulses, in frequencies of the Shumann field which are similar to human natural vibrations would keep the body and mind in balance when affected by EMF radiation. There is still more theory than practical application and we will pay extended attention to this in the *Healer's Guide*, 2008 issue.

A Faraday cage or Faraday shield is a structure made out of conductive material, or by a mesh of such material. This (shield) enclosure blocks out external static and other electrical fields.

- **Water:** The human body is approximately 70% water. The quality of the water you drink is very important for removing toxins and keeping the body hydrated. Also, the energetic properties of individual water sources make a measurable difference on one's energy level, health and well-being. Consider the properties of healthy water in nature. Not only is it free of contaminants, but it is also energetically charged by air, sunlight and natural movement. Now consider city tap water. Not only is it void of most life-giving properties, but it is recycled and cleaned. Sure it is bacteria and possibly parasite free due to the addition of anti-bacterial chemicals, but cleaning does not eliminate the energetic contamination and neither do filters or reverse osmosis systems. Tap water also flows under the ground of major cities. The ground under a city is energetically contaminated by heavy, negative radiatory fields from the past and present, as well as other forms of pollution. The best drinking water comes from a well, pristine lake or springs, containing the life-giving properties. Investigate water sources and find out more than just what the bottle says. It's a good practice to leave the unopened (air-tight) water containers in the sun for a few hours and bless, pray, or ask for your water to be blessed. If you have any doubts about the benefits of water blessing, visit your local bookstore and read Dr. Masaru Emoto's book, *The Hidden Messages of Water*. It contains the results of years of scientific research regarding the effects of exposing water to dozens of influences including cell phones, heavy metal music, microwaves, prayers, blessings and the vibration of words.

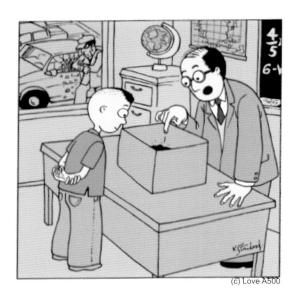

(c) Love A500

"See, Jimmy, as the population grows too dense, the rats begin to brutalize each other....."

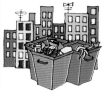

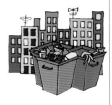

• **Chemicals in your home:** Buy responsibly and use responsibly. Don't be fooled by seemingly natural products. Read the labels. Cleaning products are one of the largest contributing factors to toxins in the home. Replace current chemical cleaners with environmentally friendly and biodegradable products, that work. Keep all dangerous products far away from bedrooms and living areas, preferably in a storage area or garage.

It is also wise to check for radon, a naturally occurring, radioactive gas, produced by the decay of uranium - radon is responsible for many cases of respiratory disease and other illnesses. Also, consider testing for mold in your environment, especially when you are trying to troubleshoot for the origin of mysterious symptoms or respiratory problems. Mold can be very toxic and causes a myriad of health-related issues. The mold may not be visible as it hides behind the walls or under the floor. Its spores are smaller than a virus and can easily travel.

☯

We all want our homes to be clean, safe places to live. The Natural Resources Defense Council (NRDC) has determined that the top, common household contaminants most dangerous to health are: cigarette smoke, radon, formaldehyde, pesticides and lead. Tips on how to minimize your exposure can be found at:
www.nrdc.org/health/home/fchems.asp

There are never-ending influences and it is impossible in a large city like Los Angeles to eliminate them all. Try to have balance and discernment. Large corporations overuse modern technology and chemicals, contribute to environmental pollution, and harm Mother Nature. Equally, there are those who dedicate an unhealthy amount of energy to their constant worries. All extremes are harmful. Use common sense. If after using the most environmentally safe biodegradable soap you could still scrape the dirt behind your ears with a teaspoon, change the soap. Sometimes products do not work, even though they are well intended. Investigate your environment, find the potential health threats, then take the necessary steps within your range of influence and correct them.

Environmental resources for health and safety:

☐ **California Department of Health Services,** Free Radon Test Kit, (800) 745-7236 - www.dhs.ca.gov/radon/default.htm

☐ **HomeStoreProducts.com,** Test kits for: Mold, Radon Gas, Bacteria, Asbestos, Radon in Water, Water Quality, Lead in Water, Lead Surface, Carbon Monoxide, Lead in Paint/Dust, Pesticides in Water, (800) 427-0550 - www.homestoreproducts.com

☐ **Less EMF.com,** Electromagnetic Safety In the Home & Office, (8 8 8) L E S S - E M F - www.lessemf.com/emf-news.html

☐ **Natural Resources Defense Counsil, NRDC,** Environmental issues - www.nrdc.org

☐ **AirNOW,** Air Quality Forecasting and Monitoring - www.airnow.gov

☐ **Clutter Busting,** Get Rid of Your Clutter and Feel Great, Brooks Palmer, (310) 903-1041 - www.clutterbusting.com

By far the most terrifying film
you will ever see.

aninconvenienttruth
A GLOBAL WARNING

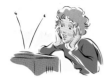

Conscious Media

The Healing Power of Television, Internet, Radio & Print

Exposure to love, abundance and joy creates a healing environment. Exposure to fear, violence, destruction, or difficulties creates disease. Each individual has the ability to choose and be in control of what they are exposed to through media, giving everyone the power to create either a healing or a diseased environment.

Conscious Media consists of information and entertainment that presents a wide variety of perspectives while encouraging awareness. Often topics are covered which are not featured on mainstream channels and if so, minimal time and attention is dedicated to their coverage. Rather than presenting information as a predigested, positioned and formulated idea or belief, conscious media educates and informs, for the most part, in an unbiased manner. The viewer is presented with the entire story, so that they may form their own personal conclusions and points of view drawn according to a proper, well-rounded understanding of the subject matter. At least they are exposed to facts which are not commonly shared. One's accurate perception of our world condition is dramatically altered after 30 minutes of evening news. The top seven or ten stories reflect the most shocking happenings or gruesome crimes. Of course, with 12 million people in Los Angeles it's not difficult to find a few tragedies. If news programs would repeatedly contain practical and inspiring information such as new knowledge or the latest breakthroughs on how to improve the quality of one's life, with an underlying theme of optimism, it would impact society positively and create a different perception of the world's future.

> The mission of conscious media is to inform, empower and discuss beneficial topics as well as to present a variety of perspectives on each subject, giving each viewer the freedom of creating a healthy opinion. By seeing things in their proper perspective and living in "truth" (even though truth is a personal choice), healthy relationships with one's environment can be established.

Conscious media, via it's holistic approach, creates a supportive atmosphere for learning, personal growth and healing, with topics related to the environment, science, metaphysics, spirituality and nature. Information is power. Informed and aware citizens are viewed as a threat to the very fabric of a market-oriented, materialistic society. This is a society which promotes democracy as its ideal, but the very channels by which it disseminates information, do little to promote this ideal. Independent opinions and thinking are encouraged, but the general public is not informed enough to stray far from the common beliefs and group thought. This is evident by the sheer amount of people living in fear vs. those living in love and peace;

"You can tell the ideals of a nation by its advertisements."
-
Norman Douglas, British writer, *South Wind* (1868 - 1952)

those living in ignorance vs. those who are enlightened. The media has a responsibility to fulfill its duty to be a healing tool for society and to eliminate those aspects of fear, chaos and destruction. Conscious media aligns their values and missions with like-minded businesses, whose common goal is to serve and heal humanity. Therefore, their audience is introduced to products or services that are harmonious and beneficial.

According to a press release from the American Medical Association (AMA) to a congressional field *(Children increasingly exposed to graphic media violence. From September 13, 2004),* children exhibit several measurable negative effects when exposed to "entertainment" violence.

● Children accept violence as an effective way of settling conflicts and assume that acts of violence are suitable behavior.

● Children grow to be emotionally desensitized to violence and will be less likely to take action on behalf of a victim when violence occurs in real life.

● Children develop an increased fear of becoming a victim of violence, with a resultant increase in self-protective behaviors and a mistrust of others.

● Children have a higher tendency for violent and aggressive behavior later in life than children who are not as exposed to violent media.

22-34% of young male felons imprisoned for committing violent crimes (homicide, rape, assault) report having consciously imitated crime techniques watched on TV (Journal of American Medical Assoc. - Studies in Violence and Television). **Be aware of how much TV your children watch. Limit viewing to 1-2 hours each day. Take time together to talk about how violence and guns are glamorized on TV and in video games.**

AMA Trustee Ronald M. Davis, MD said, when addressing the House Committee on Energy and Commerce's, Subcommittee on Telecommunications and the Internet, "As physicians, we need to counsel parents that watching violent TV shows can be bad for children." The AMA urges parents to monitor and control their children's exposure to violence through TV and other entertainment media." Also, in a study of children at five public schools near Boston, children who watched more television consumed more calories. Jean L. Wiecha, Ph.D., Harvard School of Public Health, and colleagues studied 548 children (48.4 percent females) with an average age of 11.7 years. Among participants, each additional hour of television watched per day was associated with an extra 167 calories consumed, including a larger percentage of sugar-sweetened beverages, fast foods and other products commonly advertised on TV. Authors wrote, "Although children and youth are encouraged to watch what they eat, many youth seem to eat what they watch, and in the process increase their risk for increasing their energy intake."*(Arch. Pediatr. Adolesc. Med. 2006;160:436-442., (quoted by www.businessweek.com).* It was also suggested by a series of data sets analyzed in a paper by

"Don't you wish there were a knob on the TV to turn up the intelligence? There's one marked 'Brightness,' but it doesn't work."

-
Leo Anthony Gallagher, American Comedian

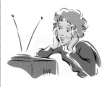

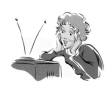

economists at Cornell University, Indiana University and Purdue University, that early childhood TV viewing may trigger autism. Authors wrote, "The medical community is increasingly convinced that something is happening in the environment that triggers an underlying biological or genetic predisposition toward autism, and these findings strongly support the need for taking a closer look at early childhood television viewing."

Replacing role models of violence with acts of compassion and peaceful methods of settling disagreements creates a more harmonious social environment that is supportive of a healthy society. In addition, it is has been observed that children who do not read, or are not read to, rapidly lose the brain capacity to imagine. When watching television, ideas are already presented in their final form, so the parts of the brain related to imagination, stagnate in development.

> Whatever is watched, listened to, or read may have a direct impact on the human bioplasmic field (aura). This field is formed by subtle vital forces, emotions and thoughts. The quality of this field determines the quality of life experiences. If the field is filled with happiness and joy, the experiences of happiness and joy will be attracted into one's life, if it is filled with pain and sorrow, life adjusts accordingly.

When experiencing ill health or in a vulnerable state, exposure to depressing, violent or plain old boring media results in even a greater loss of vital life force. Negative thoughts and emotions generated by watching a horror or sad movie, have a depressing effect on the entire system and contribute in subtle ways to the worsening of one's overall state of health. Even if healthy, it may at the very least, produce a shift in vibration or quality of energy in one's bioplasmic field (aura). Based on the law of attraction that states that like attracts like (see the chapter *Cosmic Laws*), the new or lower (negative) vibration now has the ability to attract it's equal. On the other hand, reading inspiring, uplifting and conscious material, is supportive to recovery and overall well-being. Simply watching a comedy, helps generate positive thoughts and emotions, attracting positive events in to our lives and it is clearly a much better selection.

> "You can never get all the facts from just one newspaper, and unless you have all the facts, you cannot make proper judgements about what is going on."
> -
> Harry S. Truman
> President of U.S.,
> author of
> *Mr. Citizen*

The power of choice applies not only to television, but to all aspects of media including radio, press and internet. It is a matter of supply and demand. When the viewers and readers choose media containing wholesome information instead of fear-based and destructive programming, it will diversify the advertiser's funds, resulting in a forced transformation of the entire media market. This will re-kindle the consumer interest and restore profitability. Let's practice exercising this power collectively, send a strong message and change the future of media and our future well-being. Thanks to a certain freedom of speech there are several independent internet channels to choose from. The new media market contains a selection of conscious books and magazines, films and documentaries. These are created by individuals with the common goal of raising mass consciousness and empowering humanity by presenting accurate, truthful, educational and illuminating information. High in entertainment value, this is information and thought that creates awareness and serves as a catalyst for positive changes. Messages of universal truth, life lessons, moral conduct, and eco-consciousness with an emphasis on a positive functional lifestyle are incorporated in these works.

Internet Media:

☐ **Conscious Media Network** - free video interviews on consciousness, enlightenment and human potential - www.consciousmedianetwork.com

☐ **Closer To Truth** - a new cross-media genre presenting "Knowledge Affairs" in which the fundamental questions of our times are explored by scientists, scholars and artists - www.closertotruth.com

☐ **The Natural Paradigms Channel** - presenting new, sustainable lifestyles in an entertaining format - www.naturalparadigms.com

☐ **LIME TV** - connects you to an array of experts and thought leaders as well as community members to help you lead a greener, more balanced life - www.lime.com

Falling asleep each night to the television or radio is a poor choice, from more than a health perspective. The moments when falling asleep and upon first waking up are the moments when the subconscious mind is most easily influenced. This was scientifically proven by electroencephalography *(the neurophysiologic measurement of the electrical activity of the brain)*. As we drift off to sleep, the human brain shifts into the "Theta" state *(in which the brain operates in the frequency range from 4Hz to 8Hz)* which is associated with hypnagogic states such as trance, hypnosis, deep daydreaming, lucid dreaming and light sleep. This is the exact state which is artificially induced during a hypnotherapy session. This pre-sleep state is best utilized for creative visualization and peaceful, happy thoughts. During a hypnotherapy session with a professional therapist, the commands are stated in present tense and are given with caution for the purpose of healing. However, the commands from the TV or radio heard when falling asleep can be detrimental. Falling asleep to the ten o'clock news and commercials is one of the worst habits because you never know what the last message your subconscious mind received will be. The subconscious mind is one of the strongest forces creating your life. Before falling asleep, use the time to visualize a perfect state of health, imagine your life being abundant, peaceful and joyful, and your goals being successfully achieved. But for goodness sake, turn off the TV! If visualization is challenging and music is required to fall asleep, use CDs instead.

April 23-29, 2007
National TV-Turnoff Week

What's so great about it? Turning off the television gives us a chance to think, read, create, and do. To connect with our families and engage in our communities. Turn off TV and turn on life. More than 65 national organizations, including the AMA, the National Education Assoc. and the American Academy of Pediatrics, support or endorse TV-Turnoff Week.

For more information visit:
www.tvturnoff.org

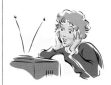

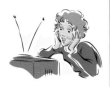

The effects of sleep on our physical well-being are well known and are a key to maintaining normal levels of cognitive skills such as speech, memory, innovative and flexible thinking. Research even suggests that sleep loss may increase the risk of obesity as the chemicals and hormones that play an instrumental role in controlling appetite and weight gain are released during sleep. From the holistic point of view, these are only fragments of the myriad of processes that take place.

Based on spiritual teachings, human consciousness, while sleeping, first shifts to the astral realm (see the chapter on the *Emotional Body*), and then "leaves," for lack of a better word, the physical body. What is created and experienced there is the direct result of the content and the state of the emotional body and subconscious mind. Sleep is the ideal time to create a positive pattern for the following day and to release negative and potentially unsupportive impressions in the subconscious mind. The intentional creation of a positive lifestyle can be enhanced by carrying over the supportive impressions from the waking state to the sleep state. When negative or destructive impressions are carried from horror movies or books, violent PC games or the evening news, the destructive pattern will be created in proportion and according to the intensity of the stimulus. Falling asleep to suggestions such as "No on proposition XY," or "Americans trust hepaflu as the #1 medicine for cold & flu," will most likely influence the next days' happenings or decisions without your even realizing it.

> ☯
>
> The power of positive affirmations was introduced to the Western medical world by Emile Coue (1857-1926), who discovered that his patient's health was improved by focusing on healing instead of fears or negativity associated with illness.
> His famous affirmation was: "Everyday, in every way, I am getting better and better." Affirmations are a highly respected self-improvement techniques validated as unequivocally effective.

"It's the repetition of affirmations that leads to belief. And once that belief becomes a deep conviction, things begin to happen."
-
Claude M. Bristol,
Author of a
Prosperity Classic
(1891-1951)

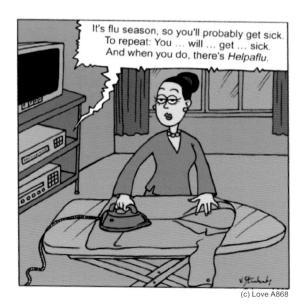

(c) Love A868

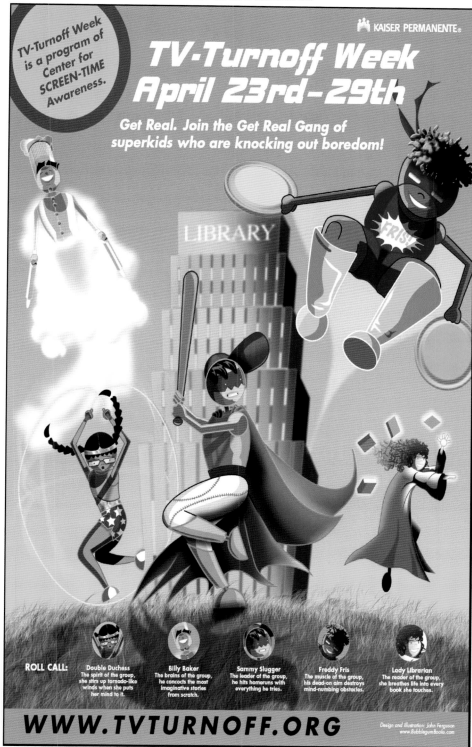

THE SPIRITUAL CINEMA CIRCLE

THE HEART & SOUL OF CINEMA... BROUGHT HOME TO YOU

Welcome to our Inner Circle. We have brought together some of the most entertaining and soul-nourishing films for you and your family to enjoy each month. Join us in transforming the heart of entertainment one home at a time.

With Love;
Stephen Simon
(co-founder of Spiritual Cinema Circle)

TAKE A CINEMATIC JOURNEY OF THE HEART, MIND & SPIRIT

4 INSPIRING NEW FILMS EVERY MONTH

Hard to find, award-winning movies

www.HealerGuide.com/movies

START YOUR
FREE TRIAL NOW!

JOIN NOW AND GET THE FIRST MONTH FREE

Recommended Movies:

☐ **A Day In The Light** - a film that spreads the message of peace of love for all people of the world - www.adayinthelight.com

☐ **An Inconvenient Truth** - offers a passionate and inspirational look at one man's fervent crusade to halt global warming's deadly progress in its tracks by exposing the myths and misconceptions that surround it - www.climatecrisis.net

☐ **Breakthrough** - a film about a new way of life through wholesome living and the raw food diet. A breakthrough to maximize human potential! - www.naturalparadigms.com

☐ **Conversations With God** - the dramatic journey of a down-and-out man who becomes a spiritual messenger and best-selling author - www.cwgthemovie.com

☐ **Eating -** The Rave Diet, a common sense approach to addressing the maladies and ailments that so many people suffer from today; an honest look at the faults of the standard American diet - www.ravediet.com

☐ **Fast Food Nation** - an ensemble piece examining the health risks involved in the fast food industry and its environmental and social consequences as well - www.fastfood-nation.com

☐ **Good Night and Good Luck** - Infotainment or courageous, hard news? Why aren't the tough stories being told? Compel the media to get back to reporting in the public interest! - http://wip.warnerbros.com/goodnightgoodluck

☐ **Icons Of Evolution** - a fascinating journey into one of the most controversial issues today, the conflict over evolution based on science, not religion - www.coldwatermedia.com

☐ **Naked In Ashes** - the bearers of a 7,000 year old legacy, yogis give up everything to seek self-realization - www.paradisefilmworks.com

☐ **Origins of Yoga** - quest for the Spiritual. Yoga as a path to the inner self - www.paradisefilmworks.com

☐ **Peaceful Warrior** - the first successful mainstream example of Personal Growth Cinema, reflects and expresses an unspoken yearning for higher wisdom. - www.thepeacefulwarriormovie.com

☐ **Spiritual Warriors** - the illuminating story of a spiritual student preparing to fight the evil power of darkness that threatens the world - www.spiritualwarrior.org

☐ **Syriana -** a political thriller that unfolds against the intrigues and corruption of the global oil industry - www.syrianamovie.warnerbros.com

☐ **The Blue Butterfly** - inspired by a true story, ten year-old Pete Carlton is diagnosed as terminally ill and his determined mother will stop at nothing to ensure that her son's dream is realized - www.bluebutterflythemovie.com

☐ **The Celestine Prophecy** - based on James Redfield's internationally best-selling novel, *The Celestine Prophecy* is a spiritual adventure film - www.thecelestineprophecymovie.com

☐ **The Humanity Ascending Series** - The Untold History of Humanity As Seen Through Evolutionary Eyes - www.barbaramarxhubbard.com

☐ **The Secret** - a groundbreaking movie that reveals The Great Secret of the universe - www.thesecret.tv

☐ **The World According To Sesame Street** - explores the drama and complexities behind producing international versions of the world's most-watched children's television program. Shows that social impact and change can come from the most unlikely sources, including a team of Muppets - www.pbs.org/independentlens/worldaccordingtosesamestreet

☐ **Unlocking The Mystery Of Life** - a documentary with the power to revolutionize our understanding of life and to unlock the mystery of its origin - www.illustramedia.com

☐ **What The Bleep Do We Know?!** - revealing the uncertain world of the quantum field hidden behind what we consider to be our normal, waking reality - www.whatthebleep.com

☐ **Who Kill The Electric Car? -** Chronicles the life and mysterious death of the GM EV1, examining its cultural and economic ripple effects and how they reverberated through the halls of government and big business - www.sonyclassics.com/whokilledtheelectriccar

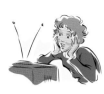

Fall asleep with a calm mind and positive emotions. Media can be utilized as fuel to success, or a source of immeasurable harm. No one appreciates websites filled with spy-ware, those annoying pop-up windows with special offers which distract our focus. When turning on the TV or radio, without a prior conscious selection of programming, it is the equivalent of opening the mind to a website with spy-ware. If there is nothing valuable on television or radio, it should remain off. If movies or television serves as relaxation after a long day of work, replace the habit of watching senseless media with an uplifting or inspiring movie.

The average child will watch 8,000 murders on TV before finishing elementary school. By age eighteen, the average American has seen 200,000 acts of violence on TV, including 40,000 murders *(Compiled by TV-Free America, Washington, DC)*. These statistics are nothing compared to violent computer games where the number of virtual murders could be hundreds per hour! Computer gaming offers other choices for both children and adults, which stimulate the mind and promote health. Conscious companies have created software supportive to wellbeing and self-improvement. See examples below.

Conscious Computer Gaming:

❏ **The Journey to Wild Divine** - step out of time and into a realm of endless possibility, where you'll practice breathing and meditation techniques, like the Heart Breath, an ancient yogic breathing technique that will help you achieve control over your mind & body - www.wilddivine.com

❏ **TheKidsOnlineStore.com** - helping your kids to grow in the physical, mental, and educational areas of their life through interaction with quality software products - www.thekidsonlinestore.com

❏ **Self-Esteem Games** - play a computer game for five minutes each morning that will help you feel more secure and confident in yourself www.selfesteemgames.mcgill.ca

Everyone has had the experience of turning on the radio, whether it be AM or FM and hearing the same 50 songs, 150 commercials and 5 topics discussed over and over again.

Conscious Radio:

❏ **KPFK Pacifica Radio for Southern California** - presenting accurate, objective, comprehensive news on all matters vitally affecting the community - www.kpfk.org - 90.7 FM

❏ **HealthyLife.Net** - internet radio, dedicated to providing all-positive radio programming to expand your mind, improve your health and lift your spirit without sensationalism or controversy. The HealthyLife.Net mission is to help eliminate fear, advance positive thought and encourage the idea that we are all one, here for the greater good of all - www.healthylife.net

❏ **KTLK LA's Progressive Talk** - Los Angeles and Orange County's Progressive Radio voice, with local personalities Stephanie Miller and Harrison combined with Air America's Randi Rhodes, KTLK is talk radio with a liberal sense of humor - www.ktlk.com - AM 1150

❏ **LIME Internet Radio** - connects you to an array of experts and thought leaders as well as community members to help you lead a greener, more balanced life - www.lime.com

"The only thing we have to fear is fear itself."
-
Franklin D. Roosevelt, U.S. President

ROBERT EASTON JSU GARCIA

IT TAKES GREAT COURAGE
TO SEE THE FACE OF GOD

DR. JOHN-ROGER PRESENTS

SPIRITUAL
WARRIORS

THE FILM

DIRECTED BY DAVID RAYNR. STARRING: ROBERT EASTON,
JSU GARCIA, SHYLA CRUIZE & LEIGH TAYLOR-YOUNG

Inspired by *NY Times* #1 best-selling author
Dr. John-Roger's book *Spiritual Warrior*

For screening information call 323-422-0002
email: zoe@msia.org

www.spiritualwarriors.com   www.john-roger.org
www.jsugarcia.com   www.msia.org   www.ndh.org

times

e life LA | FREE

whole life times

JULY 2006 | LA | FREE

spa in the sky

downsizing with style

holistic help for aging eyes

fresh

wholelifetimes.com

BER 2006 | LA | FR

wholelifetimes.com

LA's Guide to Healthy Living
Since 1978

WHOLELIFETIMES.COM

Healer's Guide offers great thanks to all the radio stations that do not match this mainstream profile. In the previous box are some progressive stations worth listening to. There are still two other important sources of media to mention. CDs and print. CDs are the most convenient method of receiving supportive information. Audio material has the ability to accelerate one's recovery or boost self-improvement goals within a few short days. Statistics show that the average Californian spends approximately 800 hours in their car, each year. This is where a Los Angeles traffic jam or a long commute to work can be used constructively. The CD player is a magic portal that will transform the driving experience into a convenient mobile classroom. It is just a matter of time before someone starts an educational CD mail delivery service. Until then, hundreds of self-improvement or self-empowerment titles may be found in major bookstores as well as online. (references below)

Print is the least invasive media vehicle. Personal exposure is well within the realm of one's control. Radio, TV and the internet have the unwelcome advantage of being able to target unprepared listeners'/viewers' conscious and subconscious minds with information that, if given a choice, would be filtered out. Even though complete control of the input received by our senses is an unrealistic hope at this time, the ability to decide what is listened to or viewed is entirely possible. When opening ourselves to receive information through media, select media outlets that carry messages of optimism, growth, support and healing.

> ☯
> **Transform your time spent in traffic into time wisely invested in self-improvement and healing. By the time you reach your destination, you will have easily and effortlessly taken care of your daily dose of self-care and education.**

Resources for Personal Development and Self Help:

❏ **Nightingale** - products for personal development, spiritual growth, wealth-building, mind development and wellness, (800) 560-5973 - www.nightingale.com

❏ **SelfHelpRUS** - an extensive collection of audio and video CDs by best-selling authors who specialize in a variety of self-improvement, career and professional development techniques, (866) 216-1480 - www.selfhelprus.com

❏ **MindPerk** - CDs, tapes and videos of world-class authorities in success and motivation - (800) 457-2523 - www.mindperk.com

❏ **Inner Peace Music** - Steven Halpern is the pioneer of the use of therapeutic music in the fields of holistic and alternative medicine. His healing music is an essential tool for relaxation, healing and wellness, and has been used by healthcare practitioners, caregivers, and hospice workers for over 30 years, (800) 909-0707 - www.innerpeacemusic.com

❏ **Luxe Vivant** - offers unique and innovative products for mind and body self improvement, 888-782-2252 - www.luxevivant.com

❏ **Wisdom Scientific** - publisher of self-help and self-improvement products and founded by family therapist Abe Kass. Based on professional experience helping thousands of clients with personal and relationship problems, (800) 771-8993 - www.wisdomscientific.com

"If you wish to achieve worthwhile things in your personal and career life, you must become a worthwhile person in your own self-development."

-
Brian Tracy,
a self-help author

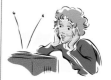

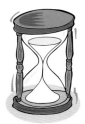

Life's Biggest Transition

Conscious Dying

A great deal of time and money goes into funeral arrangements from the casket and head stone to the will. How often does one stop to think about how to take care of his or her soul, which is eternal and which moves with us through our many journeys of life and transitions of birth and death? Many people have lived live not believing that there was a continuation of their life waiting for them when the physical body dies. And yet, when their time came, they were the first ones to call for the priest! Was it too late? What is there left for you to change or fix when you have 15 minutes left? Of course a priest is of great assistance at the time of transition. We, however believe that being conscious of everything we do, learn, think, feel and say in this lifetime, is of utmost importance. Directing our efforts to elements of ourselves, we can take with us after transition is essential. Ideas and statements in this chapter have been compiled from various traditions. Presented is a synthesis of the beliefs and understandings regarding physical death from many of the world's religions, cultures and spiritual teachings.

> According to the National Funeral Directors Assoc. "funerals are an important step in the grieving process, as well as an opportunity to honor a life lived. They offer surviving family members and friends a caring, supportive environment in which to share thoughts and feelings about the death. Often funerals are the first step in the healing process."

How many people have you made happy? Whom have you helped and what have you done to make yourself a better person? What new skills or abilities have you learned that have helped to enrich your soul in this lifetime?

> "Life is pleasant. Death is peaceful. It's the transition that's troublesome."
> -
> Isac Asimov, Science fiction writer (1920 - 1992)

This chapter sheds light on the importance of a holistic approach and on the application and fundamental knowledge of the universal *Law of Karma* or *As you give, so shall you receive*, which permeates this life and the afterlife. The Law of Karma, when understood and utilized, may be used wisely to our advantage as it relates to our healing. This is the often overlooked missing link. The information presented, might be unacceptable for some due to their belief structures. For those who are not comfortable with the information presented here, feel free to skip this chapter.

Let's start with an overview of the best known of the cosmic laws. The Law of Karma or what is sometimes known as *The Golden Rule*. Whatever you sow, you will eventually reap. If you sow a potato, will you reap an orange? No. Not only will you get a potato but perhaps a whole crop! The same thought process must be applied to all of our deeds, wholesome and unwholesome. Therefore, it would be better to plant good deeds and thoughts and reap positive rewards. If life does not end after leaving the physical body, clearly it would be better to have positive results and events to look forward to.

At the moment of death, many are unhappy with the life they have lived and are also out of time, energy and resources to make further changes. Surely those reading this book still have enough power to make changes. Call the people you have hurt and apologize. Call the people who have hurt you and tell them they are forgiven. This is usually the most difficult part, especially between family members. If you have lived a selfish life, change it! Make time to do the things you have always wanted to do or that are important to you. In this new era of technology it is possible to perform miracles just by the click of a mouse.

A very ill person was offended when encouraged to give to charity (to tithe), in order to improve his health condition. He stated, "I contributed by financing one of the military air raids during World War II. I have a presidential award and many veterans are still sending me thank you letters for my bravery. I have already contributed enough to society!" That was not exactly what was suggested. It may be difficult to predict the rewards or consequences as they relate to his particular action.

The recommended options are a little easier and have a win-win outcome. There are millions of people in need all over the world. Decide whose life or circumstances you would like to help or change. If donating to a charity is not something that resonates with you, maybe giving to an organization doing research to bring about a cure for a particular disease sounds better. You may also find ways to help someone on a more personal level. Some people use this karmic law to create wealth or opportunity. They have discovered that by helping or donating to a good cause, and improving the lives of others, their lives also have improved. Later, when asked why they gave their money to help others, they reply, "Because it was a good and noble thing to do!"

The Law of Karma, or cause and effect, works regardless of the intention behind the act of giving. The results and benefits are the same. It feels great to help others and the rewards are con-sistent. Giving automatically increases your ability to receive and your whole life begins to change. It is a much better legacy to have people remember you as a kind and generous person, who helped those in need, rather than as someone with a fancy, expensive funeral who didn't help anyone. The best part is, the

> **Six Steps for Effective Tithing:**
>
> - Set your intention.
>
> - Carefully select the organization or individual to whom you will be tithing.
>
> - Calculate your tithe - a designated portion of your net earnings.
>
> - Send your tithe to the selected organization.
>
> - Tithe on a regular basis *i.e.*, weekly, monthly
>
> - After your tithe is sent, affirm that the good karma generated is coming back to you many times!

"Be sure that it is not you that is mortal, but only your body. For that man whom your outward form reveals is not yourself; the spirit is the true self, not that physical figure which can be pointed out by your finger."

- Marcus Tullius Cicero, philosopher of Ancient Rome (106 BC - 43 BC)

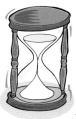

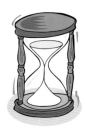

karmic rewards also carry to the afterlife and beyond.

Following a man's death, there are very few changes in his personality. Even though, there is no longer a physical body, we have another "suit" to wear, which will primarily be used at this time and it is called the Astral Body. The physical body is made out of physical cells, the astral body is made out of astral matter. This will be described further. The loss of the physical body can be compared to the removal of an overcoat. The following material pertains directly to the early stages of the afterlife. More detailed information may be studied by reading the materials listed at the end of this chapter.

There is no such thing as reward or punishment from an external power or being. The condition in which we will find ourselves after physical death is directly related to what was thought, desired or done throughout one's lifetime. Hence, the emphasis on doing wholesome deeds during the physical life. The departed individual perceives him/herself almost as they did before. The astral body is "built" during the physical life from subtle energies directly corresponding to one's emotional state. These energies are called Astral Matter. The quality of this astral matter is determined by virtues (or lack of them), passions, desires, emotions, and indirectly, by thoughts and physical habits such as the food, drink, cleanliness and conscience in which our physical bodies engaged.

A coarse and gross astral body - resulting from a coarse and gross life - will cause the individual to be responsive to lower astral vibrations and following the transition, he will find himself bound to the lower astral world (in some texts called *purgatory*) and may consequently experience an unpleasant long and slow disintegration of this coarse astral matter, before being able to move on to the higher planes of the afterlife. On the other hand, a refined astral body, created by a pure and refined life, will make a man unresponsive to the low and coarse vibrations of the lower astral worlds and responsive only to

> The prevalence of near death experiences in the adult population has been estimated by several major surveys. A Gallup Poll in 1992 led to an estimate that 13 million Americans had experienced an NDE. According to Near Death Experience Research Foundation, approximately 774 NDEs occur daily in the United States.

> "A man should not leave this earth with unfinished business. He should live each day as if it was a pre-flight check. He should ask each morning, am I prepared to lift-off?"
>
> -
> Diane Frolov & Andrew Schneider, *Northern Exposure (magazine)*, <u>All is Vanity</u> *(article)* March, 1991

After-Life and Near-Death Experience Resources:

❏ **NDERF,** Near Death Experience Research Foundation - www.nderf.org

❏ **ADCRF,** After Death Communication Res. Foundation - www.adcrf.org

❏ **OBERF,** Out of Body Experience Research Foundation - www.oberf.org

NDERF is devoted to the study of NDEs and support for those who have experienced NDE and related experiences. ADCRF is devoted to the study of after death communication and the support for those experiencing an ADC, or providing hope to those grieving from the loss of a loved one. OBERF is devoted to studying the spiritual spectrum events that do not fit into the categories of NDE or ADC. These include NDE-like events, out of body experiences, and spiritually transformative events.

[www.nderf.org/Media.htm]

its higher levels. Consequently, he will experience much less trouble in his post-mortem life. The length of time spent in certain levels of the astral world depends upon the matching amount of astral matter. Man thus makes for himself both his own purgatory and his own heaven, and these are not places, but states of consciousness.

For most, the state after death is much happier than life upon earth. The first feelings are usually ones of the most delightful freedom. Nothing to worry about, and no earthly duties remain, no credit cards or rent checks. The pain and suffering of all things relating to the physical body are gone. On the other hand, after transitioning, many souls spend time in a subtle world where coarse energies in the form of thoughts, emotions and patterns must be worked through or purified. It is simply the energies of life circumstances replaying until they are burned out. These, among others, include the non-forgiveness of self or others.

The Institute for Living and Dying offers 'Meetings at the Edge' workshops for those interested in supporting the dying, professionally or in their private life, towards a fearless and dignified death. This training is suitable for those aware that their life is coming to an end and for those who care for the dying.

Psycho-spiritual care for the dying:
www.living-dying.com

The physical body protects us from the intensity of strong unwholesome emotions. When the body is no longer present, the intensity of the emotions is felt much more strongly and is often painful. Hence, the teachings of purgatory in many religions. This is not an act of punishment as so many believe, just the natural progression of things. It is with true instinct that the Hindu religion prescribes its Shraddha ceremonies and the Catholic Church its prayers for the dead. These prayers and ceremony create powerful forces to hasten the disintegration of the coarse astral matter and thus alleviate any unnecessary suffering and speeding the person towards the higher planes or heaven-world.

"Forgiveness is almost a selfish act because of its immense benefits to the one who forgives."
-
Lawana Blackwell, *"The Dowry of Miss Lydia Clark, 1999"*

Why and how is this gross energy carried over in transition? Throughout one's lifetime, personal experiences, both positive and not so positive are accumulated along with the corresponding emotional and mental reactions. This emotional/mental charge is stored in the energy field and carried further in the time of transition. Western society, at this point, cares and understands so little about the time of transition. It is literally shrouded in mystery, pain, sorrow, fear, uncertainty, doubt, resistance or complete denial.

One's transition should be a time of joy, liberation and anticipation for the next phase of existence. Family members and loved ones need to learn all they can about the science of dying. By understanding the mechanics of the afterlife

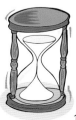

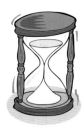

process, there is an opportunity to ease unnecessary suffering, which may naturally occur for those in transition and their loved ones. At the time of transition, our minds should be in as peaceful a state as possible and should be free of lower emotional disturbances. Family members and loved ones can help the individual in transition, by keeping extreme outbursts of grief and sorrow to a minimum, especially during the last moments and few days afterwards.

> ● **"But I am telling you this strange and wonderful secret: we shall not all die, but we shall all be given new bodies! It will all happen in a moment, in the twinkling of an eye, when the last trumpet is blown....."** 1 Corinthians 15:51-58 *(Bible)*
>
> ● **"As the embodied soul continuously passes, in this body, from boyhood to youth to old age, the soul similarly passes into another body at death. A sober person is not bewildered by such a change."** Lord Krishna, *(Bhagavad-Gita)*

"Time is very precious. Do not wait until you are dying to understand your spiritual nature. Then your death will be an experience of grace and transcendence."

Spiritual Dimension of Living and Dying, www.living-dying.com

During the transition is when all efforts to follow the holistic path during the physical life really pay off. Uncovering the root cause of symptoms during one's lifetime, instead of covering them up, generally leads to a discovery of unwholesome or suppressed thoughts and emotions, stored at deeper levels. This creates the opportunity to heal or transmute them. We are blessed to have this understanding. Now there is one less painful thing to deal with at the time of transition. You may look at earthly life as a great training field for the afterlife.

"Those who have lived a good life do not fear death, but meet it calmly, and even long for it in the face of great suffering. But those who do not have a peaceful conscience, dread death as though life means nothing but physical torment. The challenge is to live our lives so that we will be prepared for death when it comes."

-
Unknown

Experiencing or generating long term negativity - mental or emotional - manifests in one's physical life and subtle bodies in the form of illness or disease. Through our desire to heal the underlying issues, we gain the knowledge of how to heal the corresponding energetic (mental-emotional) toxicity. We have learned how to properly deal with this situation and have firsthand experience of transmuting unwholesome energetic buildup into a harmless form. This technique is important and the know-how stays with the soul forever. When the time comes and one finds oneself in the first realm of the afterlife, without the protection of the physical body, they know how to react to similar negativity and are not stuck in an uncomfortable situation. They are protected from unnecessary suffering. Of course, in the case of a person, who's energetic (astral constitution) is made from healthy astral matter, the immediate afterlife experience is quite pleasant.

For more information on how to create and maintain healthy astral matter, refer to the chapter on emotions and mind. As previously mentioned, this is only a discussion of the first experience, just after physical death. The journey of the soul is much longer and more detailed than is in the scope of this book. If you are interested in reading more on this subject, see the list of recommended books on the following page. Most are easy to order online.

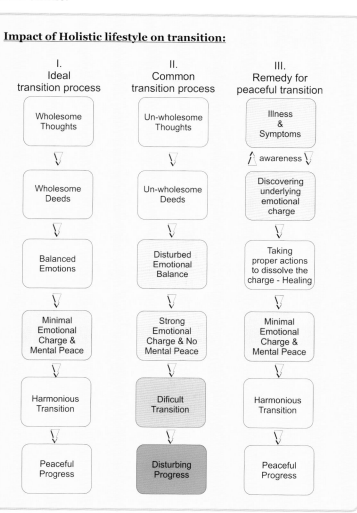

Impact of Holistic lifestyle on transition:

I. Ideal transition process	II. Common transition process	III. Remedy for peaceful transition
Wholesome Thoughts	Un-wholesome Thoughts	Illness & Symptoms
Wholesome Deeds	Un-wholesome Deeds	↑ awareness ↓ Discovering underlying emotional charge
Balanced Emotions	Disturbed Emotional Balance	Taking proper actions to dissolve the charge - Healing
Minimal Emotional Charge & Mental Peace	Strong Emotional Charge & No Mental Peace	Minimal Emotional Charge & Mental Peace
Harmonious Transition	Dificult Transition	Harmonious Transition
Peaceful Progress	Disturbing Progress	Peaceful Progress

"I am going to concentrate on what's important in life. I'm going to strive everyday to be a kind and generous and loving person. I'm going to keep death right here, so that anytime I even think about getting angry at you or anybody else, I'll see death and I'll remember."

-

Diane Frolov & Andrew Schneider, *Northern Exposure* (magazine) *All is Vanity* (article) March, 1991"

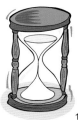

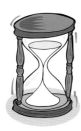

Recommended books:

❏ **On Death and Dying** - What the Dying Have to Teach Doctors, Nurses, Clergy, and Their Own Families - helps families to understand what's going on as the death of a loved one draws near, by Elizabeth Kubler Ross, M.D.

❏ **The Secrets of the Light,** Spiritual Strategies to Empower Your Life... Here and in the Hereafter - a spiritual manual for successful living and dying in the new millennium, by Dannion Brinkley and Kathryn Peters-Brinkley.

❏ **Meditations on Soul Realization** - discusses the meaning of Soul Realization and includes two advanced meditations - Meditation on Twin Hearts; and Meditation on the Soul. The esoteric meaning of the I AM in different religions and philosophies is discussed, by Master Choa Kok Sui.

❏ **Life on the Other Side** (Astara) - from the time-honored teachings of esoteric traditions and spiritual scriptures; from the writings of mystics and seers; from the dreams and psychic experiences of everyday people; and from the intuition and spiritual experiences of Dr. Robert Chaney, author.

❏ **Reincarnation, Cycle of Opportunity** - simple, straightforward answers to questions about reincarnation. A unique opportunity to understand and come to grips with your own feelings about reincarnation and what role it plays in your spiritual future, by Dr. Robert Chaney.

❏ **The Astral Body,** And Other Astral Phenomena - a study of the Astral subtle body based on the works of theosophical authors. A clear understanding of the structure and nature of the astral body, of its possibilities and its limitations, to further comprehend the life into which men pass after physical death, by Arthur Powell.

❏ **Journey Of Souls: Case Studies of Life Between Lives** - uncovers the mystery of life in the spirit world after death on earth. 29 people recall their experiences between lives as eternal spirits. By Michael Newton, Ph.D.

❏ **Esoteric Healing** - discusses the laws and rules of spiritual healing, the subtle bodies, individual and group karma, healing at the time of physical death and the basic psychological causes of disease, by Alice A. Bailey.

"The call of death is a call of love. Death can be sweet if we answer it in the affirmative, if we accept it as one of the great eternal forms of life and transformation."
-
Hermann Hesse, German-born poet, novelist
(1877 - 1962)

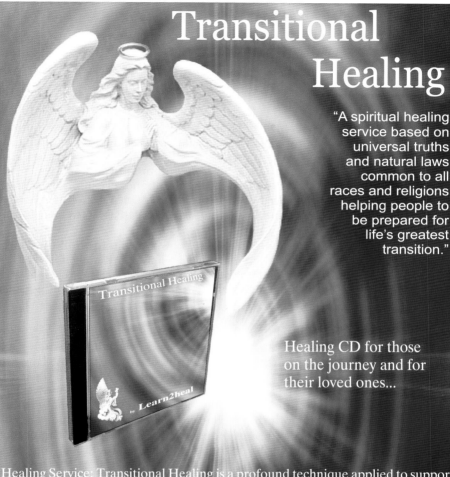

Transitional Healing

"A spiritual healing service based on universal truths and natural laws common to all races and religions helping people to be prepared for life's greatest transition."

Healing CD for those on the journey and for their loved ones...

Healing Service: Transitional Healing is a profound technique applied to support those making a journey from earthly existence to the "after-life". This technique clears the emotional weight or baggage accumulated in one's life-time. This may include suppressed emotions as non-forgivenes, traumas, anger, hatred, resentment, sadness, guilt, and most importantly fear of letting go and fear of the beyond.

Healing CD: An unique, eclectic, meditation for those in life's biggest transition and their loved ones. This guided material brings an understanding of the sacred process of dying and helps create an atmosphere of love, peace, acceptance and reconciliation.

www.TransitionalHealing.org

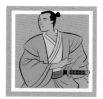

Get Your Power Back!

Your Power Comes From Within

O ffered in this chapter are a variety of suggestions to properly assess and address life situations in which you may be losing personal power. We then explain how you may take action towards optimum health and wellbeing. Often this means recognizing the abundance of internal power you have always possessed. Once you learn how to connect with this force, you can use it to create the life you want.

• Step One: to be in power means to be fully in charge of all that happens in your life. After all, it is your life. Sooner or later, it becomes evident, that allowing others be in charge means giving away your personal power.

Meditate for 10 minutes every morning in a quiet place, undisturbed, before starting the day. Ask yourself what you truly desire for the day. How will you spend your energy? With whom would you like to spend time and who would you prefer not to share time with? Which personal and professional goals are at the top of your list? This is not the time to restate the desires others want for you. It is not important what your family, or friends, or doctor would like you to do. What do you want? By outlining your desires and needs, it becomes easy to recognize when others are imposing their will or their unsuitable and unrealistic expectations. Serving others without having made a conscious choice or an agreement to do so creates uncomfortable situations. The corresponding feelings result in discord between your personal choices and others needs. This is a diversion from our life's path. The result is unhealthy mental and emotional turmoil, issues of self-worth and self-confidence, feelings of guilt, remorse, anger and frustration, and the wasting of precious life force and time.

After determining your personal goals, wants and needs, follow up with action to achieve or fulfill them. This helps to bring your power back and to take control of your life. For those who have been brought up and taught selfless service without any balance or honor for oneself, reading the above paragraph may bring up feelings of resistance. You may think, "But they need me," "I have to help them," " So and so, can't get by without my help," and so on. We are not suggesting that you are unkind and unhelpful. We merely remind you that your health and

> Lao Tzu, the author of *Tao Te Ching* wrote, "when people do not have a sense of power they become resentful and uncooperative. Individuals who do not feel personal power feel fear. They fear the unknown because they do not identify with the world outside of themselves; thus their psychic integration is severely damaged and they are a danger to their society."

> "Every time you don't follow your inner guidance, you feel a loss of energy, loss of power, a sense of spiritual deadness."
>
> -
> Shakti Gawain,
> Author and teacher in the field of personal growth

wellbeing are just as important as that of those around you. Know what your needs are and honor them. One must fill up one's gas tank before driving the car to pick up other passengers.

• Step Two: Be proactive not reactive. Those not consciously creating their lives are reacting to circumstances and events. Reacting to external situations and other's verbal or implied requests wastes your personal power. If you are not creating your life, others are, or you have opened yourself to be affected by events or circumstances which you did not choose. Whichever way the wind blows, that's where your will goes.

There is an inseparable link between honesty and personal power. It is important to say what you mean, do what you say, see things as they are and be truthful about who you are. Your self-esteem will skyrocket. Good self-esteem is an essential building block for strong personal power.

We often respond to circumstances on auto-pilot, based on habit. For example: watching something disturbing on television frequently receives an reaction of "Oh my god, this is so horrible," followed by negative feelings and thoughts about the incident for hours afterwards. This is a common, spontaneous response. It may be just as easy to react as it is to buy the advertised product following the news report, with three easy credit card payments, a free bonus and free shipping. Although most people do not react in such a manner anymore, this example demonstrates a reactive mode of operation. There will always be things in this world that are upsetting. Instead of spending time feeling sorry for others or having pity party conversations, if it is within your ability and control, take some positive action in the world to help heal it. If there is nothing that you can do about it, it is more constructive to spend the time creating something positive for yourself or those close to you.

"When I'm trusting and being myself... everything in my life reflects this by falling into place easily, often miraculously."

-
Shakti Gawain, Author and teacher in the field of personal growth

Being proactive means having control of the reigns of your life. It requires mastering control of your mental reactions, emotional reactions and your physical actions. It means thinking logically and carefully and feeling intuitively, not reacting emotionally, before arriving at a decision or taking action. Visualize the desired outcome with your heart and mind and take the necessary steps to create it. This learned and practiced ability of using a proactive approach is especially useful in extreme situations. Such is the case when given bad news or an unexpected diagnosis from a medical professional. By keeping calm, no matter what the external situation, you are capable of making rational, emotionally balanced and wise choices. Such is not the case when experiencing a reactive emotional spin. Being emotionally reactive clouds perception and wrong decisions are made. In the bigger picture, being reactive leads to making poor life decisions - whether it be with health care, relationships, or your career. Emotional reactivity is like driving a boat on the open ocean, without actually steering it. Each wave turns the boat in a different direction. It is very possible that the boat may not go anywhere. If it does, chances

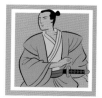

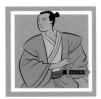

are, you are unlikely to arrive safely, until you grab the wheel.

● Step Three: Evict complaining from your life for good. Everyone complains from time to time, but if you fall into the category of a chronic complainer, stop it. Right now. If you have a difficult life situation that needs immediate attention, complaining will not make it go away and may actually make things worse. It most certainly is not a wise way to invest your personal energy. On the other hand, don't carry burdens unnecessarily. Sharing difficulties with friends in a constructive way, leads to positive solutions, but complaining is destructive. Life brings challenges and lessons, that help us to learn and to evolve. Whining about challenges sends a message to the universe that says, "I am not ready for this yet, I am failing at this test." The universe hears and responds with "okay, no problem, let's see what you're saying after a few months."

Complaining is good. It is a process of concretizing and externalizing the issue which makes it possible to identify the problem. Externalizing an issue allows one to see it more clearly and take action to resolve the situation. When people complain once or twice, it is a sign of healing. Chronic complaining is a disease. Chronic complaining is a los of power!

"Respect yourself and others will respect you."
-
Confucius, Chinese thinker and social philosopher (551 BC - 479 BC)

A patient was in an abusive relationship. She complained for months to friends, family and anyone that was willing to listen, never welcoming solutions and refusing to take action. No matter what advice was given, she slipped back into the same pattern of being abused. Time passed and her abusive relationship ended. Her live-in boyfriend left her for someone else. After a few months, she met a new man and was shocked when after only a few weeks, the relationship took on the same abusive dynamics as the previous one. Why was she surprised? After all, she had told the universe, "I am not ready to deal with this at this time." Universal laws and principles operate with precision, just think of the law of gravity. The patient received a grace period of several months before finding herself in the same position and being given a second opportunity. "Are you ready yet?" was the question she was being asked. And she was. Dealing with the situation bravely, she stood up for herself. This was all that was needed from her this time. Her lesson learned, the boyfriend moved out and a new, better relationship appeared. Her healer has not heard from her lately. She is too busy enjoying her harmonious romance and having fun. When challenges or difficulties arise, and they will, there are only two choices. Change it or accept it. Everything else is a detour away from progress, peace and happiness.

● Step Four: 'Think pink" has been humorously suggested. Having nothing to do with the color pink, it refers to keeping a positive attitude. One of the cosmic laws which has been revealed and expanded in the last ten years, is the Law of Attraction. This law simply says that whatever we repeatedly think, feel and say creates a particular frequency or vibration, drawing unto itself similar frequencies. Like attracts like. Individual radiatory fields work as magnets. The characters of these fields are directly influenced by the quality or energy of our thoughts, emotions and actions. Thinking and feeling positively, or vibrating at a higher frequency creates a magnet-like attraction to similar energies or situations. When we feel happy, the law of attraction in action has a tendency to create more happiness. When we feel and think rich and prosperous thoughts, the tendency is to attract even more richness and prosperity. When we believe that we are becoming healthier and we really feel it, the attraction is to a state of better health, often resulting in attracting a cure for our illness. Anger and sadness create a low vibration or frequency and therefore attract situations and health conditions that match them.

> ☯
> **Some people invest a large amount of their personal energy into the idea of being perfect - trying not to make mistakes. The more they try, the less friends they have. Perfection is the mastery of compassion, love, generosity and proper perception. It has nothing to do with making mistakes. We are human beings, not flawless machines. Everyone makes mistakes! Have you made your mistake today?**

Now that we have a clear picture and understanding of how the law of attraction works, it can be illustrated on a larger scale. By creating and maintaining the low vibration, mishaps, accidents or other negative circumstances are thereby attracted. It is not an easy task to continuously maintain total control over all our life situations. At least, if we make an attempt, a good habit is created. Attracting happy or positive things, not only makes life easier and more pleasurable, but your power grows as well.

• Step Five: Drop the idea of being perfect. No one is. Some people aspire to a self-created idea of perfection that is difficult, if not impossible, to reach. Each time you do not achieve your inner standards of perfection, it represents failure. When this becomes habit, the failure will manifest in other areas and things will become painful. Nobody is perfect and everyone makes mistakes. By continuing to beat yourself over the head for your lack of accomplishments, you are aiming for a big problem. You will create a negative self-image, which will affect all areas of your life. Get over it. Love yourself, respect yourself and when you make a mistake, acknowledge it (or apologize if it was harmful to someone else), then immediately visualize the correct thing to do. This will prepare you for the next time you face a similar challenge. If you are responding to the will and desire of someone else who is trying to make you perfect, consider their motives and if necessary get out of their reach as soon as possible.

"Generosity is giving more than you can, and pride is taking less than you need."
-
Kahlil Gibran,
Lebanese artist, poet and writer
(1883 - 1931)

• Step Six: Follow a dream. Do what you love to do or have always wanted. Be honest with yourself and follow your heart. There are aspects of your life which were predestined. These are the things that you feel a strong calling to do. If you ignore that call, you will miss a great experience and an opportunity to grow. If you have never listened to your heart, now is the time. Dedicate a portion of your free time to your dream and trust the process. If you decide to wait for the right time to invest in your dream, it may not happen. Make the time!

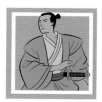

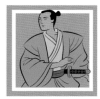

If you always wanted to be a painter, sign up for a painting class. Go for it! Your power and self-confidence will grow.

● Step Seven: Set your boundaries. If you are a "yes" person, learn to say no. Be in charge of your personal time and energy. Do not allow others to expect extra work or favors if it is not your desire to offer them. You do not have to please anyone. It is common that when children are young, parents are too demanding. Children feel that they will be loved only by meeting the parental expectations and they go overboard to please. This behavior carries into adulthood and manifests as trying too hard to please a supervisor or someone in a position of authority. A similar pattern emerges when children do not receive enough parental attention, so they go out of their way to please Mom and Dad to secure their love and attention.

With every yes you say to another's request, you may be saying no to your own priorities or to a commitment you have already made. It often happens when one has too many commitments and a new request is made. This pattern inevitably leads to a breakdown. Learning when to say no is an important step in recovering your personal power.

Pleasing others results in a loss of power. Learn to say NO. Also, schedule time for work, and time for studying, and pleasure. After setting your schedule, don't let others cross your boundaries by calling you after hours. Let the answering machine pick up. Start enforcing personal boundaries now and have fun. In the beginning it may be difficult and there will be many tests. Hold your own as best as you can.

● Step Eight: Connect to your higher self. If you do not believe in God, guardian angels or guides simply imagine that there is a part of your brain, which oversees your life and always knows the right thing to do. Consciously connect to this unconscious part of yourself. For some, it is through meditation. For others, it is through prayers or invocations. Find what feels right and do it. Stories or parables found in religious texts, regardless of background, contain guidance, truth and wisdom. The wisdom they offer can be applied to daily life. If you are unable to decode them, find a spiritual organization where you can learn. Spiritual organizations teach with a universal approach and provide examples from the religious landscape to communicate wisdom to their students. Studying the mysteries and the lessons behind the teachings helps you to navigate through life and helps to establish your connection to your guidance or intuition, fostering self-reliance and personal strength.

"Most powerful is he who has himself in his own power. "
-
Seneca,
Roman rhetorician and writer
(54 BC - 39 AD)

● Step Nine: Be present. There is nothing besides or beyond the present. The greatest loss of personal power happens when energy is stuck or invested in the past or future. The law of subtle energy (see *Healer's Guide,* Part 2) states, "Wherever your attention goes, that's where your energy follows," so by thinking about something which happened twenty years ago, you lose megatons of energy. The past is the past and you cannot alter it, no matter what. If you are always planning for events in your future, they may not even come to be. You know the saying, "If you want God to laugh, tell him your plans."

By focusing entirely on the unpredictable future, you loose the opportunity to experience the now and make the most of it. Be in the moment. Be present. This is the best investment of energy.

• Step Ten: Start networking. Create a personal database of friends and acquaintances. Each time you meet someone, ask for their business card or contact information. Enter it in your database or your Rolodex with as much information as you know about the person. Within a few months you will be surprised by how many people you know. And people know people. If you know just one person, you have access to at least an additional 50 people they know. This step is very important. When you need assistance or advice, access your network. This will not only help you in your business life but in your personal life, as well.

No one is born with a strong sense of personal power. It must be developed. Our society often confuses personal power - the power which comes from within - with the power to control others, or external situations. The biggest loss of personal power happens when we try to control others.

• Step Eleven: Control your control. It is very tempting to try to control others. Especially with family or close relationships. But there is only one person you can control, and that is you. By trying to control others, you lose your energy (power). If you feel that your input is necessary, first determine if it is possible to influence the situation and whether those involved would like your help. If not, leave it be. The mistake of trying to change people and situations that are beyond one's circle of influence is quite common. Be in charge. Be in power. You always have a choice. Assess what is within your realm of influence and what would be just a loss of time and energy.

• Step Twelve: Be honest. Not only with others, but especially with yourself. Honesty is the most important ingredient when it comes to creating positive changes and taking your power back. If you are dishonest with your family, friends or acquaintances, sooner or later you will end up alone. Dishonesty to oneself, creates immeasurable damage. It hinders the healing process because dishonestly hinders our growth. Life becomes boring, empty and miserable, unless, of course issues are faced head on and dealt with. Those who are not brave enough to stop lying to themselves live stale and empty lives and attempts to cover this emptiness end in disaster. The Law of Evolution, pushes us forward and if we don't participate willingly, we will be dragged forward, kicking and screaming. It is like consuming junk food daily and pretending perfect health can be maintained on such a diet. The Universe will slap us, so that we may grow. The first slap will probably be an illness caused by unhealthy food, such as diverticulosis. If the lie continues and health problem are blamed on everything else but the food you are eating, life may slap you harder, with cancer perhaps. And if the Law of Evolution still goes unheeded, the next destination may be six feet under where it doesn't actually end. That's where it really starts, again. (See chapter *Conscious Dying*).

"Honesty is the single most important factor having a direct bearing on the final success of an individual, corporation, or product."
-
Ed McMahon, announcer on the *Tonight Show*

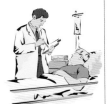

Why People Do Not Heal

The Hidden Issues

This would seem to be a logical question in the forefront of the minds of all medical professionals, but more often than not, the opposite is true. Patients who do not heal include those with chronic or reoccurring illnesses as well as those who always seem to "have something," be it a cold, sinusitis, a bladder infection, PMS, acid reflux or any other chronic health challenge. In looking beyond the symptoms, consider the reasons for illness. If a physician has not been trained in basic psychology or does not make the time to ask questions that further investigate their patients' psychologically, then it would be advisable to work with a psychologist, hypnotherapist or healer who understands how to uncover and address core issues. If you happen to be one of the above-described patients, then the points below, outlining both the conscious and subconscious mental/emotional reasons for illness, may lead you to an epiphany or two.

● Attention: When a baby is born, she requires non-stop attention from her parents. Throughout adolescence and even after becoming an adult, attention is often still an issue. Every baby quickly learns that the most powerful tool to get attention is crying. First the crying is for food or a diaper change and babies learn that crying is very efficient. Later, babies learn to cry even when nothing is wrong as a means of calling the parent - to get their attention. When crying no longer works, other more powerful attention-getting tools are developed. Children may do something really stupid or that which is considered wrong in the eyes of the parent. A child may do the opposite - something unexpectedly good. In psychology books this is referred to as negative or positive attention. If the child does something bad, do they get attention? Of course, even though the response may be unpleasant. Energy systems function effectively regardless of the quality of attention - negative or positive. In the case of the child, negative attention is still better than no attention. Oftentimes, children who want or need more attention will become psychosomatically sick or fake an illness. In return, they receive attention and care. The mind is very strong and has the ability to create illness if survival is threatened and lack of attention is a real threat to a young child. This habit, if it is not eliminated by proper parenting and social influences, may

The Adverse Childhood Experiences (ACE) study by the Department of Preventive Medicine at Kaiser Permanente, compares current adult health status to childhood experiences. The study reveals a relation between emotional experiences in childhood and adult emotional health, physical health, and causes of mortality in the United States. 22% of their Health Plan members were sexually abused as children which directly related to an increase in long-term medical consequences.

http://xnet.kp.org/perman entejournal/winter02/goldt olead.html

"When an elderly woman was asked why she was standing in line to buy stamps from a teller when she could have used a stamp machine she replied: The machine won't ask me about my arthritis!"

-
Source Unknown

become an unconscious habit in adulthood, creating illness or preventing a person from healing. Of course, the attention from friends, co-workers, a partner or doctors is a perfect substitute. You can see this pattern in people who complain non-stop and share their health problems with everyone they meet. This pattern, which is often unconscious by this point, prevents the body from employing its mighty healing powers and prolongs illness. The longer the illness endures the more suffering experienced, the more complaining; which equals lots of attention. This pattern can be conscious or subconscious and is one of the strongest obstacles on the road to healing.

> When illness repeatedly serves as a convenient shield to avoid work responsibilities or pressure, a powerful pattern is set in motion. Each time a responsibility arises, a cold or flu may be evoked, subconsciously. This can become a serious issue when later, the same individual starts their own business. The subconscious pattern will continue to react to work pressures, and will often induce illness sabotaging their efforts and projects.

• Protection: Children often create or pretend illness so that important issues related to their bad behavior or low grades are overlooked or go unaddressed due to the parents' sympathy. This habit is brought forward from childhood to adulthood. If it worked as a convenient shield against reaping bitter rewards, or as a way to escape responsibilities, then as an adult they may assume illness will work the same way for them when they are older. Illness creates a shield from dealing with the responsibilities of adulthood and protects, to a certain extent, against the hostility and severity of life. This thinking or acting out is often fear-based and unconscious.

• False Identity: Poor health and frequent visits to medical facilities may become such an inseparable part of, or habit in one's life that ill health creates a seemingly integrated part of one's identity. Every step towards better health becomes a direct threat to the personality ego. Individuals with this problem will most likely not be seeking the help of an alternative or independent health care specialist where insurance compensation can not be used. The recovery from such a state is a long and difficult process.

• Laziness: For those in management positions of large corporations this pattern is not a surprise. There are always individuals who will try to stay on the payroll as long as possible without any signs of work effort. When the pressure to perform increases, they simply disappear home for health reasons and come back to work later, when the spotlight has shifted to another person or subject and it is safe to return. This is also often seen in dysfunctional families where one or more of the family members are not contributing and being served by other family members due to their "poor state of health," which prevents them from actually doing something. This can create real health problems because of the power of the human mind. This problem requires a different approach to healing that includes the willingness of the patient.

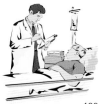

• Blind belief and acceptance in the western medical system: It may become impossible to recover when you are diagnosed

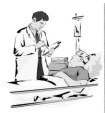

with only six months to live and the opinion is accepted as a final verdict. A verdict is only a formulated judgment based on the experience of others with the same illness at the same stage of development. At this point, it is necessary to ask yourself if you really believe that this is true. Does your intuition tell you something completely different? If there truly is a desire to live or a recognition of unfinished business, it is time to search for alternative methods while working to strengthen your soul connection in order to bring forth the vital energy necessary for healing. This shifts one's perception from, "what has to be done before I die?" to "what new and unforseen remedies or treatments may I try to heal this illness?"

- Drug Dependency: Certain health conditions may have required medication for a time and the patient becomes addicted - physically or mentally - even though the health condition has improved and the medication is no longer needed. This usually requires treatment in the form of rehabilitation.

- Lack of Self-Worthiness: When a calcified idea of one's self as being worthless or undeserving is present, healing may take a long time due to an inability to accept any improvement. The underlying thought, "I do not deserve get well," or "I am not worthy of healing," blocks the attempts of the body to repair itself. For the most part this is a subconscious choice, but a choice nevertheless.

- Escape: When the pressure of an environment (family, work, friends, etc.) increases and expectations exceed a tolerable threshold, illness is an easy solution that allows one to brush off responsibilities and expectations. It is a socially acceptable reason for stepping out of the action and it isn't perceived as a show of weakness. This may also go hand in hand with the aforementioned childhood habit of getting sick. This often shows up later in life as getting sick before an important event, even if it is a pleasant one *i.e.*, an expensive vacation, a prominent work promotion. These events have no obvious reasons to make someone ill, but when one is not able to withstand additional input, the body reacts with the old, effective habit. It is mistakenly believed that the triggers that lead to illness are exclusively unpleasant happenings, but it has been proven by clinical hypnotherapy, neurofeedback and other scientifically based therapies that these triggers fall on either end of the spectrum - negative as well as positive. Sudden, unusually joyful moments may be unconsciously perceived as a terrible trauma. This is evident when someone is stuck in a rut and a positive shift suddenly occurs. If they are inclined towards this sort of psychosomatic illness, something terrible will happen that prevents them from moving forward to their new level of success or happiness. This must be addressed on the neurological and habitual levels.

"Job stress can be defined as the harmful physical and emotional responses that occur when the requirements of the job do not match the capabilities, resources, or needs of the worker. Job stress can lead to poor health and even injury."

[Stress at work, United States National Institute of Occupational Safety and Health, Cincinnati, 1999]

"You cannot run away from weakness; you must some time fight it out or perish; and if that be so, why not now, and where you stand?"

-
Robert Louis Stevenson, Scottish novelist, poet
(1850 - 1894)

• **Religious Beliefs:** This is a delicate subject. Inasmuch as the *Healer's Guide* staff could have been burned at the stake a mere few hundred years ago, for the text of this book, dogmatic or extreme beliefs are often the cause of ill health and must be addressed. When religious beliefs such as, "I must suffer for God as he suffered for me," or "God wants me to suffer because I am a sinner," or "I have to suffer in this life so when I die I will go to heaven," or "I am being punished for my sins," are deeply ingrained, consciously or subconsciously, it is difficult to heal. Religious texts and scriptures are subject to interpretation and have also been subjected to intentional misinterpretations by man. Read a wide variety of texts, read theosophical literature, study with spiritual teachers and make your own conclusions. When, you are ready to heal destructive beliefs, hypnotherapy will help to extract unsupportive ideas from the conscious and subconscious mind.

• **Environmental Factors:** What good are expensive treatments administered to a lung cancer patient who still secretly smokes in the bathroom? What is achieved by visiting an energy healing specialist for help with chronic fatigue, if the client returns to an apartment with walls full of toxic mold? How effective would treatment for diverticulosis and acid reflux be when shredded animal patties, soft drinks and fries are consumed daily? Take a look at your environment and personal habits to determine if any are contributing to illness. Rule out hidden environmental influences.

• **Addictions:** This refers to all known addictions - alcohol, street drugs, coffee, cigarettes, junk food, sex, television watching, money, and more. Addiction is the state of physiological or psychological dependence on a potentially harmful substance. However, everything which is used in excess may be considered an addiction and is harmful. Overuse or abuse of anything creates problems. It is of no use attempting to heal someone whose illness is compounded by an addiction. Unless they make a wholehearted effort to eliminate the root cause, there is no hope of becoming healthy. The addiction must be conquered.

• **Karma:** The Law of Karma has been referenced throughout history by all world religions and spiritual teachers. Many attempts to explain this Universal law have been made. The Law of Karma is described as a law of cause and effect and suggests that whatever we do will result in a corresponding situation returned to us. It is also known as "The Golden Rule" and has been incorrectly portrayed as a law of punishment. For further information see the chapter called *Natural Laws*. For now we will simply say that if the health situation of individual is not improving and there are no obvious or hidden reasons for its manifestation, it is quite possible that there is a personal lesson

> "Formaldehyde is second only to gas stoves and pesticides as a cause of chemical overload. Gas stoves cause a lot of depression and arthritis, pesticides cause brain dysfunction, neuropathies, heart problems, lung problems, almost anything. Then comes formaldehyde, which can be found in any synthetic fabrics, carpets, any foam rubber found in furniture or mattresses, and any house that has press board or plywood in it. If people are sensitive, they need to get rid of that stuff or move out."
> **John R. Lee, M.D.**
> **interview with William J. Rea, M.D**
> **www.ehcd.com**

> "I hold this as a rule of life: Too much of anything is bad."
> -
> Publius Terentius Afer,
> a comic playwright of the Roman Republic
> (170 - 160 BC)

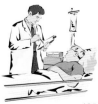

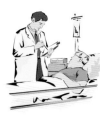

and/or karmic obligation involved. Until the lesson is learned, the healing is not probable. It is an exact law but it is also subject to change under certain influences. Healers who are accustomed to working with the Law of Karma as it relates to their patients are able to advise them on appropriate measures.

● Social Benefits: Illness often allows social benefits, compensation, or relief from a job which is emotionally or mentally draining. Sometimes this benefits abuse is done unconsciously and illness remains, as in the case when the individual believes that they are unable to support themselves without the assistance. More often than not, this abuse is conscious. In rare cases, benefits abuse takes place for simple gains such as a blue lane parking spot or being able to be first in line.

● Improper application or incorrect healing method chosen: It is possible that the healing method selected was not the right match (needed a physiotherapist, not a chiropractor, wrong medication), applied incorrectly (treatment or medication was too strong or not strong enough) or simply was not the appropriate tool (energy healing instead of a cast for a broken bone), to address the illness at hand. If you haven't been able to loosen a 2" bolt with 1" wrench for the past two years, try the 2" wrench instead. The body knows how to heal itself and the only way to facilitate that healing is to supply it with the modality it responds to.

It is possible that 75% or more of illnesses are unresponsive to treatment due to one or more of above mentioned reasons. Determination and a strong will, coupled with introspection to uncover the reasons why an illness may not be healing, is an absolute necessity for improving one's health. In our busy society, personal health care falls around the 6th or 7th position in a list of our priorities, right after paying the mortgage, taking care of family needs, business responsibilities and social obligations. Out of one hundred people surveyed it appeared that 78% stated that health was the first or second most important aspect of their life. When investigated thoroughly, however, the reality of the survey was that only 21% actually treated health as a most important aspect of their lives. There is a significant difference between what people think is a priority and what they actually do. It is human nature to take our health for granted until we have a health crisis and even in the midst of one, there are often more important situations which require our immediate attention at the expense of our health. Take the time for regular tune-ups from holistic health professionals to keep your body, mind and spirit in tip top shape. When it is necessary to take a few days off to repair the body and recover, try to honor this as best as you are able. Often, after a band-aid is put on a health crisis, as is the case with a physical, emotional or mental strain, it is common for one's attention to immediately shift back to other important life issues and health is taken for granted again, going unnoticed until the time when

"To get rich never risk your health. For it is the truth that health is the wealth of wealth."

-
Richard Baker,
English chronicler
(1568–1645)

the body requires its next emergency attention. After any critical health situation is resolved, the focus must shift back to a regular program of prevention and well being.

When someone does not heal, find out if there is an intention to heal or if it is just a superficial desire to feel better as soon as possible and return to the old life routine? If the wish of getting well is so strong, that one would do anything, including getting rid of addictions, working with the right professionals, being willing to look at conscious and subconsciously destructive patterns and making positive changes to their lifestyle, healing will occur most of the time. When self-care is neglected and the only time one directs their attention to health is in the case of a medical emergency, the chance of irreparable damage increases exponentially.

> The intention to heal is absolutely essential. It is the starting point for all recovery. Do not allow others' negative opinions to sway you. Support is very important - enlist the love and support of family and friends.

Carpal tunnel surgery is an example of a quick operation that often leaves irreparable damage or scar tissue; herniated discs are surgically fused together leaving unexpected constant pain that results in a lifetime of prescription drugs; intestinal tracts are cut shorter in the case of digestive problems and there are many other quick-fix solutions that promise fast relief and a rapid return to the regularly scheduled program. When routine surgical procedures are unsuccessful and leave unexpected damage or postoperational problems, the real damage is to the integrity of the human system (physical and energetic). Once the physical and energetic systems have been traumatized, further repair by surgical or alternative methods is impossible. The only solution that remains is medication to suppress the body's response and pain.

When people do not heal, it is because they are not listening to what their body needs in the language that the body speaks. No one would choose a Chinese translator for a French meeting, but choosing a tarot reader to attract new love partner seems normal. If the language the body speaks is too foreign to understand, there are always healthcare professionals who speak your body's language. If your situation has not improved, the following questions should be asked:

> "Health is a state of complete physical, mental and social well-being, and not merely the absence of disease or infirmity."
> -
> Unknown

☐ Is there a sincere willingness to heal and to discover the true cause of illness?

☐ Was there any previous physical damage done to the body that makes healing impossible?

☐ Is the chosen method the right fit for the particular illness and the person?

☐ Is the health care professional a healer with direct knowledge and know-how or is his/her approach based on ifs and guesses?

☐ What is the #1 priority of your life?

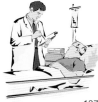

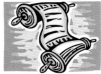

The Cosmic Laws

Laws of Nature Unveiled

All events in time and space are governed by Cosmic laws. Cosmic laws are unchangeable. Upon understanding the mechanics of the cosmic laws, one may use them for personal benefit, to eliminate suffering, attain health and abundance, and to overcome or avoid unnecessary struggles in life. The cosmic laws may also be thought of as the laws governing the Soul, for the Soul, over time, learns to work advantageously with them to promote spiritual growth and evolution. Ignorance or denial of the Cosmic laws does not change the fact that they exist. Choosing not to believe in the Law of Gravity does not affect its existence, as anyone who would jump off a ten story building would discover.

Modern science has a good handle on most of the natural laws, physics and chemistry, but most in the west have not yet fully accepted the existence of the parallel paths of spiritual science. The ancient rishis and spiritual seekers from a variety of races and cultures have performed experiments to validate the cosmic laws.

Hermes Trismegistus (ancient Egyptian sage), said it best: "That which is below is like to that which is above," or as it is better known, "As above so below." Cosmic Laws are as valid in our physical world as they are in throughout the Universe. All of the laws are interrelated. For example, one may override The Law of Karma by praying or invoking the Law of Grace or Mercy. A person suffering from a severe karmic-related illness, may ask for the Law of Mercy to relieve them from their suffering and teach them the lesson quickly, if they offer to work off this "karmic debt" by helping others. The Law of Mercy often kicks in by apologizing to someone we have hurt and truly learn the lesson to not make the same mistake again.

Through right understanding and the application of these laws it is possible to master life and support spiritual growth. Those unaware of the laws, attribute their life circumstances to destiny or chance when in fact, chance and destiny depend largely on the individual. A healer might try to determine if a client is in violation of certain laws and therefore responsible for their difficulties. Some clients may be instructed on how to work with the laws to actively co-create their healing.

> "Universal Laws are the basic principles of life, which transcend the diversity of individual beliefs and philosophies. These laws apply to whatever one's individual belief system or philosophy is. When applied correctly the Universal Laws allow anyone to reach their maximum spiritual potential and greatly enhance the experience of our manifestation in the physical."
>
> *Flowing with Universal Laws*,
> **Margo Kirtikar, Ph.D.**

> "What is below is like that which is above, and what is above is similar to that which is below to accomplish the wonders of one thing."
> -
> Hermes Trismegistus, Egyptian Sage

Illness is often the result of being unaware of the fact the we have subtle bodies. If you are not aware of your emotional or astral body, how can you even begin to know what is detrimental to it or how to heal it? By understanding the nature of the subtle bodies and the cosmic laws and how to work with them, you can be in control of your life.

- **The Law of Karma:** This is the law of cause and effect or "as you sow, so shall you reap." Whatever we think, say and do has direct consequences. The Law of Karma does not judge as all cosmic laws are neutral, impersonal and exact. It does not punish and it does not distinguish between good or bad. It goes hand in hand with the Law of Evolution.

Cosmic Laws are not limited to the accepted and suggested moral conduct of man. They extend above and beyond. Meditating on and following the Cosmic Laws results in a more harmonious, stress-free life, and the expansion of wisdom for the achievement your desires.

In order to evolve, lessons must be learned. Events and circumstances are often incorrectly labeled good luck, bad luck and coincidence, when it is actually the Law of Karma in action. Personal karma may be changed, enhanced or neutralized, via specific actions as mentioned in the example above. One simple example that demonstrates an aspect of karmic law - action and reaction - is punching a wall. If you punch the wall with your hand, the wall will be damaged and your hand will be hurt in proportion to the intensity of the hit. If you hurt someone intentionally or unintentionally a corresponding penalty will be set in motion. If a deed of good will is performed, a corresponding reward is set in motion. Sometimes people who wish to evolve quickly and follow the spiritual path set in motion a quickening of their karma, preferably under the guidance of their Guru. Both extremes of karma are then experienced in a shorter time. Try your best to not create negative karma and to neutralize or minimize past negative effects by service and goodwill.

"For it is in giving that we receive; It is in pardoning that we are pardoned; And it is in dying that we are born to eternal life."

- Saint Francis of Assisi

- **The Law of Evolution:** Everything is evolving. It is nearly impossible to go backwards. The typical rate of evolution is very slow. Humans are the only species who may consciously undertake the fast track program. Choosing to work actively with the Law of Evolution by working on personal growth and spiritual development, allows one to attain rapid movement forward, creating a more peaceful and satisfying life.

- **The Law of Mercy or Grace:** Invoking or praying for the Law of Grace may ease one's negative karma. Whether or not Grace intercedes depends on whether the lesson has been learned. If you find yourself in a difficult situation and believe that you have fully understood the lesson, invoke the Law of Grace. A thief who is reaping the karma of his unwholesome deeds by being robbed repeatedly, finally understands the impact of his past behavior and he learns that it is not okay to steal. If you are experiencing difficulties try to understand the

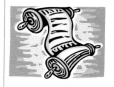

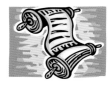

lesson before going to sleep, silently ask that it be revealed through the Law of Grace.

● **The Law of Forgiveness:** This law is the cornerstone of many religions. Learn to forgive others who have trespassed against you. This entitles one to forgiveness for the things they have done and is the key which will fully allow the Law of Grace to manifest. Forgiveness of others and oneself results in mental, emotional, spiritual healing and inner peace.

● **The Law of Motion:** Everything is in motion and motion is life. Change is an inevitable part of life. Living life in a state of inertia, results in stagnation and illness. Expressing creativity, helpful action or service is the remedy for illness caused by inertia. Change is constant. It is foolish to believe that things will stay the same.

● **The Law of Reincarnation:** It is irrelevant whether one believes in it or not, the law will continue to function. Reincarnation is a law taught in the world religions of Taoism, Hinduism, Buddhism and others. There are very few religions whose interpretation of Holy Scripture differs. In the gospel, the Master Jesus hinted on the Law of Reincarnation when he referred to the past incarnation of John The Baptist and said that he had come again.

> "For all the prophets and the law have prophesied until John. And if you are willing to receive it, he is Elijah who was to come." (Matt 11:13-14) "And the disciples asked him, saying, 'Why then do the scribes say that Elijah must come first?' But he answered them and said, 'Elijah indeed is to come and will restore all things. But I say to you that Elijah has come already, and they did not know him, but did to him whatever they wished. So also shall the Son of Man suffer at their hand.' Then the disciples understood that he had spoken of John the Baptist." (Matt 17:10-13)

Incarnating is for the purpose of evolution, to gain experiences on earth one cannot attain without a physical body. This is frequently suggested to explain the varied states of human consciousness and the level of suffering throughout the world. The earth and humanity cannot evolve past a certain point until progress has been made collectively. Spiritual development or mystical experiences are good, but they are not much use unless they are translated and shared with humanity.

"The people's good is the highest law."
-
Cicero
(106 BC - 43 BC),
lawyer and philosopher of
Ancient Rome

● **The Law of Correspondence:** Or more commonly referred to as "As above, so below." Every part contains the whole. None of our bodies are separate. You are not separate from your soul. By changing your inner world - thoughts, emotions and virtues, you create corresponding changes in your outer world of health, success, abundance. Whatever you think and feel, both consciously and subconsciously, creates your reality. Be a conscious creator and not subject to whatever comes your way.

● **The Law of Oneness:** Everything, throughout all time and space, is connected to everything else. There is only one essence and every manifestation in the universe is an expression of God.

Almost all world religions recognize oneness at some level. You are one with God. Jesus and Buddha were living examples of the potential within each and every human being. This is self-realization. Everything is interrelated and interdependent. What you think, feel and do, affects the whole - or everyone else - on some level. Understanding and experiencing oneness is part of the foundation for building good virtues. People often act as though they live in a bubble and their actions only affect them. The understanding that everything one does affects all of humanity, the earth and the universe may change one's actions. One becomes more accountable for their actions and as a result experiences an expanded state of awareness.

• **The Law of Attraction:** States that "Like Attracts Like." Our thoughts are merely energy and all visible material objects begin as thoughts. When a thought is strong enough or held repeatedly it tends to manifest. Focusing on what you do not have, from a position of *lack,* creates a thoughtform of lack, which because of the law of attraction means you will attract even *more* lack. Correspondingly, by focusing on what you have, you will attract more of the same. When you are under the impression that there is something missing in your life and it becomes the focal point of your desire, constantly re-affirming it in a state of non-having-ness, ensures that it will not be attracted into your life. Also, focusing continuously on what you do not want, has a tendency to attract exactly that. All thoughts must be held with certainty. You must believe and feel that the things you desire are already present - a strong feeling of having-ness. All situations in your life, positive and negative, have been attracted by you, based on your thoughts and feelings. The Law of Attraction works in the realms of thoughts and emotions which is the manifesting force for the physical reality. In the physical world it happens that opposites may attract *i.e.,* male vs. female or negative vs. positive in magnetism. This is not a demonstration of The Law of Attraction in action as we are referring to. For more information on working with this law, refer to *Healer's Guide,* Part 2.

> "By the powerful Universal Law of Attraction, you draw to you the essence of whatever you are predominantly thinking about. So if you are predominantly thinking about the things that you desire, your life experience reflects those things. And in the same way, if you are predominantly thinking about what you do not want, your life experience reflects those things."
>
> Ester and Jerry Hicks,
> *"Ask and It Is Given"*

> "The Law of Attraction is kind of annoying, unless one has mastered it. You get that which you put out."
>
> -
> Flemming Allan Funch,
> founder of New Civilization Network (NCN)

Cosmic Law resources:

❑ **Autobiography of a Yogi** - explains with scientific clarity the subtle, but definite laws by which yogis perform miracles and attain self mastery, by Paramahansa Yogananda - www.yogananda-srf.org

❑ **Esoteric Healing** - discusses the laws and rules of spiritual healing, the subtle bodies, individual and group karma, healing at the time of physical death and the basic psychological causes of disease, by Alice A Bailey

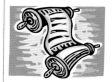

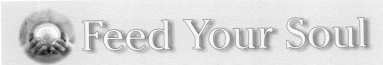

Feed Your Soul

Feed Your Soul is a grass roots non-profit organization dedicated to helping those in need. It originally started as a feeding program in Santa Monica, California and has since spread throughout Los Angeles, other areas of California, and several other states. Since its inception, it has fed over 100,000 people and has placed over 75 people into permanent housing.

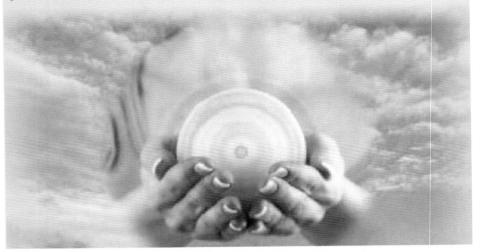

Feed Your Soul is now looking to help where government aid has failed.
We are a bridge between public resources and private aid.

It is in giving that we receive...

A minimum of 85% of all money donated goes to
those in need directly!
We are a charity, not an organization.
We aim to help where society, government or relatives
have overlooked.
We feed the hungry and help those in need.
We offer food, rental deposits, and emergency assistance.
This is the new face of charities, helping where the need is directly.

You make a difference...

www.feedyoursoul.org

Feed Your Soul, 23852 Pacific Coast Highway #543, Malibu, CA 90265, info@feedyoursoul.org

The Integration

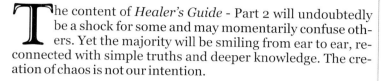

Part 2

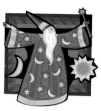

The content of *Healer's Guide* - Part 2 will undoubtedly be a shock for some and may momentarily confuse others. Yet the majority will be smiling from ear to ear, reconnected with simple truths and deeper knowledge. The creation of chaos is not our intention.

We are all creatures of habit. History has shown that when a belief has been accepted by society and new or more complete information is presented that challenges what we have long believed to be true, we are slow to accept a new vision or understanding of the world. Historically, there has been opposition to new information, especially when the information has threatened or shaken deeply ingrained beliefs or when the information challenged those with a financial interest in the status quo. This is an old story that never stops being current.

Even though certain information about health and the nature of our existence as humans has been around for eons, often, the dissemination of this information was controlled. The reasons for control have varied over time. At one time, religion sought to consolidate its power by restricting the flow of information. Today, certain institutions and economies are invested in the corporatization of our identity and our care. At the same time, as our society grows its technological muscles and brain, many of the simple things are forgotten or get lost along the way.

Much of the information shared in this section (Part 2) has been known for thousands of years. This knowledge is comprised of ancient wisdom, universal and natural laws that govern the Universe, and principles that dictate and define our earthly existence. Humanity's rapid rate of evolution and the assistance of numerous conscious media vehicles are ensuring the dissemination of this *new* information. By knowing how to use this knowledge, with integrity and wholesome intent, personal empowerment and vibrant health are just two of the ultimate and beneficial results.

"The mind can assert anything and pretend it has proved it. My beliefs I test on my body, on my intuitional consciousness, and when I get a response there, then I accept."

-

D. H. Lawrence, English novelist (1885 - 1930)

Scientific discoveries have lead to phenomenal breakthroughs in the area of healthcare. Recent discoveries in the area of psychology have lead to a deeper understanding of the complexity of the origins of disease and the development of new methods of care and treatment. Progress aside, the remaining missing links in the western healthcare system, are an understanding

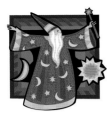

of the healing power of the human spirit and the knowledge of how to work with the human energetic anatomy and its affects on the physical body.

Success in life depends upon many things, but most of all upon balance and harmony. The trinity of the energies bursting forth from the universe encompass divine will, divine intelligence and divine love. By living a life in alignment with the universe, we are able to embody all three aspects in our microcosm, or individuality, as part of the macrocosm, or the whole. When we talk about the body-mind-spirit connection, it can be compared to the individual embodiment of the holy trinity in mankind. All three aspects are interconnected and inter-dependent and health depends not only on the health of the three aspects individually, but also how they function or integrate as a whole.

When we look at the three aspects of a holistic health care system - the functional system introduced in this book - we also recognize the three components of this system. First we have physicians, providing their knowledge of physical anatomy and of specific treatments for disease and the holistic medical and alternative practitioners, striving to achieve balance and harmony through herbs, lifestyle management, the application of scientific techniques, specific to their modality and the education of patients as to the wisdom of their body-mind. (Let us call this Divine Intelligence in action). Secondly, we have the patients who possess, the strength of their spirit, the innate healing ability of their physical body and a soul-level understanding of the timelines of their life, which translate into a desire, or lack of desire, to live. (Let us call this Divine Will in action). Thirdly, we have the esoteric and energy healers who understand the universal laws and principles and know how to work with them, and with spirit to increase the soul connection. These healers guide others to self-awareness, while working with subtle energy and the energetic anatomy. Their work affects the physical body via the endocrine system and leads the patient to the knowledge that their energy body is the pattern or blueprint that their physical life follows. (Let us call this Divine Love in action).

"So divinely is the world organized that every one of us, in our place and time, is in balance with everything else."
-
Johann Wolfgang von Goethe
German dramatist, novelist, poet, & scientist
(1749 - 1832)

Now that we have an appreciation for the role that each plays, it is easy to see the importance of accepting and acknowledging the gifts which each divine expression, or aspect of the healing equation brings. Each healthcare practitioner serves humanity with their unique expression of divinity. One must also look within to rediscover the divine power within themselves. Realize its limitless abundance and have faith in your healing ability along the road to self-discovery and vibrant health.

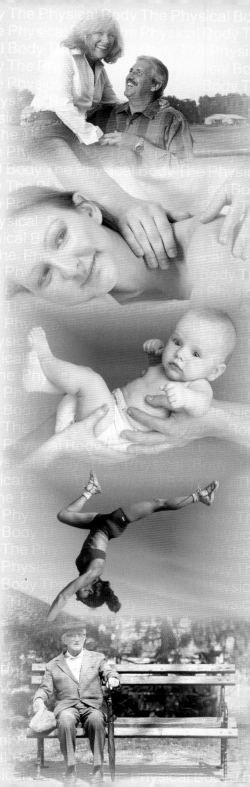

The Body

Your Temple

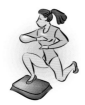

The Physical Body

The Temple

The human body is a beautiful, precisely designed machine, possessing extraordinary, innate wisdom. It is completely automated and performs thousands of functions in any given second. The heart doesn't need to be told to beat, the lungs to inhale and exhale or the tissue to repair itself. A common school of thought states that the body is designed to last 120 years or more, yet few but a handful of humans have been able to reach that potential, due to disease, infections and lifestyle choices. Through improvements in hygiene, the progress of western medicine, and the shift in self-care and spiritual awareness, the average life span has been extended to 70+ years. Now it's time to overcome the final hurdles and take it to the next level.

Our enemies are the physical, mental and emotional stressors of the modern lifestyle. Poor living conditions, crowded cities, EMFs, pollutants, contaminants, acid rain, the U.S. burger diet, the side-effects of medication and the daily use of household chemicals and poisons, all of which are man-made, have taken their toll on our health. At the same time, science races to find the cure for the illnesses the American lifestyle creates. The whole scenario can be likened to a salmon swimming against a current. They do make it up the river to spawn, but at what cost?

Breaking news in 2004 informed us that scientists had identified the first link between stress and aging. A finding which may explain why intense, long-term emotional strain makes people get sick and grow old faster. Chronic stress appears to hasten the shriveling of the tips of the bundles of genes inside cells, which shortens their lifespan and speeds the body's deterioration. Elissa Epel, a psychiatrist at the University of California at San Francisco, who helped conduct the research said: "This is the first time that psychological stress has been linked to a cellular indicator of aging in healthy people."

Nowadays, caring for the body requires more thought and attention than it did in the past because the environment grows more polluted and toxic by the year. How many can say their body feels truly well year-round? Although wellness may seem like a pipe dream, reuniting with nature by following natural laws and performing a few simple tests to identify and eliminate the most common health killers will go a long way toward reaching the goal. At the very least it will make the experience of being in your physical body much more pleasant.

"There is but one temple in the universe and that is the body of man."

- Novalis
German lyric poet
(1772 - 1801)

146

Food

This will be a huge wake up call and for some, very tough. Here are the things that no one wants to hear, things that make people plug their ears and sing "lalala." For the general public adhering to a healthful diet means changing comfortable habits. For the food companies it could mean the loss of profits. Hundreds of diseases are caused every year by what people put in their mouths. Is it possible that most obesity, heart disease, diabetes and a large percentage of cancers are self-inflicted? It is reported that close to 30% of cancers are genetic, the rest are lifestyle-imposed. Human beings are suckers for punishment. Heart disease is almost entirely preventable. The five daily servings of fruits and vegetables in the food pyramid is a joke. The over-consumption of meat and dairy are leading people to their graves. *[see page 155 for the movie, "Eating"]* two-thirds of Americans are overweight and 40% of children aged 5-8 are obese or have high blood pressure, or both. According to the American Diabetes Association, there are 20.8 million children and adults in the United States, or 7% of the population, who have diabetes. While an estimated 14.6 million have been diagnosed, there are 6.2 million people (or nearly 1/3) who are unaware they have the disease *[www.diabetes.org]*. Something's gotta give because these conditions are creating a strain on society.

> ☯
>
> Open your refrigerator and cupboards and quickly assess the nature of your food supply. If you realize, that more than 50% of your food is processed, fake or junk food, consider taking a simple pH test of your body fluids to avoid possible health problems. For pH testing information see page 153.

Eat to live vibrantly, don't live to eat. Eating patterns established due to lack of time, stress, commercial advertising and general misconceptions about food rule the American lifestyle but with a little practice can be transcended.

● **Processed Food** - made from real food that has been put through devitalizing chemical processes. The food is then infused with chemicals and preservatives. Beef jerky, jam, hot dogs, and low-fat yogurt with sugar or aspartame are a few examples of processed food.

● **Junk Food** - contains very little real food. Junk foods are made of devitalized processed food, hydrogenated fats, chemicals, and preservatives, and include anything made with refined white flour. Canned breakfast drinks, cold/sugary cereals, doughnuts, take-out fast foods, and soda are examples of junk foods.

● **Fake Food** - is made primarily of chemicals, and often contains gums and sugar fillers. Food containing artificial coloring, flavoring or aroma *i.e.*, certain candy, sugary snacks. The synthetic chemicals are used to make artificial flavorings.

> "The goal of life is living in agreement with nature."
>
> Zeno,
> Greek Philosopher
> (335 BC - 264 BC)

The body requires a variety of foods provided by Mother Nature, in their natural state, as often as possible. Nature's food was designed for every living species on the planet, humans included. Good food is perfectly balanced for optimum digestion and health and does not include MSG, Acesulfame-K,

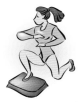

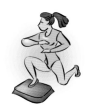

Green #3, Blue #1, Blue #2, Yellow #5, Yellow #6 and Red #3 (all are carcinogens), BHA & BHT (banned in England), potassium bromate (banned worldwide, except in the U.S. and Japan), nitrates, propyl gallate, artificial sweeteners, and other chemicals. Nature's food is designed for the body. It is plant food – nuts, fruits and vegetables which supply a body with vitamins, minerals and LIVE enzymes to maintain optimum health. Cooking, pasteurizing and chemical processing destroy the enzymes which are crucial for proper body functions. Learn how to create simple meals with live plant foods and substitute 25% or more of cooked foods for raw. (See resources on page 149) Those who have healed their diets report dramatic increases in energy overall, not being tired after eating, the disappearance of chronic aches and pains, spontaneous remissions from severe diseases, better quality of sleep, increased libido, lowered cholesterol, regular menstrual cycles, no PMS, clarity of mind, improved memory and more. You wouldn't dream of putting low quality gas and burned oil in your $40,000 car, but most people don't think for an instant before putting chemically stabilized, microwaved, devitalized, genetically modified food in their far more valuable body. Miracles happen when we eat food that was designed for our bodies.

If cooked foods are recommended by your practitioner, then follow the instructions until the healthy integrity of the digestive tract is regained, then slowly add more live foods. When cooking vegetables, never boil or microwave. Steam vegetables lightly, cook soups for a short time or stir fry for a minute or two on

Dr. Edward Howel, a physician, biochemist, and author of *Enzyme Nutrition & Food Enzymes for Health and Longevity* says, "When we eat cooked, live enzyme deficient food, the body is forced to produce enzymes needed for digestion. This stealing of enzymes from other parts of the body sets up a competition for enzymes among various organ systems and tissues of the body. The resulting metabolic dislocations may be the direct cause of many chronic incurable diseases such as obesity, heart disease, Cancer, and other degenerative problems."

"Nothing will benefit human health and increase the chances for survival of life on Earth as much as the evolution to a vegetarian diet."

-
Albert Einstein
(1879 - 1955)

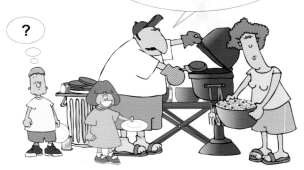

...Hurry up kids! I made some very healthy, vitamin-fortified, genetically-modified, irradiated, cloned, antibiotic-treated, industry-approved burgers!!!

medium-high temperature. Frying meats in a pan or grilling on high temperatures has been linked to many cancers. The World Health Organization states that Heterocyclic Amines (HCAs) - cancer-causing substances, a family of mutagenic compounds, are produced during the cooking process of many animal products, including chicken, beef, pork, and fish. Even meat that is cooked under normal grilling, frying, or oven-broiling produces large quantities of these mutagens. [www.americancancersocietypromotesdisease.org]

Healthy cooking - workshops and classes:

- **Sivananda Yoga Vedanta Center** - Prepare a delicious wholesome, vegetarian meal with all the nutritional elements needed for optimal health - www.sivananda.org/la/CookingWS.htm

- **The Cancer Project** - Food for Life Nutrition and Cooking Classes for Cancer Prevention and Survival - www.cancerproject.org/resources/cooking_class.php

- **Leaf Cuisine** - An in depth, hands-on, and practical introduction to the art of making raw, vegan foods - www.leafcuisine.com/courses.html

- **Matt Amsden's RAWvolution** - Chef Matt teaches raw food preparation classes and offers consultations to students converting to a raw foods diet - www.rawvolution.com

- **Melisa Ward, Organic Gourmet** - Learn to prepare meals with an emphasis on using organic produce and products. www.mwardonline.com

Here is a list of basic guidelines for healthy eating:

- Organic whenever possible.
- No processed foods.
- Limit packaged foods to healthier choices such as pastas made with rice flour and brown rice.
- Meat, dairy in moderation. Chose a product which is labeled "Organic."
- Coffee, sugar, white flour products and alcohol in moderation, if at all.
- Unnatural sweeteners - never!
- No chemical additives, nitrates or food coloring.
- Select the following oils: olive, flax and borage to supplement or add to salads.
- Reduce convenient microwavable* meals.

If you never thought that it would be possible to make a shift to include more raw food in your diet, see the movie, *Breakthrough,* a documentary film featuring a raw vegan family. The Garden Diet company offers e-books with recipes and instructions on how to prepare delicious raw food meals.
www.HealerGuide.com/ GardenDiet

There are a myriad of studies proving that it is safe or unsafe to use microwave ovens, and it is hard to decide which study to trust. It is recommended to think twice before you "nuke" your food. Use the electric stove instead when possible.

*In a Comparative Study of Food Prepared Conventionally and in the Microwave Oven, published by Raum & Zelt in 1992, at 3(2): 43, it suggests that the production of unnatural molecules is inevitable. Naturally occurring amino acids have been observed to undergo isomeric changes (changes in shape; morphing) as well as transformation into toxic forms under the impact of microwaves produced in ovens.

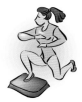

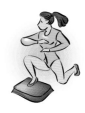

Organic food is important on so many levels. If you eat meat and dairy products, produced by organically raised animals it is much healthier. These animals are fed a healthier diet, treated humanely, and they were not cloned, given antibiotics or hormones. Organic fruits and vegetables are never genetically modified, treated with chemicals, pesticides or waxes.

Some may argue that there is no visible difference between GMO, or non-organic and non-GMO, organic food. Think of it this way, if you have two identical, unlabeled DVDs, but one is R-Rated and the other one is a fairly tale and you give them to a child to watch, is there a difference? Others will argue that the prices for healthier food are too high in comparison to conventional produce. The consumer demand for organic foods went up 20% in 2005 alone. This translates to lower prices in the supermarket and as the demand continues to rise, there will soon be little difference in the prices, if any.

The easiest way to shift one's perception about food and to welcome new tastes is to try cuisine from restaurants that specialize in its preparation.

Mission Organic 2010 is a campaign to encourage all Americans to make more organic food choices. If you join Mission Organic 2010, you pledge your commitment to make at least 10% of your eating choices organic through the year 2010 and receive a Free Organic Starter Kit. Here you will find peer-reviewed scientific evidence on how organic produce benefits health and the environment.
www.organic-center.org

Suggested restaurants:

❏ **Solar Harvest -** natural cuisine, 242 S. Beverly Drive, Beverly Hills - www.solarharvestfood.com

❏ **Real Food Daily Organic Vegetarian Cooking** - vegan cuisine, 514 Santa Monica Blvd, Santa Monica, & 414 N. La Cienega Blvd. Los Angeles www.realfood.com

❏ **Leaf Cuisine -** raw vegan cuisine, 11938 West WashingtonBlvd., West Los Angeles, CA 90066 - www.leafcuisine.com

❏ **Euphoria Restaurant -** raw food cuisine, 2301 Main Street, Santa Monica - www.rawvolution.com

❏ **Vegin' Out** - simple, affordable, cooked, vegan meals delivered to your home or office - www.veginout.com

❏ **Juliano's Raw Planet -** gourmet raw vegan food and catering, 609 Broadway, Santa Monica - www.planetraw.com

❏ **The Spot -** a natural food restaurant, 110 Second Street, Hermosa Beach - www.worldfamousspot.com

"No matter what it's called - a soft drink, soda or pop - drinking too much can cause tooth decay and harm your health. Sugar and acid in soft drinks, juices and sports drinks can set up the perfect environment for tooth decay. Drinking too much of these beverage likely contributes to other health problems, such as osteoporosis, kidney stones, and especially overweight and obesity, which are prime risk factors for type 2 diabetes in teens and adults."

-
Missouri Dental Association

If sauces, artificial flavors, sugar and processed food are eliminated and food is eaten in its natural state, it would be surprising if obesity existed at all. If meat were cooked without savory sauces and spices, it would be interesting to see how few people would really enjoy or eat meat in large quantities. It is virtually impossible to overeat fruits and vegetables and would take truckloads to create obesity. The easiest foods to indulge in are pasta, fried potatoes, cheese, soft drinks (one can of popular soda contains approximately 10 packets of sugar or 10 teaspoons), sugary snacks and desserts. The healthy functioning of the hormones and glands, especially the thyroid, (when it is under active is responsible for a slower metabolism) is maintained naturally, by eating a balanced natural diet. Hormonal irregularity or an under-functioning thyroid would rarely be responsible for weight problems.

It is hard for people to believe that a plant-based or raw food diet is more supportive to health. So many misconceptions around food exist. "I won't get enough protein," "I'll be deficient in calcium and increase my chances of osteoporosis," "I need meat to be strong." The advertising campaigns of the meat and dairy industries have been very effective!

In one study, funded by the National Dairy Council, a group of post-menopausal women were given three 8-ounce glasses of skim milk every day for two years, and their bones were compared to those of a control group of women not given the milk. The dairy group consumed 1,400 mg of calcium per day and lost bone at twice the rate of the control group. According to the researchers, this may have been due to the average 30 percent increase in protein intake during milk supplementation. The adverse effect of increases in protein intake to one's calcium balance has been reported by several research laboratories (they also cite ten other studies).

"The association between the intake of animal protein and fracture rates appears to be as strong as the association between cigarette smoking and lung cancer."

Dr. T. Colin Campbell

"Milk, it now seems clear, is not the solution to poor bone density. To the contrary, it's part of the problem."

Dr. Charles Attwood

According to Dr. Neal Barnard, president of the Physicians Committee for Responsible Medicine, "Milk, in particular, is poor insurance against bone breaks ... the healthiest calcium sources are green leafy vegetables and legumes. ... You don't need to eat huge servings of vegetables or beans to get enough calcium, but do include both in your regular menu planning."

[re-printed with permission PETA & www.milksucks.com]

"The ratio of calcium to magnesium in dairy products is 10:1, way too high. In nations with high rates of osteoporosis, the ratio of total calcium to magnesium intake is at least 2:1, usually over 3:1. South Africa, with a ratio of 2 parts calcium to 3 parts magnesium in the average diet, has an osteoporosis rate of 7. In the USA, the ratio is 4:1 and the osteoporosis rate is 144."

www.health-reports.com,
How To Beat Osteoporosis & Build Stronger Bones

Did you know that the causes of osteoporosis are attributed to a sedentary lifestyle with no weight bearing exercise and the leaching of calcium out of the bones due to an improper diet and stress?

It is convenient to stick with accustomed eating habits because they fit easily into the normal daily schedule; wake up, grab a coffee, hurry to work, breakfast at the drive-thru or vending ma

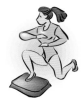

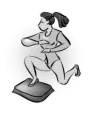

chine, daily stress, quick restaurant lunch or fast food, snack on an energy bar in the afternoon, grab a bucket of chicken or pizza on the way home (in a traffic jam), catch up with domestic duties, watch evening news and fall asleep, exhausted. If the above example were the only available lifestyle choice, some would rather choose death. A large percentage of the world's population would perceive the way Americans treat their bodies and choice of lifestyle as human slavery and self-abuse. This has nothing to do with the expression or care of the human spirit. The standard American diet and lifestyle can be compared to the destiny of a malnourished hamster on a wheel who can't stop running because the wheel is spinning too fast. Our lifestyle is the wheel and society does not stop spinning it. By taking the time to acknowledge that we are in control, we can slow down and set our own pace, make the right choices and finally be liberated from the wheel.

Proper pH is Crucial for Health and Vitality

Many practitioners understand that disease often results from an internal acid/alkaline imbalance, weakening body systems, creating an ideal environment where bacteria and viruses can thrive, making it difficult for the body to resist disease. Over-acidity is easy to test for and almost as easy to reverse. Over-alkaline environments create their own problems as well, but are quite rare these days. An overly acidic PH (or potential of hydrogen), can be identified by testing body fluids such as blood, saliva and urine. The body works hard to maintain a blood pH of 7.365 and will do so at all costs. Chronic acidity hinders all cellular activities and forces the body to borrow minerals, including calcium, sodium, potassium and magnesium from vital organs and bones to neutralize the acid resulting in mineral deficiencies. Mineral supplements may help one feel better for a time, but they act only as a Band-Aid, hiding the deeper problem. Symptoms of acidosis may include acid reflux ("GERD"), migraine headaches, constipation alternating with diarrhea, fatigue, poor digestion, bad breath, mouth sores, lactic acid buildup and weight gain. Acid related diseases include diabetes, obesity, bladder and kidney stones, premature aging, osteoporosis or weak, brittle bones, chronic joint pains, chronic fatigue, immune deficiency problems, and more.

Eating habits, stress, toxicity, improper elimination, most prescription medications and the inability to excrete acids all contribute to an over-acidic state. The biggest factor is a diet with acid-producing foods such as meat, eggs and dairy, white flour, fried foods, coffee, soft drinks, alcohol, sugar and artificial

People who drink diet soft drinks don't lose weight. In fact, they gain weight. The findings come from eight years of data collected by Sharon P. Fowler, MPH, and her colleagues at the University of Texas Health Science Center, in San Antonio. "What didn't surprise us was that total soft drink use was linked to overweight and obesity. "What was surprising was when we looked at people only drinking diet soft drinks, their risk of obesity was even higher." In fact, when the research-ers took a closer look at their data, they found that nearly all the obesity risk from soft drinks came from diet sodas.

[www. naturalsweetenernews.com]

"Every time we sit down to eat, we make a choice. Please choose vegetarianism. Do it for ... animals. Do it for the environment, and do it for your health."
-
Alec Baldwin, Actor

sweeteners. The lower the pH, the more acidic the body fluid, the higher the pH, the more alkaline. You can easily test your saliva and urine with inexpensive pH test strips (litmus paper) that are available in the fish section of pet stores or simply order at: *www.Healer Guide.com/phtest* to prevent serious unforeseen health problems.

Saliva & Urine Testing:

The saliva and urine pH test is a simple, painless way to monitor your body's pH. With this test you can measure your susceptibility to osteoporosis, and many other degenerative diseases. The pH of saliva and urine are affected by digestion and other bodily activities. It is suggested that the test be taken first thing in the morning (even before your morning routine and hygiene) for the best results.

● Taking the pH of your saliva:

1) Tear off a small piece of litmus paper (pH paper) from the roll, an approximately 2" long strip.
2) Gather the saliva on your tongue and place the pH paper in the saliva for a few seconds, just to make it wet.
3) The pH strip will change color.
4) Compare the color to the color chart on the litmus paper box.
5) When you find the color which is the closest match to the sample PH strip, the number on the color chart will indicate the pH of your saliva.
6) Testing should not exceed more than 35 seconds or reading may be inaccurate.

● Taking the pH of your Urine:

1) Tear off a small piece of the litmus paper (pH paper) from the roll, approximately 3" long strip.
2) Place the portion of litmus strip into your median flow of morning urine. Do it quickly, you need only a couple of drops not the whole waterfall.
3) The pH strip will change color.
4) Compare the color to the color chart on the litmus paper box.
5) When you find the color which is the closest match to the used sample, the number on the color chart below will indicate the pH of your urine.
6) Testing should not exceed more than 35 seconds or reading may be inaccurate.

The pH of morning saliva should read between 6.0 – 7.4. The saliva pH of those with chronic degenerative diseases or someone who is unhealthy will read 5.5 or lower. Both extremes (below 6.0 or above 7.4) should be considered a warning and lead to a consultation with a medical professional. For urine measurements you would like to see a urine pH above 6.0. If you get a dangerously low or high reading, do not panic, it is possible that the reading was not accurate and that you should re-test the next day. Many people may find alkaline saliva pH and an acidic urinary pH reading. This means that alkaline minerals are not being eliminated and that the body may be pulling minerals out of reserves to maintain the current body pH. This could be a sign that you are not getting enough alkalizing minerals and becoming acidic. Also consider, that if you have been under stress magnesium and calcium are often eliminated which can lead to a false reading. Certain medications can do the same.

The goal is to get your urine pH close to 7.0 and your saliva pH above 6.0. Correcting the pH balance is fast and easy and is accomplished by eating alkaline-forming fruits and vegetables.

Water is the most important element in establishing and maintaining proper pH. Your body is 70% water and loses approximately 2.5 liters of water per day. To effectively hydrate your body it is necessary to drink water that is alkaline. Alkaline water helps to neutralize acids, remove toxins from the body and it acts as a conductor of electrochemical activity between cells. Test the pH of your water. If it tests acidic, you may want to change your water source.

"The countless names of illnesses do not really matter. What does matter is that they all come from the same root cause...too much tissue acid waste in the body!"

-
Theodore A. Baroody, N.D., D.C., Ph.D.

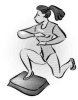

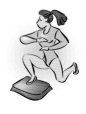

Make an effort to continuously maintain a balanced state. Make a list of foods and beverages you consume on a regular basis and replace a minimum of 50% of the most acid-forming foods, with alkaline-forming ones. The most acid-forming foods are sweeteners, coffee, alcohol, drugs and meat. The most alkaline-forming are fresh vegetables, green juice drinks, figs and lemons.

A quick overlook of Alkaline-forming and Acid-forming food:

● Alkalizing:		● Acidifying:	
Alfalfa sprouts	Kelp	Artificial	Pasta
Almonds	Kiwi	sweeteners	Pastry
Apple cider vinegar	Leafy Herbs	Bananas(green)	Pickles
Apples	Leeks	Barley	Plums
Apricots	Lemons	Beans(processed)	Pork
Artichokes	Lettuce	Beef	Poultry
Asparagus	Limes	Beer(most brands)	Rice
Avocados	Mango	Blueberries	Seafood
Bananas	Melons	Bran	Soft drinks
Beans(green)	Mushrooms	Butter	Soy sauce
Beets	Nectarine	Cereals	Sugar
Bell peppers	Okra	Cheese	Table salt
Broccoli	Onions	Chocolate	Tea (black)
Brussel sprouts	Oranges	Coffee	Tobacco
Cabbage	Papaya	Crackers	(cigarettes)
Cantaloupe	Parsley	Cranberries	Vinegar
Carob	Peaches	Drugs (street)	(processed)
Cauliflower	Pears	Eggs	Wheat bread
Celery	Peas	Fish	Wine
Cherries	Pineapple	Flour(white, wheat)	Yogurt (with sugar)
Coconut	Plums	Fructose syrup	
Cucumbers	Potatoes	Jams	
Dates	Pumpkin	Juices(with sugar)	
Eggplant	Radishes	Ketchup	
Figs	Raisins	Lamb	
Garlic	Raspberries	Liquor	
Ginger	Seaweeds	Milk(pasteurized)	
Grapefruit	Squash	Molasses	
Grapes	Strawberries	Mustard	
Honey(raw)	Turnip	Oats	
	Watercress		

For more information and a detailed list of alkaline or acid forming foods visit: www.naturalhealthschool.com/acid-alkaline.html or Download FREE Acid-Alkaline Food Chart & Recipes at: www.ph-ion.com

"We are indeed much more than what we eat, but what we eat can nevertheless help us to be much more than what we are. "

-
Daisie Adelle Davis, nutritionist
(1904-1974)

Start with simple things. Have a glass of water with a few lemon slices at each meal. Make one meal a day an alkaline-forming one. A food's acid or alkaline-forming capacities have nothing to do with the actual pH of the food itself. Lemons are alkaline forming in the body, but they test acidic before eaten. Cooked meat tests alkaline, but is highly acid-forming when digested.

How to Troubleshoot for Vitamin & Minerals Deficiencies

Vitamin and Mineral Deficiencies have a wide variety of symptoms and there are several causes:

■ Too much cooked foods - lack of fresh fruits and vegetables.

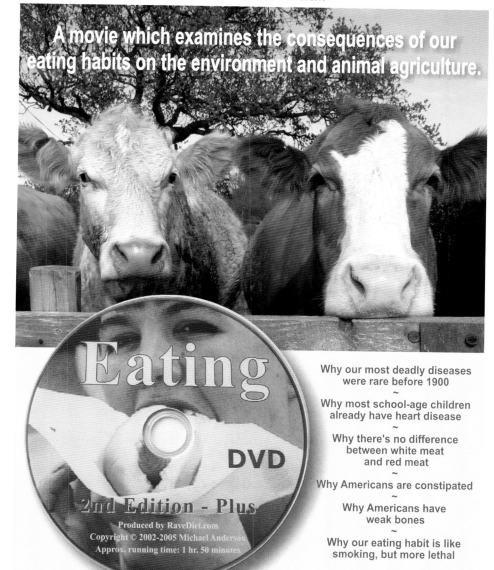

A movie which examines the consequences of our eating habits on the environment and animal agriculture.

Eating

DVD

2nd Edition - Plus

Produced by RaveDiet.com
Copyright © 2002-2005 Michael Anderson
Approx. running time: 1 hr. 50 minutes

Why our most deadly diseases
were rare before 1900
~
Why most school-age children
already have heart disease
~
Why there's no difference
between white meat
and red meat
~
Why Americans are constipated
~
Why Americans have
weak bones
~
Why our eating habit is like
smoking, but more lethal

Produced By: RaveDiet.com

The Eating Plus DVD covers a lot of ground very comprehensively - and all within 110 short minutes. Among the many highlights are interviews with Dr. Caldwell Esselstyn, Dr. Neil Pinckney, Dr. Ruth Heidrich and Dr. Joseph Crowe from the world-famous Cleveland Clinic Foundation, on the topic of our eating habits and its consequences.

Testimonials from people who have reversed a wide range of diseases, including genetically-based high cholesterol, gout, arthritis, chest pains/acid reflux, high blood pressure, asthma and adult-onset diabetes with the help of a change in their diet.

www.HealerGuide/Eating

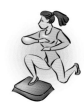

- Chronic illness or stress, uses an excessive amount of vitamins and minerals for continuous repair.
- Lower levels of nutrients from conventionally grown produce, not enough organic.
- Acidic pH imbalance.
- Malabsorption. Typically seen in the elderly or resulting from alcohol or drug abuse, thereby impairing nutrient absorption.
- Anorexia or Bulimia
- Heavy metal toxicity

Most people know that vitamin C is not being stored in bodily organs and has to be supplied on regular basis because it is essential for life and for maintaining optimal health. The cooking of vegetables and fruits can reduce the vitamin C content by 40%. C will be be completely lost if foods are frozen for longer than two months (frozen concentrate) Vitamin C is also destroyed when it is exposed to air. All bottled juices should be consumed right after opening.

The average U.S. diet supplies enough nutrition to prevent most deficiencies, but is insufficient to sustain vibrant health. Organic produce, when available is a must. Use supplements only as an intermediate remedy, while gradually implementing healthy dietary changes. Foods contain hundreds of compounds vital to your health, but they are not present in supplements. Choose wisely. Ask your health care professional, not a supplement seller, for an unbiased recommendation.

A quality iron source during pregnancy or for vegetarians and vegans is often recommended. Buying vitamin supplements solely based on advertising without consulting a qualified Nutritionist or

"Vitamins such as A, E and D are fat-soluble which means that excess quantities can accumulate in the body. A person who eats a vitamin-rich diet and simultaneously consumes multivitamin supplements could be overdosing."

-
Healer's Guide 2007

Common Symptoms of Mineral Deficiencies:

- **Calcium** - muscle aches and pains, muscle twitching and spasm, muscle cramps and reduced bone density.

- **Chromium** - glucose intolerance or insulin resistant hyperglycaemia (excess sugar in the blood), raised serum lipids and weight loss.

- **Cobalt** - bad circulation, migraines and spasms.

- **Copper** - an anemia that is unresponsive to iron therapy, abnormally low numbers of white blood cells, improper nerve function, improper metabolization of protein, increased cholesterol levels.

- **Iodine** - enlargement of the thyroid gland, during pregnancy can result in cretinism in newborns, involving mental retardation.

- **Iron** – cracked lips, fatigue, dizziness, irritability, headaches, difficulty concentrating, shortness of breath, brittle nails, anemia.

- **Magnesium** – neurological and muscular tremors, anxiety, depression, loss of appetite, nausea, vomiting, personality changes, muscle spasms, low calcium.

- **Manganese** - skeletal abnormalities, impaired glucose tolerance, and altered carbohydrate and lipid metabolism, impaired growth, impaired reproductive function, slow wound healing.

- **Zinc** - allergies, hair loss, skin trouble and weight problems.

When unusual symptoms appear, such as tiredness, weakness, depression or anxiety, irritability, nervousness, skin irritations, dehydration from vomiting or diarrhea, it should be immediately reported to a qualified medical professional. No one should attempt to diagnose and treat deficiencies on their own. Excess mineral or vitamin levels can cause serious health problems.

Naturopath should be avoided. Every body is different and therefore every body needs its own customized vitamin and nutritional program. Symptoms caused by vitamin and mineral deficiencies can be misdiagnosed as a more severe illness.

Vitamin & mineral testing will confirm a deficiency. Minerals are easily measured by hair analysis, a very accurate and inexpensive method of testing, which also quantifies the level of certain toxins. Blood tests are able to identify most vitamin deficiencies. The test must check the levels of <u>all</u> vitamins and minerals, not just a select few. Both tests are quick and easy to perform. Following, are samples of pages with hair analysis results plus a list of centers for testing.

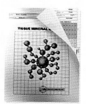 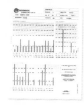 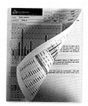

Photos courtesy of Trace Elements, Inc. Trace Elements is a leading laboratory in providing hair tissue mineral analysis (HTMA) for healthcare professionals worldwide since 1984.

Hair-analysis Resources:

Burbank

● **Paramount Herbs**
707A Main Street
Burbank, CA 91506
(818) 848-7414
www.paramountherbs.com

El Segundo

● **Body Doc Healing Center**
1924 B East Maple Ave.
El Segundo, CA 90245
(310) 546-6863
www.bodydocchiropractic.com

Encino

● **Randy Martin, Ph.D. O.M.D. L.Ac.**
17000 Ventura Blvd, Suite 220
Encino, CA 91316
(818) 905-6171
www.drrandymartin.com

Los Angeles

● **Illumina Healing Center**
1157 South Robertson Blvd.
Los Angeles, CA 90035
(310) 798-8082
www.illuminahealing.com

Manhattan Beach

● **Illumina Healing Center**
1713 Artesia Blvd. Suite C
Manhattan Beach, CA 90266
(310) 798-8082 - www.illuminahealing.com

Santa Monica

● **Holistic, Complementary and Integrative Medicine**
1752 Ocean Park Blvd.
Santa Monica, CA 90405
(310) 433-5249 - www.dralomar.com

West Los Angeles

● **Randy Martin, Ph.D. O.M.D. L.Ac.**
1444 Camelina
West Los Angeles, CA 90025
(310) 979-6495 - www.drrandymartin.com

West Hollywood

● **Holistic Medical Center**
8264 Santa Monica Blvd
West Hollywood, CA 90046
(323) 650-1789

Woodland Hills

● **Center for Wellness and Longevity**
23161 Ventura Blvd, Ste. 209
Woodland Hills, CA 91364
(818) 222-2080 - www.wholistichealer.com

"Health is a blessing that money cannot buy."

-

Izaak Walton, an English writer (1593 - 1683)

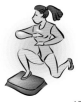

157

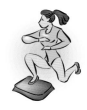

After discovering vitamin/mineral deficiencies, let the professional assess the cause. Mega-dosing with supplements on your own is not the best solution, especially if the cause is malabsorption. Malabsorbtion can be determined by the "Intestinal Permeability Test." A solution of two non-metabolizable sugars are consumed. One sugar is normally absorbed by the intestinal mucosa, the other is not. When the non-absorbed sugar is later found at a high concentration in the urine, it indicates Leaky Gut Syndrome. If the normally absorbed sugar is found to be lacking in the urine, it indicates malabsorption. The intestinal mucosa, or lining, can be compared to skin, a one-cell layer thick barrier between the contents of the intestines and the body's tissues. The mucosa facilitates the absorption of nutrients and also acts as a barrier to prevent parasites, fungi, bacteria and all of their metabolic waste products, viruses, toxins, and inadequately digested food particles from entering the bloodstream. This toxic condition is often referred to as" leaky gut syndrome."

Many laboratory tests for mineral deficiencies, intestinal permeability or parasites. These tests can be ordered through healt hcare professionals and range in prize from $70-$120. The information gained from these inexpensive test is priceless.

Stress and Fatigue

Who is without fatigue these days? The biggest culprit is stress. The body is in a constant state of "overdrive" due to job pressures and responsibilities, paying the bills or debts, getting things done, serving family needs, etc. The body rarely gets to relax and this results in an overstimulated nervous system, elevated hormones and heart rate and a brain which is often referred to as "fried." Over 60% of doctors visits are due to stress-related symptoms.

Top Stress Related Symptoms:
- headaches and digestive disorders
- muscle tension and pain
- sleep disturbance and fatigue
- chest pain, irregular heartbeat
- decreased sex drive, irregular periods
- immune system suppression
- problems with memory and concentration; confusion
- repetitive or continual thoughts
- less interest in hobbies or fun
- sudden shifts in mood, frustration, anger, resentment
- quick to irritability, oversensitivity
- sense of being overwhelmed or swamped; anxiety

"Two step formula for handling stress. Step number one: don't sweat the small stuff. Step number two: remember it's all small stuff."
-
Anthony Robbins

Your practitioner may recommend the Adrenal Stress Index Test to rule out over-exhaustion and the depletion of the adrenal glands. The results will show how the body's stress response system is functioning by checking the balance and level of two stress hormones, cortisol and DHEA.

Adrenal imbalance results in increased levels of cholesterol and triglycerides, impaired thyroid function resulting in decreased metabolism, lowered body temperature, and insomnia, PMS, infertility or cessation of the menstrual cycle. Glucose and insulin function are altered, blood sugar increases, fat is stored - especially around the mid-section, salt and water are retained, decreased immune function, diminished mental and physical regeneration due to low levels of growth hormone, accelerated aging, protein breakdown is increased leading to premature wrinkles, muscle loss and weakness. The extent of the symptoms depends on the level of adrenal depletion. Your specialist will read the results to determine the level of your insufficiency and suggest that you reduce stress and implement glandular/nutritional supplements to rebuild your adrenal function.

Household products stored under your kitchen sink, in your bathroom, on your laundry room shelves and in your garage can be toxic and potentially harm-ful to your health. See the information in the House-hold Products Database for health effects. For a guide and the safe-handling of household chemicals, log on to:

www. householdproducts.nlm.

The second test we recommend for fatigue is the Carbohydrate Challenge Test or Glucose Tolerance Test. Swings in blood sugar levels are very stressful for the body. If you have frequent energy highs and lows throughout the day, have yourself checked. The specialist will have you eat a high carbohydrate meal of white bread, a banana, and orange juice, after taking your blood and saliva sample. During the next three hours, additional blood and saliva samples are re-taken and glucose, insulin and cortisol levels are measured. If you are found to have difficulty metabolizing sugar, eating light frequent meals and avoiding white flour, caffeine or sugary foods is typically recommended.

"It is only the liver that can purify the bloodstream and we only have one liver."

-
Sandra Cabot, M.D.,
In-depth report about the liver and related diseases,
www.liverdoctor.com

Another common source of fatigue is liver toxicity. A daily dose of toxins from household chemicals, processed food, chemically treated water, etc., are broken down into metabolic waste which taxes the liver and kidneys. A good liver or kidney cleanse may help to skyrocket personal energy. There are a variety of liver cleanses, flushes and herbal products to assist the process [as a quick reference visit: *www.drhuldaclark.org/ therapy_liver.asp]* Ask your alternative care professional for their advice as to which methods are appropriate for you and to help determine if your body is strong enough to do a cleanse.

Parasites, Yeast, Fungus and Mold

These four play havoc with health in a really big way! Great Plains Laboratory, a provider of testing services for medical practitioners explains, "Excessive yeast produces toxic metabolites, which can pass through the blood-brain barrier causing brain fog, behavior problems and learning difficulties. Excessive bacteria byproducts can interfere with neuro-

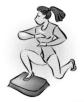

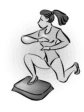

transmitters and cause chronic fatigue." If you are suffering from a chronic health problem characterized by fatigue, digestive difficulties and lowered immunity, make it a priority to check for these sneaky invaders. Parasite infections can lead to a variety of symptoms, *i.e.*, bloating, weight loss, abdominal cramping and pain, nausea, vomiting, loss of appetite, fever, rash, itching anus, and bloody or foul-smelling stools. A comprehensive stool test quantifies the presence of pathogenic yeast parasites, bacteria, beneficial bacteria levels, intestinal immune function, inflammation markers and overall intestinal health. The intestinal tract is home to many kinds of bacteria and yeast, some beneficial and some not. It plays a key role in immunity. Parasites further hamper health and immunity.

The treatment process of tap water doesn't remove all contaminants and parasites. Single-celled organisms such as cryptosporidium and giardia can often slip through water purification treatments unharmed. These parasites are protected by a tough outer coat and the chlorine added to municipal water systems has little effect on them. Tap water should always be boiled before drinking.

Awareness regarding human parasites has mistakenly been reduced to searching for big worms or flukes acquired in exotic countries. In actuality, there are dozens of smaller parasites. The most common parasites that infect humans in the United States and Canada are giardia (Giardia lamblia), Entamoeba histolytica, cryptosporidium (Cryptosporidium spp.), roundworm (Ascaris lumbricoides), hookworm (Ancylostoma duodenale and Necator americanus), pinworm (Enterobius vermicularis), and tapeworm (Taenia spp.) that can be picked up from the family pet, undercooked meat or even an infected person handling your food. It is a common misconception that parasites stay confined to the intestinal tract. Certain parasitic species can attack internal organs such as the liver, pancreas, lungs, heart or even the brain. These cases are often initially misdiagnosed. The pork tapeworm is the most common disease-causing brain parasite. A leading cause of brain seizures, it is usually contracted from undercooked pork. After becoming attached to the intestine, it can grow to the length of several feet. When this worm invades the brain, they don't grow as large but cause severe neurological problems. The overgrowth of yeast, toxic bacteria, and parasites, are all possible causes of fatigue, easily identified by the stool analysis.

"During the past few years, the field of medical parasitology has seen some drastic changes, including newly recognized parasites and an overall increased awareness of parasitic infections. We have seen organisms, like the microsporidia, change from "unusual parasitic infection" to being widely recognized as one of the most important infections in a compromised patient."

-
1997 edition of
Diagnostic Medical Parasitology

If you suspect parasites in your system and they have not been identified by other testing methods, then the Organic Acid Analysis Test will identify which bio-chemicals or metabolic waste produced by parasites and yeast are present. Metabolic waste can circulate throughout the system and cause a low grade, chronic poisoning of sorts. Sometimes a stool test will not pick up on all organisms, especially those in the small intestine. This test does not replace the stool test, but it will give more concrete evidence. More information (with illustrations) about human parasites can be found at:

www.drnatura.com/parasites.php

Heavy Metals

Toxic metals such as mercury, lead, aluminum, cadmium and arsenic can impede development, cause neurological disorders and impair normal brain functioning. Symptoms of heavy metal poisoning can be identical to neurological and psychiatric disorders. Toxic metals have been indicated in cases of autism, ADHD and multiple sclerosis. Besides hair analysis, toxic metals can be tested in urine, blood and stool. The blood test detects recent metal poisoning and the hair analysis proves long term toxicity from, for example: silver-mercury tooth fillings, the presence of lead wall paints in household, aluminum in cosmetics, or home chemicals. The hair test also shows the ratio between nutrients and toxic metals. Chronic high levels often lead to mineral depletion.

> Mercury toxicity is often linked to leaking silver-mercury tooth fillings. Some countries, like Sweden, Canada and Germany, have either banned or imposed serious limitations on amalgam usage. But it is important to know that every time you remove one filling and put another in its place, as is the case when replacing silver-mercury with composite fillings, you run the risk of killing the nerve of the tooth and then needing a root canal or extraction! The lifespan of a composite filling is 3-5 years, therefore it is wiser to choose a longer lasting filling material (*i.e.*, gold - 30+ years).

HAIR ELEMENTS

The Great Plains Laboratory, Inc.

LAB#:
PATIENT:
SEX: Male
AGE: 2
CLIENT#: 24510

POTENTIALLY TOXIC ELEMENTS

TOXIC ELEMENTS	RESULT µg/g	REFERENCE RANGE	PERCENTILE 68th 95th
Aluminum	31	< 8.0	
Antimony	0.11	< 0.066	
Arsenic	0.11	< 0.080	
Beryllium	< 0.01	< 0.020	
Bismuth	0.16	< 0.13	
Cadmium	0.075	< 0.15	
Lead	0.74	< 1.0	
Mercury	0.32	< 0.40	
Platinum	< 0.003	< 0.005	
Thallium	< 0.001	< 0.010	
Thorium	0.001	< 0.005	
Uranium	0.095	< 0.060	
Nickel	0.30	< 0.40	
Silver	0.33	< 0.20	
Tin	0.75	< 0.30	
Titanium	32	< 1.0	
Total Toxic Representation			

ESSENTIAL AND OTHER ELEMENTS

ELEMENTS	RESULT µg/g	REFERENCE RANGE	PERCENTILE 2.5th 16th 50 84th 97.5th
Calcium	556	125- 370	
Magnesium	120	12- 30	
Sodium	41	12- 90	
Potassium	43	12- 40	
Copper	60	8.0- 16	
Zinc	170	100- 190	
Manganese	0.34	0.20- 0.55	
Chromium	0.43	0.26- 0.50	
Vanadium	0.24	0.030- 0.10	
Molybdenum	0.16	0.050- 0.13	
Boron	0.77	0.60- 4.0	
Iodine	7.7	0.25- 1.3	
Lithium	0.011	0.007- 0.023	
Phosphorus	184	160- 250	
Selenium	0.63	0.95- 1.7	
Strontium	2.8	0.16- 1.0	
Sulfur	52600	45500- 53000	
Barium	1.2	0.16- 0.80	
Cobalt	0.028	0.013- 0.035	
Iron	19	8.0- 19	
Germanium	0.037	0.045- 0.065	
Rubidium	0.048	0.016- 0.18	
Zirconium	2.8	0.040- 1.0	

The Hair-analysis chart on this page is courtesy of The Great Plains Laboratory, Inc.

-

www.greatplainslaboratory.com

SPECIMEN DATA

COMMENTS:		
Date Collected:	Sample Size:	0.198 g
Date Received: 11/15/2006	Sample Type:	Head
Date Completed: 11/18/2006	Hair Color:	
	Treatment:	
Methodology: ICP-MS	Shampoo:	

V06 99

RATIOS

ELEMENTS	RATIOS	EXPECTED RANGE
Ca/Mg	4.63	4- 30
Ca/P	3.02	0.8- 8
Na/K	0.953	0.5- 10
Zn/Cu	2.83	4- 20
Zn/Cd	> 999	> 800

The Great Plains Laboratory, Inc. · 11813 W. 77 Street, Lenexa KS, 66214 · Tel: 913.341.8949 · Fax: 913.341.6207

Analyzed by: ©DOCTOR'S DATA, INC · ADDRESS: 3755 Illinois Avenue, St. Charles, IL 60174-2420 · CLIA ID NO: 14D0646470 · MEDICARE PROVIDER NO: 14945.1

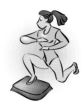

Common illnesses attributed to metal toxicity:

● Mercury can cause depression, fatigue, developmental disorders. A mouth full of mercury can cause a multitude of problems. If the levels of mercury in your body are high, visit a holistic dentist specializing in mercury filling removal. They will replace the mercury fillings with another, less toxic material. Ask your dentist for alternative tooth fillings of the highest quality. Certain white replacements corrode quickly, progressing to inevitable root-canal procedures within the next few years.

● Aluminum has been linked to Alzheimer's disease and is found in deodorants, shampoos, regular table salt, aluminum foil and aluminum cookware.

● Lead can cause depression, nausea, fatigue, communication, developmental and concentration problems and is found in older lead-based paints, or old water pipes. Water pipes can also leach other toxic metals into your home's water supply.

> Metal toxicity is highly underestimated yet highly dangerous to human well-being. Although the complete cure of acute or chronic heavy metal toxicity is possible, many people suffer liver or brain damage which may not be fully reversible. It is a common misconception that toxic metal has to be swallowed or digested. The majority of heavy metal toxicity is caused by absorption through the skin and the inhalation of polluted air.

Certain laboratory tests require a pre-authorization beforehand from a medical practitioner. Test kits can be ordered by phone and then taken to a health professional for their signature. The samples can be shipped overnight by courier and the lab or health professional will file for reimbursement from your insurance company. The results must be interpreted by your health professional.

Food Allergies

Food Allergies can show up in a number of different ways. Symptoms may range from fatigue, digestive problems, rheumatoid arthritis, depression, anxiety, psychosis, seizures, hyperactivity, learning difficulties, attention deficit disorder(ADD) and more. Allergy testing is done by a blood sample and 96 common foods are tested in one shot! The days of the old fashioned skin scratch testing are thankfully behind us.

For metal, parasite & allergy testing contact:

❑ **Dr.Randy Martin,** West Los Angeles & Encino, (310) 979-6495, www.drrandymartin.com

❑ **Dr.Wael Alomar,** Santa Monica - (310) 4330 5249, www.dralomar.com

❑ **Dr.Michele Cohen,** Los Angeles & Manhattan Beach (310) 798-8082, www.illuminahealing.com

❑ **Dr.Emil Levin,** 8264 Santa Monica Blvd., West Hollywood - (323) 650-1789

❑ **Dr. Marylin Snow Jones,** 23161 Ventura Blvd, Ste. 209, Woodland Hills, (818) 222-2080, www.wholistichealer.com

❑ **Dr. Paul D'Alfonso,** 1924 B East Maple Ave., El Segundo, (310) 546-6863, www.bodydocchiropractic.com

❑ **Dr. Jon Buratti,** 1914 W.Alameda Av., Burbank, (866) 572-6984

Keep Your Circadian Rhythms In Line with Nature

Circadian rhythms refer to the 24-hour cycle of the physiological processes of living beings. They are the natural cycles that control appetite, energy, mood, sleep and libido. When the body is out of sync with nature, these rhythms are affected, manifesting as sleep and mood disorders. Other rhythmic cycles include the menstrual and ovulation periods. The pineal gland and hypothalamus are suspected of being the actual clock of the body. Hundreds of scientists worldwide study our biological clock and its existence is universally accepted. The interest of science was sparked following the discovery that certain disease patterns were experienced at different hours of the day and times of the year. For example asthma is generally worse during the night when hormonal secretions decrease. These rhythms affect our health, safety, performance and productivity. The pharmaceutical industry is now trying to time drug delivery to realize greater effectiveness with lower dosages.

Nature's rhythms or cycles include the four seasons and the twenty-four hour rotation of the earth. The physical body responds to these cycles by utilizing the earth's signals and cues for the proper timing of secretions of hormones, chemicals and neurotransmitters. Morning light sends the message to produce neurotransmitters which then signal when it is time to wake up. The neurotranmitters then prompt the body to produce cortisol and serotonin, elevating the blood pressure and raising the body temperature. At sunset, the body secretes melatonin and blood pressure drops, in preparation for sleep.

The night shift, fluorescent lights, frequent traveling and lighting late into the evening have disrupted our connection with the sun, the primary circadian rhythm regulator. People used to follow the sun by waking up at dawn, working outside during the day and going to sleep when the sun set. Now people are lucky if they get 30 minutes of sun on a lunch hour or the drive to work.

Disorders which may be indicative of disrupted rhythms include: depression, bipolar disorders, PMS, mood and sleep disorders, low libido, prenatal/postpartum depression, fatigue, seasonal affective disorder, ADD/ADHD. Chronic fatigue syndrome sufferers usually have affected circadian rhythms. Simple corrections in lifestyle habits are all it takes to shift the body back to the correct pattern. If difficulties persist, light therapy sessions will reset the circadian clock, restoring the body's timing and levels of melatonin and serotonin. Some researchers believe that depression sufferers have an unresponsive body clock.

The benefits of light therapy have not been chemically understood. After much scientific experimentation, the NIH concluded that winter depression exists in about 35 million Americans, as a result of the lack of sunlight. It seems the citizens of Los Angeles are literally hooked on sunlight and more than 2 days of cloudy weather can cause signs of depression for some. It seems that Light Therapy may be an antidote to the winter blues.
For more information, visit:

www.apollolight.com

The term "circadian", coined by Franz Halberg, comes from the Latin words circa, "around", and dies, "day", the literal translation is "about a day." The formal study of daily, weekly, seasonal and annual biological temporal rhythms is called chronobiology.

Resource: Smolensky, M., L. Lamberg. *The Body Clock Guide to Better Health.*

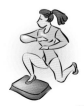

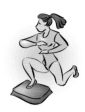

Wake therapy 'reboots' the body clock, by waking the patient up several hours earlier than usual. Wake therapy only needs to be used for one night followed by waking up the patient every morning with a bright light. This reverts the rhythms back to an active day cycle, alleviating symptoms of depression.

Light therapy is usually administered (or recommended for home use) by a physician, physical therapist, or psychologist. Look for a well-trained, experienced clinician.

Water

Probiotics are small organisms that help maintain the natural heathy balance of the gastro-intesntinal tract. Taking antibiotics or antiparasitic herbs kills the good bacteria along with the bad ones, so supplementing with probiotics such as Lactobacillus and Bifidus is a must, following the course of treatment. Supplementing with probiotics is a safe and natural as these bacteria are already a normal part of the digestive tract. A decrease in beneficial bacteria can cause diarrhea, urinary tract infections and yeast infections. Ask your doctor.

The importance of quality drinking water is expanded upon in *The Environment* chapter. Water is essential for life. Many people don't drink enough water resulting in headaches, tiredness, poor skin, muscle pain, depression and other problems. The U.S. National Research Council recommends 1 ml of water for every calorie you eat which is about 2.5 QTS per day. Too much water may create strain for the kidneys. Drinking distilled water is viewed by some as another potentially dangerous habit. *[www.miraculewater .com/WaterLibrary/Distilledwater.htm]*

Great uses of water for personal health include salt baths, healing mineral springs and colonics. Colonics clean the intestines and flush out accumulated mucus, gallstones, non-elimated toxic waste, parasites, yeast and other undesirables. Toxins accumulate in the colon after many years of even the healthiest diet. Several treatments are usually required in order to change the state of your health. Be sure to repopulate the colon with healthy bacteria (probiotics). Be sure to ask your specialist if a colonic is recommended or appropriate for you. Cleansing programs and undertaking short one day water fasts regularly is important for colon health. Get permission from your physician before doing water fasts. Often, it is contraindicated for those with certain health conditions or on some medications.

"Physical fitness is not only one of the most important keys to a healthy body, it is the basis of dynamic and creative intellectual activity."

-
John Fitzgerald Kennedy, Thirty-Fifth President (1961-1963)

Another great way to detoxify the body using water is with ionic foot baths, available in holistic spas (see page 167). You can also purchase one for home use. Heavy metals and other toxins, by the law of gravity, settle in the feet. The action of the ionized water with salt crystals draws the toxins out. After 30 minutes in a foot bath, the water is gray and you feel great.

Exercise

Exercise often brings up negative feelings and images. Those who can't find the time may experience feelings of guilt.

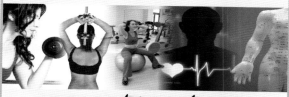
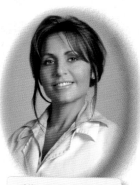
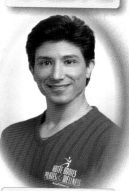

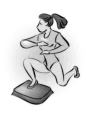

Prioritizing is the key. There is no time or energy left for exercise if you are in the habit of living the previously mentioned Los Angeles lifestyle model. Priorities must change. The health of the citizens of our country is at stake. According to recent surveys, 60% of adult Americans are not physically active, 50% of youth between 12-21 do not participate in regular physical activity, 25% of second graders can't touch their toes, 76% of elementary kids can't do a chin up, 50% of boys and 33% girls can't walk up and down stairs for six minutes without straining their cardiovascular system and 30% of boys under 13 can't run a mile in less than ten minutes, 40% of kids age 5-8 are obese and have high cholesterol. Do it for yourself and for the health of your children. Set a good example.

All it takes is 30 minutes, 4-5 times a week. Walking, taking a yoga or tai chi class, doing any physical activity. If you have an abundance of energy or have excessive frustration or anger, something with more intensity such as aerobics, running or kick-boxing will help to move that unhealthy energy out of your system, but be sure to pair this up with meditation and other self-improvement tools to get you to calm emotional equilibrium. Whatever it is, make it enjoyable and have some variety. If you consider exercise boring, play tennis one day, swim the next and golf the day after. Talk to your physician before embarking on an exercise program. Ask for suggestions and advice on how to properly implement your plan. If your New Year's resolution was to start exercising call a health club close to you.

Many body-care products labeled "natural" may contain petrochemicals. Study the labels of your personal care products. These toxic substances can cause allergic reactions: Sodium Lauryl/ Laureth Sulfate, Petrolatum (petroleum jelly), Methyl, Propyl, Butyl, Ethyl Paraben, Synthetic Fragrances Diethanolamine (DEA), Triethano-lamine (TEA), Diazolidinyl Urea, Imidazolidinyl Urea, Propylene Glycol, PVP/VA Copolymer, Stearalkonium Chloride, Synthetic Colors or FD&C or D&C.

"Beauty is not in the face; Beauty is a light in the heart."

Kahlil Gibran,
Poet, philosopher, artist
(1883-1931)

Skin Care & Beauty

The skin is the body's largest organ and it is one of the primary organs of elimination. The skin can be considered like an extra set of lungs and kidneys. Help it by skin-brushing with a loofah 3-4 times a week before showering or bathing. This opens the pores and helps detoxification while easing the strain on the kidneys. So does deep breathing. Several times a day, be aware of your breath. Most people breathe in a very shallow manner, using only the top portion of their lungs. Take deep breaths throughout the day, filling the bottom portion of the lungs deeply before exhaling. This will oxygenate and bring more nutrients to the cells, including the skin. Omega Fatty Acids 3, 6, and 9, found in olive, flax seed and borage oils are extremely important for healthy skin - take them internally and use quality oils for moisturizing. Salt baths are great for cleansing and detoxifying while softening the skin (see Salt Bath in *The Vital Body*). Use natural, organic, pH balanced soaps, creams,

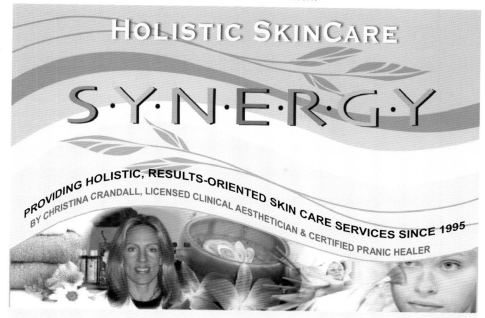

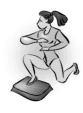

lotions and hair care products. *Dr. Bronner's Magic Soap* is a great all-purpose body cleanser. The Whole Foods and Wild Oats stores carry several different product lines. Why use products with chemicals? There are much better alternatives. Chemicals are commonly absorbed through the skin and pollute the environment. Many skincare and beauty services/spas use natural products. Look for these when going to the spa or having facials. Sunbathe regularly, Sun supplies us with vital energy, but do not overexpose to avoid the appearance of early aging, wrinkles and the possibility of skin cancer.

There is a branch of Ayurvedic medicine which focuses on beauty, confidence, posture and skin care. Their practitioners offer entire treatments that focus on this area of health.

● **Dancing Shiva** - providing blissful ancient Indian therapies and ayurvedic medicine - 7466 Beverly Blvd - 2nd floor Los Angeles, CA 90036 - www.dancingshiva.com

● **Surya Spa -** 563 Muskingum Avenue, Pacific Palisades, CA 90272 (310) 459-7715, an ayurvedic clinic offering personalized therapy and treatments - www.suryaspa.com

Touch and Bodywork

Bodywork is extremely important for those with a sedentary lifestyle. Typical areas affected by desk jobs include the upper back, neck, shoulders and lower back. Work-out injuries occur from muscles that are too tight due to lack of activity. Joints and muscles lose flexibility and strength, creating pain which fosters more inactivity. Stay limber & pain-free with regular massage and chiropractic.

The healing power of touch is nothing short of miraculous. A simple hug is so powerful, it can change someone's mood and their entire day in an instant. Receive bodywork as often as possible. Massage is unparalleled in its ability to loosen tight muscles, relieve stress and quickly move toxins toward the proper channels for elimination. Cranial Sacral therapy, Rolfing, Osteopathy, Physical therapy offer unique advantages in the area of bodywork, depending on the structural issues at hand. Chiropractic is invaluable for its ability to correct subluxations, more commonly known as spinal misalignments while improving nerve connection to the organs and tissues. Keeping the physical body in alignment improves health and helps it function more efficiently.

"Look at sex realistically and in a light mood. Sexual energy is needed to upgrade your brain cells. Sex, sweetness and intimacy are good but you must also have a functional brain"

-
Grand Master Choa Kok Sui, scientist, spiritual teacher, author of *Experiencing Being*

Sexual Energy

Healthy sexual expression and the correct use of sexual energy promotes physical, mental, emotional and spiritual health. Sex energy is one of the most powerful forces in the human body. Unfortunately, two extreme conditions are commonly prevalent. One is suppression, resulting in unhealthy sexual fantasies, perversions and horrible crimes involving innocents. The other is overuse. Sexual energy in ancient civilizations was utilized as a force for longevity and rejuvenation. It was observed that partial celibacy or retaining sex energy during illness increased the body's ability to heal by ten times or more. It was understood that not properly conserving and transmuting sexual energy resulted in weakness, disease and early death, while hindering creativity, spiritual development and evolution.

> ❏ **Healing Love** – Taoist Sexual Secrets for Health & Bliss by Michael Winn & Joyce Gayheart. The secrets of transforming sexual energy into radiant health. Specific sexual cultivation practices for men & women, solo & pairs. DVDs, CDs - www.healingdao.com/healinglove.html
>
> ❏ **Taoist Secrets of Love** - Cultivating Male Sexual Energy by Mantak Chia & Michael Winn, ©1984, published by Aurora Press, P.O. Box 573, Santa Fe, New Mexico
>
> ❏ **Spiritual Essence of Man** - by Grand Master Choa Kok Sui, discusses the transmutation of sex energy into love and spiritual energy to accelerate mental and spiritual developments, among other topics.

A portion of the sex energy is distributed to vitalize the legs and the brain. By observing elderly folks this is easy to see. As their sexual energy declines with age, so do their mental faculties and the strength of their legs. Those who choose partial or total celibacy as part of their life's path must know how to properly transmute sexual energy, otherwise the excess or pent up energy may lead to discomfort or unwholesome actions. If sex energy is suppressed and psychological addictions or other unhealthy behaviors are present, psychotherapy and/or counseling is called for. Sex energy can be transmuted into love, intimacy, artistic expression and used for spiritual development. For those who would like to pursue higher artistic and spiritual goals or divine union with their partners, there are classes, and workshops which teach the proper use of sex energy.

> When transmuting sexual energy into the spiritual, the same vital energy, prana, is at work in both. "Any sense activity or sense experience consumes a lot of prana. The highest of all goals in human life, spiritual attainment, requires the maximum available pranic energy on all levels - mental, intellectual and emotional."
>
> -
> His Holiness
> Sri Swami
> Chidananda
> Saraswati Maharaj

A summary of the care of the physical body:

- ■ Test and maintain proper pH of saliva or urine regularly.
- ■ Test for toxins and heavy metals. See your practitioner for testing and a recommended elimination method.
- ■ Test and eliminate bacteria, parasites and fungus. See your practitioner for testing and recommended elimination method.
- ■ Eat organic, nutritious, enzyme rich foods-minimum 25% raw.
- ■ Reduce meat and dairy consumption. Eliminate sugar, sweeteners and processed foods. Limit microwaving. Limit frying and grilling of meat.
- ■ Regular, adequate exercise especially yoga and cardiovascular conditioning. For those with health conditions, check with your physician.
- ■ Sunshine, clean water and clean air.
- ■ Cleanse your colon regularly with colonics or occasional water fasts. Do herbal cleanses for your internal organs, including the liver and kidneys.
- ■ Sleep 8 hours, between 9pm - 7am to keep circadian rhythms in balance.
- ■ Balance and conserve sexual energy, with healthy sexual expression.

After incorporating the above pointers, to free the body from all its unnecessary burdens and to increase its vitality, your body will use its new surplus of energy to heal its major and minor or chronic health conditions. If you are already in good health, just think of what you'll be able to do with all that extra energy!

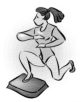

Dr. Tea Says "Drink to Your Health With Tea"

By Mark "Dr. Tea" Ukra, & Julie Jackson

Just to set the record straight, I am not a medical doctor and I don't have a PhD. I am an expert on tea. I have been called a tea guru, a tea junkie, a tea connoisseur, authority, specialist - even a tea evangelist. But today, I am simply known around the world as Dr. Tea. Tea is my passion and has been for my family dating back some 250 years. Upon opening the Tea Garden & Herbal Emporium in Los Angeles, my friends and clients appointed me Dr. Tea as I speak of tea as a Dr. would speak of medicine. I carefully guide my clients toward the integration of the body, mind and spirit with optimum health and vitality through tea – the second most consumed beverage in the world behind, you guessed it, water.

When tea found me, it changed my life and health. It will change yours too, one cup at a time. Caffeine addiction, afternoon snacking, late night binging, depression, insomnia, aging, obesity, chronic illnesses and more. We all experience it, and yet we all have the power to fight it by integrating tea in to your everyday life.

To understand why your body needs tea as a staple in your everyday life, you must understand tea. All tea comes from one plant, camellia sinensis. There are not separate white, green, oolong and black tea plants. There is only one tea plant. The only difference in the tea you drink is the process by in which it is produced. However, all four teas, whether bagged or loose leaf, will provide you with health benefits that can help you realize your full potential in a healthier lifestyle.

Let's start with caffeine. Medical research has shown that caffeine addiction can trigger a multitude of health issues and compound those I mentioned above. Those trying to shed a few pounds have probably hit a wall after a few weeks on their diet. Why? The common culprit is often the caffeine in their diet. You see, caffeine from coffee places your body into a state of shock and actually increases appetite. Further, there is an acid in coffee which increases your insulin levels which in turn increases your blood sugars and which traps your body fat so you can not loose weight. Tea lowers your insulin levels. Have you ever seen a heavy Asian?

Now let's compare tea to coffee. When preparing a pot of tea, you have the ability to remove 90% of the caffeine in any tea by rinsing (the process of brewing and throwing away) the first steep. The four teas stack up like this: Black tea, the most common in the states, already gives you 50% less caffeine than a cup of coffee. Moving on to oolong, one of my favorites, you will get an astounding 70% less caffeine. Current media darling, green tea, will top out at 80% less caffeine than coffee. And the winner? The budding superstar in tea, white tea at 90% less than a cup of coffee!

So why, Dr. Tea, you ask, is the caffeine in tea not as harmful to my body?

The answer lies in the fact that caffeine's effect in tea is entirely thwarted by a friend of ours by the name of L-Theanine. L-Theanine is an amino acid found only in tea leaves. It stimulates the pro-duction of alpha brain waives which create a state of relaxed, focused, energized thought. Coffee, however, does not contain any L-Theanine.

Still not convinced you should be drinking tea everyday? Tea contains an anti-oxidant called epigallocatechin

Cont'd on page 172

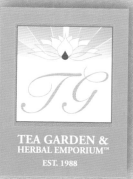

TEA GARDEN &
HERBAL EMPORIUM™
EST. 1988

DEDICATED TO THE TEACHING AND GUIDANCE TOWARDS THE INTEGRATION OF THE BODY, MIND AND SOUL!

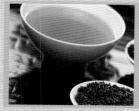

Take care of your body, relax and nourish with one of our Custom Blended Teas. We offer over 100 varieties so that you'll be sure to find the ones that are just right for you.

There is nothing more calming than a clear mind. Our Teas and Herbs are made of the finest ingredients on earth to help you relax and rejuvenate.

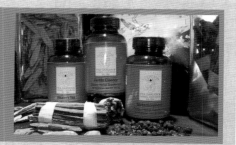

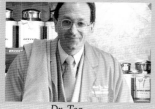

Dr. Tea

Seize the time to connect to the depths of your soul, to lift your spirits and to appreciate peace and calm.

IT IS OUR PASSION TO HELP YOU ON THIS JOURNEY

Tea Garden & Herbal Emporium ™
800.288.HERB (4372)
www.teagarden.com

For Store Location or
FREE Samples, visit out website
and enter Promo Code **HEALER'S GUIDE**

gallate (EGCG) which has been medically proven to fight against cancer cells, reduce risk of heart attack, lower cholesterol, reduce weight and strengthen skin cells. It's a fact, tea drinking societies live longer happier healthier lives. Unlike coffee which is steeped only once, tea is meant to be brewed over and over. The effects of L-Theanine and the EGCG will continue to be felt in each subsequent steep.

Let us not forget the herb-based tea blends. Most people are aware of the benefits of a nice cup of chamomile tea at the end of a long, stressful day. We at the Tea Garden specialize in providing our clients with herbs from the Orient and our master herbalists are dedicated to finding the right regimen to fit your personal needs. By incorporating herbs into your daily diet, whether it be an herb-based tea or tonic, you will realize the deep wisdom

that forms the basis of this incredible Asian life art. You will find the need to become more cognizant of the call to protect ourselves naturally from pollution, stress, and other detrimental factors in our environment. Hundreds of millions of people a day from around the world rely on these powerful tonic herbs to improve their lives. I encourage you to do the same.

On behalf of the Tea Garden, I commend you for taking the first step in seeking out a healthier body, mind and spirit through tea and herbs. Drop me a line anytime and let me know how you are progressing. We love to hear from you.

And don't forget, let tea be your guide to good health, one cup at a time!

Tea Garden & Herbal Emporium
8612 Melrose Avenue
West Hollywood, CA 90069
310-205-0104
800-288-HERB
drtea@teagarden.com

Yoga

The Body Mind Connection

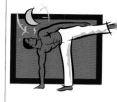

Yoga is an ancient art and science originating in India. It fosters the development of the body-mind connection and awareness of oneself as a being fully connected and a part of the universe and all of creation.

The Yogic physical exercises or postures are called asanas. Yoga exercises focus on the health of the spine and result in flexibility which keeps the body youthful. By taking care of the spine's flexibility and strength, circulation is increased and the nerves housed in the spine are bathed in nutrients and oxygen. The more challenging asanas offer the student an opportunity to discover and control their emotions, improve concentration, strengthen their will, and to unify the physical and etheric bodies. Asanas often uncover hidden mental attitudes and emotions and enable the release of unsupportive patterns.

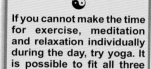

If you cannot make the time for exercise, meditation and relaxation individually during the day, try yoga. It is possible to fit all three into a one hour session!

The foundations of the philosophy of yoga are contained in Patanjali's sacred text, *The Yoga Sutras*, written in approximately 200 AD. The book is an assembly of the loosely written text from over 4,000 years ago. It outlines the limbs of yoga - eight-steps that comprise the complete practice of yoga.

1) Yamas - Universal morality. These are the moral virtues which purify the human vehicle and, more importantly, the soul. The result is personal happiness, a joyous society and greater connectedness with oneself. There are five:

• **Ahimsa** - Compassion for all living things. Literal translation: non-injury or cruelty to any creature or any person. Non-violence is practiced on oneself and others, both in actions and thoughts. Ahimsa also means kindness and thoughtful consideration of others. Do no harm.

• **Satya** - Commitment to Truthfulness. Translation: "to speak the truth." It is not desirable to speak the truth in all situations as it may be harmful. If this is the case, then it is better to say nothing. It is tied in with Ahimsa. Deliberate deception and exaggerations are harmful to others.

• **Asteya** - Non-stealing. Take nothing without permission that does not belong to you. This includes other's mental property, creations, time or attention.

"Most people think that aging is irreversible and we know that there are mechanisms even in the human machinery that allow for the reversal of aging, through correction of diet, through anti-oxidants, through removal of toxins from the body, through exercise, through yoga and breathing techniques, and through meditation.

-

Deepak Chopra

173

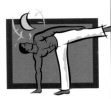

- **Brahmacharya -** Sense control. Translation: abstinence, self-restraint, responsible behavior, particularly regarding sexual activity. It does not mean celibacy unless one chooses it. It means not harming others and using sexual energy to regenerate our connection to our spiritual self.

- **Aparigraha -** Neutralizing Greed. Translation: Take only what is necessary, what one has earned. It also means letting go of attachments. Hoarding implies a lack of faith in oneself and God to provide.

There are two popular teachings of the science of yoga.

- Kriya Yoga is a specific system brought to the west by Paramahansa Yogananda. It consists of yogic techniques that hasten the practitioner's spiritual development and bring about a profound state of tranquility & God-communion. *[www.yogananda-srf.org]*

- Arhatic Yoga taught by Master Choa Kok Sui, synthesizes and integrates all yogas. After the purification of the physical, etheric, astral, and mental bodies, the chakras are substan-tially activated in a secret sequence to safely and effectively awaken and then circulate the Kundalini energy throughout the body.

[www.pranichealing.com]

2) Niyama - Rules or Laws. They are personal observances. These refer to the internal view of oneself and of behaviors. There are five:

- **Isvara Pranidhana:** Surrender to God, the realization that one is not in control of one's existence. The contemplation of God in order to align oneself to God and God's will. Spend time each day honoring the omnipresent force which guides and directs our lives.

- **Samtosa:** Contentment with one's life. Accept peacefully what happens and realize the higher purpose in everything. Yoga calls it Karma. Be happy with what you have instead of longing for what you do not have.

- **Sauch:** Cleanliness, purity of the body and thoughts. Both inner and outer aspect. Outer cleanliness simply means keeping ourselves clean. Inner cleanliness is about the health of bodily organs and of the mind. Practicing asanas and pranayama are the essential means for achieving Saucha. Cleansing the mind of hatred, passion, anger, lust, greed, delusion and pride is even more important.

- **Svadhyaya:** Inquiry or examination. The study of sacred texts and to study oneself through personal reflection with self-awareness in all activities. Eliminate unwanted or self-destructive habits.

- **Tapas:** A disciplined use of energy. Literally it means to heat the body, which cleanses it, directing energy to achieve the ultimate goal of union with the Divine. Being disciplined burns away unnecessary desires. Tapas include spiritual austerities, respect for the body, and keeping the body fit, as well as observing the food eaten, posture and breathing patterns.

3) Asanas - Body postures. Improves health, strength, balance, flexibility and prepares one for deeper meditation by opening the channels in the physical body. Results in a quieting of the mind and is a valuable preparation for meditation and the expansion of consciousness. Asanas tone the body.

4) Pranayama - Breathing exercises, and control of prana. Prana means breath or life force and Yama means control. It also involves the directing of that breath. Asana and Pranayama

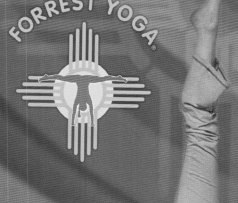

Forrest Yoga

Committed to
"mending the hoop of the people"
—creating in each of us a sense of freedom,
a connection to our spirit
and the courage to walk
as our spirit dictates.

International Workshops,
Teacher Trainings,
and Conferences

(888) 453-5252
www.forrestyoga.com

Breath, Strength, Integrity, Spirit, Go Deeper

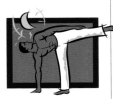

create heat. The result of this heat purifies the nadis or nerve channels. One learns control of the body and mind, while increasing energy and sense of peace. On the physical and mental levels, yogic breathwork helps one focus, creates balance, increases lung capacity, oxygenates the blood, purifies the nerves and decreases the stress of body and mind.

5) Pratyahara: Control of the senses or literally "to withdraw oneself from that which nourishes the senses." It is the withdrawal of attachment to external objects and the practice of non-attachment. Emotional imbalances result from attachment to the senses or outer circumstances. One easily influenced by sensations and external happenings cannot have inner peace. Withdrawing from the five senses helps to reach the meditative state of Samadhi, or enlightenment. This is done by shifting awareness away from the outer world to the inner self. In this state, one is able to discover their true nature.

6) Dharana: Concentration and cultivating inner perceptual awareness. One steadies the mind by focusing their attention upon an object. The object is not as important as the purpose - to stop the mind from wandering, and is essential to being able to properly meditate.

7) Dhyana: Devotion, meditation on the Divine. This is one step past Dharana and is a state of awareness. It involves concentration, while being aware of everything. The other limbs are important to practice regularly in order to arrive at this state. Here, both the mind and body are quiet and receptive.

8) Samadhi: Union with the Divine Samadhi is a state of union or yoga with everything - with the universe - and a divine state of ecstasy. It is oneness realized, bliss and interconnectedness. In Samadhi, the body and senses are at rest, yet the faculty of the mind is alert and a state of expanded consciousness results. It is very difficult to achieve Samadhi and careful study and practice of the above are necessary preparation.

"The more yoga you practice, the more your own body tells you what and when to eat. If you honor this inherent wisdom, you'll find over time that your body knows best."

-
Steve Ross,
yoga teacher,
Maha Yoga

Although the true yoga practice is quite extensive and in-depth, it is possible to fit yoga into a busy schedule in a half hour or one hour a day. One must learn the limbs of the practice from a knowledgeable teacher. It is not necessary to practice all of the above steps to gain the health benefits of yoga. Simple Hatha Yoga poses and breathing exercises are enough to maintain good health. Yoga is extremely beneficial for those recovering from injury or accidents. One can practice the postures to the extent that they are able. Flexibility and strength will increase with practice. The health benefits such as stress reduction are often immediately visible upon commencing practice and are unparalleled by any other form of exercise or practice.

"A Healing Journey Through Yoga" Expert Insight with Ana Forrest

By Venetia Carotenuto

My intent in teaching yoga is to do my part in mending the hoop of the people; to inspire people to clear through the stuff that hardens them and sickens their bodies, so they can walk freely and lightly on the earth in a healing way, in a Beauty Way."

Ana Forrest, creator of Forrest Yoga and the founder of the Forrest Yoga Institute in Santa Monica, California developed her own style of yoga after many years of dealing with unresolved emotional and physical pain. She had frequent migraines, was epileptic, sexually and physically abused, and suicidal. She struggled with bulimia, drugs, alcohol, and tobacco. Yoga was the first tool she experienced that made a difference. It saved her life, gave her a reason to live, and a purpose for living. Through experimentation with yoga she found that a key component to personal healing was finding out how each yoga pose works for a particular individual. This taught her to throw away what didn't work and find out what did.

The style of yoga she designed, Forrest Yoga, specifically addresses contemporary physical and emotional stresses and challenges. It concentrates on individual needs and emphasizes personal awareness of your body, breath, and your pain. Intense pose sequences, compassionately taught, develop skills in awakening each of the senses. Experiencing yoga in this way is a deeply rewarding and exhilarating practice. It becomes a very empowering tool for self-exploration and a road to freedom.

Educating people to bring aliveness and breath into every cell of their body is Forrest's passion. "When I look around in our world, I see craziness and atrocities and tragedies everywhere. My vision is to do my part in mending "the Hoop of the People. To teach people the tools I've developed in Forrest Yoga in order to bring them healing."

Ana Forrest inspires people to learn how to embody their spirit (spreading their spirit and breath through every cell of their body) and transform their past experiences into wisdom for daily living. "When people start to get centered and know their own truth, they aren't as swayed by fears or by authorities that don't necessarily have the authority to define the truth for you or me."

Ana Forrest lives her life the way she teaches – by honoring and celebrating the beauty of life and the power of spirit. She is an inspiring individual with a unique approach to an ancient practice. Forrest Yoga is a breath of fresh air, a challenge, and an incredibly powerful yoga workout that builds not only flexibility, intelligence, and strength but also helps deepen the relationship with your authentic Self. "Accessing your intuition -- the voice of your Spirit – builds personal strength and ushers integrity into your daily interactions with all beings. I invite you to heal, grow, and welcome your Spirit home."

Anna Forrest
Forrest Yoga
www.forrestyoga.com

See Ad on page 175

Inspired Instruction | Intimate Atmosphere

Kundalini

yoga

The Blessings Center

founded by Gurutej Kaur

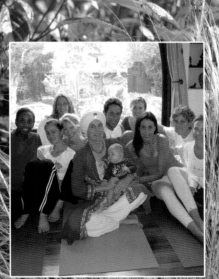

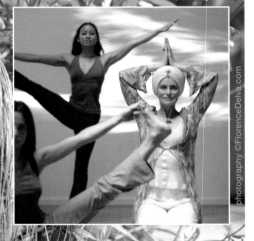

photography ©FlorenceDelva.com

kundalini

anusara

meditation

323.930.2803   < for info & schedule >   www.gurutej.com

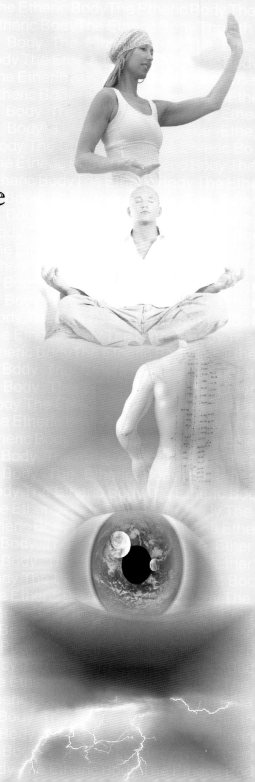

The Vital Force

Your Etheric Body

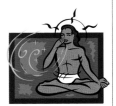

The Vital Force

Your Etheric Body

The following words have something in common: "hond", "chien", "cane" and "pes." Even though they look and are pronounced differently, they express the same thing. They all mean "dog" when translated into English. Similarly, the energetic structure directly vitalizing (sustaining life) the physical body is called by different names in different languages. Scientists have made it even more confusing with their effort to label new discoveries as accurately as possible. They recently gave birth to such words as zero-point energy, bio-physical energy, vacuum energy and a few others which point to the same subject labeled otherwise as Ether, not to be confused with the well known Ether, or $(CH_3CH_2)_2O$ used for anesthesia. It is the term used to describe the all, pervasive energy found virtually everywhere throughout the universe. *"The established wave nature of light and other radiation eliminates every doubt about the authenticity of the existence of ether. The ether waves come to us both from the remote areas of the universe, from the depth of atoms, and from atom nuclei. Thus, all of macro and microcosmic space is filled with ether."* The Cognition of Reality By The Methods of Classic Physics © 2002 Sukhorukov G.I., Sukhorukov E.G., Sukhorukov R.G.

> **Zero Point Energy (ZPE), or vacuum fluctuation energy** are terms used to describe the random electromagnetic oscillations that are left in a vacuum after all other energy has been removed. If you remove all the energy from a space, take out all the matter, all the heat, all the light... everything - you will find that there is still some energy left. One way to explain this is with the uncertainty principle from quantum physics that implies that it is impossible to have an absolutely zero energy condition.
> *[NASA, www.nasa.gov]*

"Vacuum energy is an underlying background energy that exists in space even when devoid of matter."
-
Source: Wikipedia, Free Encyclopedia

This energy with all its aspects shaped and formed, works as a matrix or a non-physical blueprint for all physical objects, the human body included. Simply said, before something appears in the physical world, the corresponding form has to first be created in the ether.

For example, if you decided to create a statue, the shape and form of the statue must first appear in your mind via your imagination before you can form it. This means that the statue already existed in your, mind (it was created), before it could materialize. The strong intention of the mind and will, followed by physical action, resulted in the creation of the statue. Your thought process can actually form or influence the ether in many ways. The physical body also has an energetic matrix and its pattern/shape is similar to the physical body. It will be referred to as the *Etheric Body*.

The human Etheric Body is a complex mechanism. As mentioned, the Etheric Body is the source of energetic support for our physical body and without this quality of subtle energy, physical objects tend to break down and the physical body tends to die. If the energy is not completely missing from the matrix, but is severely reduced, the physical body does not die, but a corresponding physical manifestation of breakdown will appear. In other words, the body becomes ill or injured.

Our ancestors knew about the energetic matrix and discovered that when repaired, the physical body followed suit and repaired itself, as well. They discovered that the energy in our Etheric Body is distributed through a network of energetic pathways. The physical counterpart of the pathways is the human nervous system.

One healing system based on this principle is acupuncture. Acupuncturists mapped the energetic pathways and called them "meridians" or "nadis." They also learned how to influence the level of energy in these meridians, increasing or decreasing the amount or flow of energy by inserting tiny needles, correcting the imbalance. Each organ is related to a specific meridian. This "needle-poking" has been proven to influence the energy flow, vitalizing particular physical body organs, resulting in healing. In several countries, different healing techniques or styles were developed including Ayurveda, Pranic Healing, Reiki, Qi-gong, all with the same underlying principle. This principle is based on directly influencing the Etheric Body to bring about physical results.

The Etheric Body is so close to the physical realm that for some people it is even possible to see it with the naked eye. This method of seeing, called *clairvoyance*, is very rare and unless born with the ability, one must be trained. The more common method of validating or perceiving this subtle energetic field is through the sense of touch and is called *clairsentience*. Based on the direct experience of alternative medicine teachers, approximately 90% of people are able to feel their own energetic field on the first attempt and the rest usually learn within the next few days. Once it's felt, this knowledge of how to feel it always remains. It is like a small initiation.

Clearsight offers comprehensive studies in clairvoyancy and energetic medicine. The student learns to access their innate clairvoyant ability to read auras and the chakras and to be able to perceive energy as colors, pictures, images and pure energy of all types. This reading procedure allows the student to become an intuitive counselor, an energy healer, and to perceive the energy changes in the essence of all living things.

www.clearsightaura.com

"The future of acupuncture will to some degree depend upon our ability to reconcile the old and new within a new science of energy medicine. This can only be accomplished if we honor both our traditional roots and the challenge of building on the foundation provided by scientific research."

-
Dennis Tucker, Ph.D., L.Ac.

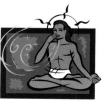

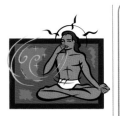

The exercise I would like to share with you was first introduced to me about 15 years ago. I was reading a book which claimed that trees have a lifeforce and an energy field, which humans can utilize for empowerment and healing. It sounded good, but due to my scientific background I wanted to know what kind of energy it was and where is it coming from. So, I asked my energy healing teacher and he instructed me to do following:

1)

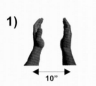

Rub your palms together vigorously, contact and extend your fingers at least 12 times then clap your hands and shake them to relax. This sensitizes the hands and frees them of stale energy.

Now, sit or stand comfortably and breathe deeply and slowly. Your breathing should be deep and at least 5 to 7 times before returning to your normal rate of breathing. Raise your hands in front of you with your palms facing each other. *Pic. 1*

2)

Keep a distance of about 10 inch. between your palms. With your hands in this position take another 5 deep breaths, Pic.2. (Just relax, there is no hurry) Every time you exhale, focus on your palms and the space between them. When you have finished with the deep breathing, focus on your palms and move them slightly closer to each other and then apart again. *Pic.3 - 5.*

3)

You can also move them in a circular motion back and forth. Every time you move them, the motion should be gentle and should not exceed a couple of inches. *Pic. 6-7.*

4)

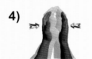

First, you will feel a subtle tingling, vibration or heat in your palms. The more you experiment, the stronger it will get. Some may feel a sensation similar to invisible cotton candy on your fingertips. The first common reaction (if trying this for the first time) is suspicion that this could be your own body heat, a illusion or autosuggestion. When you keep practicing this (moving your palms back and forth), your doubts will fade and you will realize that the feeling of tingling and vibrating is caused by something other than just your physical hands or body heat. This is the lifeforce which wraps around your palms. By consciously creating this gentle motion, the energy fields of your palms interact with each other causing the tingling. Have fun with it. If this was your first attempt to acknowledge your own energy field (clairsentience), with time your awareness will increase. If you have already mastered this exercise and can feel your own field strongly on each attempt, try to perform the same exact exercise in front of the mirror in a darkened room. You may see a light bluish glow surrounding your palms but this is a more advanced exercise. You may want to consider professional training for this ability (clairvoyance).

5)

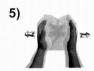

6)

7)

This exercise is probably the easiest way of to feel your own energy field. Its purpose is not to just create a *wow* effect for those who feel this for the first time. This is simply the easiest way to understand the force upon which most alternative healing modalities are partly or fully based. This will help you to have a more open mind when you are in a session with a healer or holistic practitioner. It is also a reminder for those who have already gone through similar experiments that what we see (the physical world) is only a fragment of what truly exists.

M.Polak - Healer's Guide 2007

The Etheric Body, in certain texts is frequently referred to as the *Etheric Double* or *Vital Body*. In ancient scriptures, it is said to be the first essential component of the human being and is an inseparable part of our existence throughout our physical life. It is unfortunate that after thousands of years of knowing this information, this subtle structure has been overlooked by conventional medicine. Nevertheless, the positive effects of conventional medicine can be seen every day regardless of the lack of knowledge regarding the human Etheric structure. By combining these two fields of expertise in the future, disease won't have much of a chance!

> The etheric body is recharged and energized by sleep, exercise, sun, wind, water and earth. Pay attention to your connection to Mother Nature. Revitalize your etheric body often.

Sleep is the most important time for recharging this subtle field and getting our energy back. When we miss a night of sleep we feel that we have no energy. If we were to miss three nights of sleep without a nap, the feeling of weakness and listlessness is alarming. After five or six days without sleep, the physical body may simply die. Please do not try this at home, it has already been scientifically tested! A strong and healthy Etheric Body, recharged during sleep is absolutely essential for physical health and vice versa, ill people have an unhealthy Etheric Body. Once the concept of the etheric body is grasped, there are other ways to re-charge, but none other than deep meditation are as effective as sleep.

The concept of Etheric matter is not limited to the physical body. There are other sciences which are based on this principle. One of the ancient sciences that works directly with the Etheric aspect is Feng Shui. It is an environmental art and science which investigates the flow of supportive or unsupportive Etheric matter in the environment (*i.e.,* home or business) and suggests remedies for the correction of any problems or obstructions to the energy field. The result is often minimizing the interference of the environment with the human Etheric structure, due to its harmonizing effect. Thus minimizes the risk of illness due to unsupportive environmental factors. When certain locations have the reputation of being problematic (*i.e.,* people get sick often, accidents always happen in the same place), it is referred to as a place with bad energy. It is a common mistake to label the energy good or bad. Energy isn't good or bad but

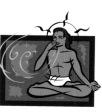

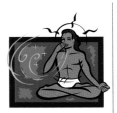

it is supportive or non-supportive for our bodies and our efforts to live in harmony with the natural laws. Similarly, fire is not necessarily bad until you, in moment of ignorance, step in it. "Feng Shui" translated from Chinese means "wind and water" and is a simple explanation of how unformed Etheric matter behaves, constantly in motion and unbridled until manipulated by will and consciousness.

Recharging your energy field can be done by drinking special teas. According to ancient Ayurvedic wisdom, tea has an energetic aspect and it is a great way to move your prana, or lifeforce.

Tea is healing on many levels; aiding digestion and eliminating toxins. Reducing the body's burden of excess toxins, will increase your energy level.

For more information on the healing power of tea, see page 170.

Some people have learned how to influence their Etheric field in less scientific ways. With the use of certain energy-influencing hand movements, crystals or even correct pronunciation of sounds and words called *mantras*, they have discovered how to bring the Etheric field back to its natural balance to create optimum physical health. By applying these methods on others they became healers and these healings were incorrectly labeled "miraculous." Bringing a portable radio into the era of King Arthur would have also been perceived as a miracle because radio technology was not yet known. We now know that radio waves travel through the ether. The Etheric Body and its direct influence on physical health was seen as miracle by many, until the technology behind it was explained. Thoughts also travel through the ether. Everyone at some time has had the experience of thinking about someone and a moment later, the phone rings and it's them. Prayer and distant energy healing work on a similar principle. Schools teaching this subject have often been labeled as esoteric or mystery schools for lack of standardized modern scientific terminology.

"Once we recognize that all matter is actually energy, we can begin to form a new vision of ourselves and the world around us. We begin to realize that our surroundings are not what they seem."
-
William Buhlman, author
The Secret of the Soul

Schools offering studies in energy healing:

❑ **Barbara Brennan School of Healing** - combines hands-on healing techniques with spiritual and psychological processes. The Healing Science Workshop is offered globally -www.barbarabrennan.com

❑ **Inner Cosmos** - energy healing classes and workshops. Kriyashakti training available - www.innercosmos.com

❑ **Integrated Energy Therapy**® Certification Training - Learn how to safely release limiting energy patterns. CEUs - www.energywellbeing.com

❑ **Lionheart West Institute of Transpersonal Energy Healing** - professional training with certification or personal growth and learning - www.lionheartinstitute.com

❑ **Learn2heal** - introductory Pranic Healing workshops, clinics and basic training. Step-by-step application of energy healing - www.learn2heal.com

❑ **The Reiki Center** - training are conducted by Master Teachers in the True Usui Lineage. First degree to mastership - www.reiki-center.org

❑ **US Pranic Healing Center** - basic, advanced, psychotherapy and higher courses in Pranic Healing. CEU's available - www.pranichealing.com

❑ **Yuen Method** - combining Chinese Energetic Medicine with energetic techniques, quantum physics, Qi and Shen Gong - www.yuenmethod.com

The Etheric Body is a complex mechanism distributing the life-force (chi, prana, biophysical energy) to the physical body. The next logical question is where does this lifeforce come from and how is the etheric body vitalized? What generates the energy? This is the job of energetic generators. They are tur-bine-like etheric components that draw vital force from the available, unlimited ocean of all-pervasive etheric energy of one's surroundings. This free energy cannot by absorbed by our bodies, so the energetic gen-erators - *chakras* - exist to absorb and transform the free energy into a more digestible form for our bodies to use. The chakras can be seen as a quickly spinning vortex of lifeforce. The easiest way of visualizing this is to remember how water shapes itself when the plug is pulled from the bathtub drain. It creates a whirlpool. Similar whirlpools are formed when the life- force is being drawn in and utilized. (picture below)

The human energetic anatomy is comprised of major and minor chakras. The major ones support the endocrine glands and organs. Dozens of minor chakras support the other areas of the body - hands, feet, jaw, elbows, knees, etc. The book, *Miracles through Pranic Healing*, by Master Choa Kok Sui dis-cusses, in-depth, all major and minor chakras, their locations and functions.

Everything in the universe will break down sooner or later unless energy in some form is added to it. If you do not feed your physical body, it will break down. If you do not care for your car it will break down too. Similarly, the chakras also need maintenance. When they are not properly cared for, the quality and amount of lifeforce in our etheric system diminishes. The result is an undervitalized phys-ical body. In its weakened state such a body will break down with disease.

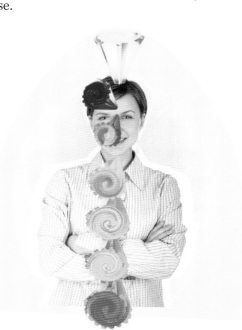

"Please open your eyes now, but keep attention in the inner energy field of the body as you look around the room. The inner body lies at the threshold between your form identity and your essence identity, your true nature. Never lose touch with it."

-

Eckhart Tolle, contemporary spiritual teacher and writer on spirituality

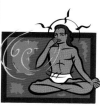

Approximate shape and position of several energy centers (chakras) in the human ener-getic anatomy. This picture shows only a few of the chakras on the front side of the body. For a more complete chart and location of centers, including the back of the body, refer to the resources listed at the end of this chapter.

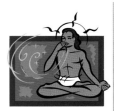

It is from this understanding that another wave of healing modalities sprouted. Sometime referred to as New Age modalities, those with only a little knowledge about the chakras attempted to influence physical wellbeing by applying incomplete techniques on them. The interesting thing is that, even with limited knowledge such attempts actually produced results, although somewhat inconsistent, for those who did not fear to try.

When the lifeforce is flowing through our human energetic system of nadis and meridians, some of this energy radiates into the surroundings. This was best described by Master Stephen Co from AIAS *(www.yourhands canhealyou.com)* when he compared lifeforce passing through the meridians to an electric current. When electricity is passing through metal wiring, it emanates an electromagnetic field. This is why it is unwise to build a house under or next to high-voltage power lines. In the case of lifeforce, the field emanating from our bodies is not electromagnetic but is a *bioenergetic* field of lifeforce, referred to as the *Aura*.

The aura is another important component of the Etheric human anatomy. It can be likened to a protective bubble, that prevents potentially harmful energies from entering our field to be absorbed by our chakras, which could possibly be further distributed into the physical body, causing illness.

The strongest portion of our aura can be perceived as a 1-2" thick layer of light-blue/light-gray field outlining the shape of the physical body. It is easily seen in the head area even by an untrained individual. The actual reach of the lifeforce field extends to a greater distance, generally 3-5 feet. The exact size cannot be determined because the field is continuously in flux, corresponding to the amount of energy running through the body at a given moment. The more energy, the bigger the field. The Etheric Body

A person's aura contains information about them. Their moods, personality, emotions, health. Your aura is constantly interacting with other energy fields. It acts like a transmitter and receiver. If you have ever taken an instant dislike or like to someone after just meeting them, this is your aura in action. The information passes from your aura, to your etheric body, through the meridians to your central nervous system. It is then received by the conscious or subconscious mind - depending on your level of awareness.

With the auric field, you can perceive how every decision and everything you experience in your life affects your body." according to healing expert Barbara Brennan. "It all shows in the auric field, every thought, every feeling and so forth."

-
At Play In The Auric Field From Science To The Sacred, Pathways Jounal Articles, Interview with Barbara Ann Brennan

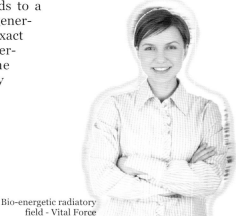

Bio-energetic radiatory field - Vital Force

also has additional components which are not in the scope of this book but can be studied in detail in specialized literature (resources on the next page).

As people began to perceive this energetic aspect, it was assumed that by influencing the Aura of a person, healing or some physical improvement could be affected. Those who study human energy, learn how to keep the Aura strong and uniform so the protective abilities of this natural shield are maximized, as their first lesson. This could be considered energetic disease prevention. There is a new technology called the *Aura Video Station* which can actually scan and show the shape and condition of human auric or bioenergetic field on a TV monitor. It is quite exciting to see it with your own eyes and we highly recommend the experience. This technique is in its infancy and still limited, but it is fascinating nonetheless. There are several pioneers who have scientifically mapped our subtle human anatomy and translated it into modern terminology. Credits are given in the back of the book.

"Energetic hygiene is the practice of keeping your energy body as clean and charged up as possible through emotional regulation, dietary recommendations, special physical exercises, the use of salt as an energetic cleansing agent and numerous other techniques. Most people feel their personal energy surge when they begin practicing energetic hygiene regularly."

Master Stephen Co,
U.S. Pranic Healing

Cutting edge technology for measuring subtle energy:

Reimar Banis, M.D., N.D., has developed a new system of energy-medicine that he calls Psychosomatic Energetics. The new technology combines quantum technology, EEG and energetic homeopathy. The newly invented test device (Reba) is the heart and soul of this system and emits a broad spectrum of frequencies onto the patient. This device enables practitioners to measure the four levels (etheric, emotional, mental, causal) of the subtle energy field (Aura). This method uncovers important soul issues hidden in the depths of the subconscious, which up until the invention of this technology could only have been reached by methods such as hypnosis.

For more information regarding the Reba: www.terra-medica.com

source: *How Emotional Conflicts Block the Flow of Energy* by Reimar Banis, M.D., N.D., Switzerland, translated by Ulrike Banis, M.D., N.D.

Energetic self-care is not common knowledge but if we consider our life from a holistic point of view, it is an inseparable aspect without which a permanent improvement seems impossible. It is similar to the concept of physical hygiene. Everybody washes their hands, takes a shower or bath daily and wears clean clothes to prevent infection. The subtle bodies need care and hygiene too. This is called energetic hygiene, the term describing the process of keeping one's energetic system and energetic environment clean. It is common for people to assume that everything in their energetic field belongs to them. Actually, every one of us can, or does, at times, suffer from energetic contamination from unclean places or unhealthy individuals.

There are several easy steps which will prevent an accumulation of harmful etheric energy in one's system. The following practices are simple, but relatively unknown.

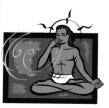

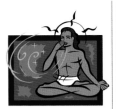

A summary of the care of the etheric body:

● **Take a salt bath with essential oils:** A salt bath facilitates healing by keeping your energy field and physical body clean. Prepare the salt bath with 3-4 lbs of sea salt or table salt that contains no added aluminum (see the container label). Often regular table salt contains aluminum as a anti-caking agent. Pour the salt in to a warm bath. Add 20 drops of an essential oil to boost the cleansing properties of the bath and remain in the bath for 25-35 minutes (no longer) and then shower off. The essential oils commonly used are lavender (relaxing, good for stress), tea tree (very cleansing), eucalyptus (extremely cleansing - good for cold and flu and when bronchial/lungs are affected), do not mix different oils together unless you know how to do this safely. The stronger the cleansing action of the salt and oil used, the more vital energy will be extracted as a by-product of cleansing. For that reason, try to have the salt bath at night, so you can re-charge while you sleep. Swimming in a clean ocean is even better! This is highly recommended two times per week.

● **Physical exercise:** When your physical body moves, especially during aerobic activity, the subtle energetic structure (meridians, chakras & aura) are partially stimulated as well. This results in the release of energetic blockages, congestions or stale energies produced by sedentary work. People often feel more energized following the after-work workout because their energetic anatomy is able to breathe again.

● **Good sleep:** A good night's sleep is absolutely essential for the physical body to function and it is primarily during sleep that the energetic body is recharged. Also, a short power nap during the day keeps the energetic level high which manifests as a strong life force (Auric) field. A strong field prevents the absorption of energetic contaminants and minimizes the possibility of being affected by an energetically unclean environment.

● **Meditation:** Its influence on the etheric body manifests as stimulation to all components of the energetic anatomy. The flow of subtle energies throughout the meridians and chakras rapidly increases during meditation. The Etheric body becomes highly energized and strengthened. The push of increased energy flow forces stagnant energies or blockages to leave the body and areas which lack energy are re-energized. Meditation can be considered as a cleansing energetic shower.

Resources on the structure, function and properties of the Etheric Body:

"Energy is the essence of life. Every day you decide how you're going to use it by knowing what you want and what it takes to reach that goal, and by maintaining focus."

-
Oprah Winfrey,
O Magazine, July 2003

❏ **The Etheric Double** - a study of the etheric body; its nature, appearance, functions, its relationships to the other vehicles, its connection with prana, or vitality, and with certain methods of healing, by Arthur Powell

❏ **Hands of Light** - an understanding of how the human energy field looks, functions, is disturbed, heal and interacts with friends and lovers. A guide to healing, by Barbara Ann Brennan

❏ **Your Hands Can Heal You** - Pranic Healing energy remedies to boost vitality - provides practical instructions for managing your pranic energy, by Master Steven Co, Eric Robbins, John Merryman

❏ **The Book of Chakras** - explores the nature of subtle energy, the chakras - where they are and how to use them, by Ambika Wauters

❏ **Man Visible and Invisible** - describes the function of etheric body, function and colors of the aura under the influence of different emotions, by C.W. Leadbeater

Recognize and Release
Energy Vampires
By Master Healer Satish Dholakia

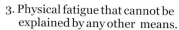
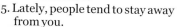

Sometimes you meet someone and you feel very energized and connected with life. You feel joyous energy all around you in their presence. You want to spend more time with such people. And sometimes it also happens that you meet someone and immediately you feel drained, exhausted and confused. Often, those who do not have a strong connection with their own source or inner light, have a tendency to drain your energy. They are frequently referred to as energy vampires. They survive by "stealing" other's light; their life force. This could be very energetically draining for you.

The interesting thing to notice is you cannot satisfy a vampire. No matter how well you behave, or how much you give of yourself, there is a black hole that is never satisfied, never happy, always hungry for more.

Vampires come in many forms. One common thread you may notice is they cannot connect with the source of light within themselves. Their basic agenda is to consume your lifeforce. Another name for this game is *psychic warfare*. The two chakras that vampires source for energy and commonly "attack" are the solar plexus chakra and the third eye chakra. The solar plexus chakra is used for draining the lifeforce and third eye chakra is used for draining the will force.

The following are some common signs you may notice when your lifeforce is being drained :

1. Feelings that something is just not right.
2. Your "gut" tells you that the feelings you are having are not normal, or come from an external source.

3. Physical fatigue that cannot be explained by any other means.
4. Unexplained lack of concentration.
5. Lately, people tend to stay away from you.
6. Things are constantly going wrong.

And there could be many more variations of these signs of psychic energy interference. Protect yourself from energy vampires! Your body has all the intelligence to guide you, protect you and tell you the difference between what's right and what's not right. Your gut - your stomach - is the most accurate psychic on the planet. The challenge is to connect with this accuracy within. Just a little practice of this skill and you will be empowered for the rest of your life. Just stay aware of your body.

Where are you?
Maybe your feet touch the ground. Be aware of your feet.
Maybe your hand is holding the phone. Be aware of your hand.
Maybe you are sitting on a chair. Be aware of your derriere.

And so on. Simply being aware of your body, where you are, is the first step, and a very powerful one, to protect yourself from energy vampires. May you be free from all energy vampires!

Love and Blessings,

Satish Dholakia, Master NLP, Spiritual Healer, Inner Cosmos

See Ad on page 190

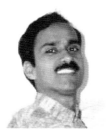

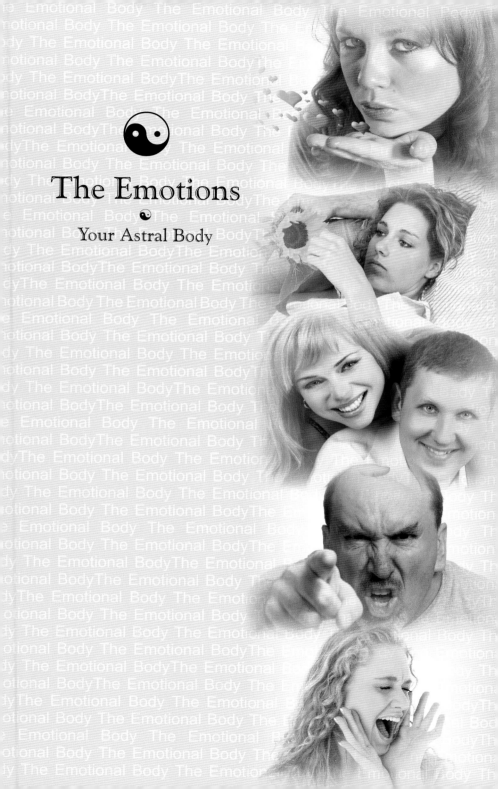

The Emotions

Your Astral Body

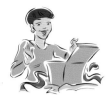

The Emotions

Your Astral Body

Pioneering research done by Dr. William A. Tiller recently revealed the following information; Tiller and his colleagues at Stanford University developed a subtle energy detector. It is described as an ultra-sensitive Geiger counter-type device that demonstrates the existence of energy fields. The device does not detect the frequency of electromagnetic waves, but rather detects subtle energies. With this special detector, Dr. Tiller demonstrated that subtle energy fields respond to the outer stimulus of intentional human focus. Soon it will be possible to identify what human focus is made of and to deconstruct its various energetic aspects including the etheric, emotional and mental subtleties. It is possible that with the refinement and further development of this new technology, scientists will be able to demonstrate that emotional energies originate from the human energetic structure called the Emotional Body. Reference to this body appears in ancient scriptures under different names; kama-rupa, bardo-body, astral body, etc.

The emotional body refers to a subtle structure comprised of energies corresponding to one's emotions. This structure exists alongside the etheric body and among its many functions, it is designed to carry a man's full consciousness after physical death. It is frequently referred to as the Astral body. Everyone possesses an astral body, but few are aware of its existence and far fewer are able to consciously develop and control it during their physical life. Just by knowing of its existence, one can become more aware of it. Taking time away from a big city can give you the experience of knowing what belongs to your emotional body and what is really an experience of the emotions inherited

Arthur Powell in his book Astral Body explains that the functions of the astral body may by roughly grouped under three headings:

● **To make sensation possible**

● **To serve as a bridge between the mind and physical body**

● **To act as an independent vehicle (body) of consciousness and action**

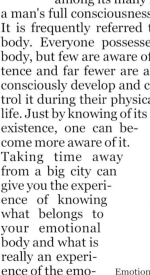

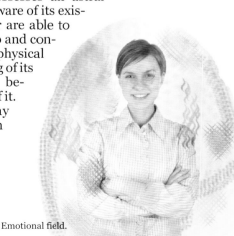

Emotional field.

from a collective field of emotional bodies. During the few moments after waking, one may remember a dream that was vivid or seemed too real. This actually may be a fragment of memory from the night's astral experience. The physical body exists in the physical world and the astral body exists in the astral worlds - the worlds or planes of existence in which one finds oneself periodically during sleep and after the death of the physical body (see the chapter *Conscious Dying*). When speaking of astral realms, it is more appropriate to refer to them as a condition of nature, or state of consciousness rather than a specific place. The awareness of the different states can be likened to the life of a caterpillar. When the caterpillar is born, it is unaware that its future destiny is to become a butterfly, although this information is inherent in its nature. It eats, sleeps and lives the caterpillar life. One day, the time arrives and the transformation called metamorphosis begins. The butterfly is born to its new life; a seemingly different butterfly world. We assume that the butterfly is without recollection of its previous caterpillar "world." Another comparison may be made to radio signals. There are hundreds of radio stations broadcasting different shows in the air, or ether, as we now know. Even though they occupy the same space at the exact same time, they cannot interfere with each other because each has a different frequency. Similarly the physical body and the Emotional body have different bio-frequencies and occupy the same space.

An encyclopedia says that "Astral projection (or astral travel) is an inter-pretation of out-of-body experiences (OBEs) achieved either awake or via lucid dreaming, deep meditation, or use of psychotropics. Proponents of astral projection maintain that their consciousness or soul has transferred into an astral body." There are schools who teach students to achieve this experience step-by-step. The book *Astral Body*, first published in 1927 and reprinted until today should provide enough necessary knowledge before one decides to experiment.

The nature of the Emotional Body corresponds to the quality of the psychoemotional energy one possesses. Positive and happy thoughts/emotions will produce a light energetic mass with a light vibration. Thoughts/emotions of negativity will produce a heavy energetic mass or a denser frequency. Both are the building blocks which compose the Emotional Body.

"It is sown a natural body; it is raised a spiritual body. There is a natural body, and there is a spiritual body."
-
Corinthians 15:44

It is therefore important to pay attention to the nature and quality of the psychoemotional energetic mass we generate daily throughout our physical life. Doing so improves the quality of life while in the physical body and ensures a pleasant transition during the physical death. When listening to a radio show which broadcasts in the AM mode (low frequency), the sound quality is considerably worse than when the broadcast is received in the FM mode (high frequency). Similarly, following one's transition, it is explained in many religions and esoteric texts, that the experience of an individual in an astral body comprised of low frequency energies (negative psychoemotional mass), will attract a corresponding frequency and the quality of afterlife in which conditions and experiences are incomparably worse, than the conditions and experiences of an individual with an astral body comprised of highly vibrating energies.

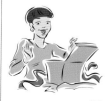

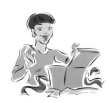

During intensive training in certain martial arts schools, students learn to intuit the actions of their opponent beforehand. They are taught how to perceive their opponents' intentions by reading the bio-energetic aspects of their focus. This is usually practiced in pairs. One student sends out his focused intention while the other attempts to recognize what the intention is. This practice is rather lengthy and requires special instructions. On a smaller, personal scale the following exercise derived from the above practice helps to understand how one can validate the energetic presence of thoughts and emotions directed to a part of the physical body.

Step 1 - wash your hands thoroughly

Step 2 - shake them and then clap them together

a)

Step 3 - raise your hands in front of your body at your solar plexus level as shown on the picture (a).

Compare their weight and find out which palm feels heavier. If one seems heavier than the other, shake and clap them together again and repeat the process until the weight in both palms feels equal.

b)

Step 4 - focus on your right palm (b) and silently affirm the following: "my right palm is very sad, my palm is very depressed, my palm is angry." Do this for NO more than 10 seconds!

Step 5 - Compare your hands again (c) and feel if there is a difference between them. If the right hand feels heavier, the exercise was performed correctly and it should serve as validation of how "heavy" negative thoughts-emotions can be.

c)

Step 6 - wash your hands with soap under cold water to remove any residues of the negative energies. If you do not wash your hands, you may experience pain in your right palm!

Step 7 - This can be considered the most important step. Now focus on your clean right palm again and silently affirm: "I love my right palm, I am very happy with my right palm" now focus on your whole body and say "I love my whole body. I am very happy, healthy and I am full of joy!"

"To be angry is to revenge the faults of others on ourselves."
-
Alexander Pope, English poet
(1688 - 1744)

Thoughts and emotions are merely energy. This energy is measurable and palpable. Wherever your focus is, that is where your energy flows. Negative thoughts and emotions are destructive. Over time they affect the physical body and therefore should not be projected towards oneself, others and especially children. The harm caused to someone else from an unwholesome outburst of negativity whether intentional or unintentional, may not only result as difficulties for the person on the receiving end, but by the Law of Karma, will result in direct harm to the person who caused it. It isn't worth it! It pays to maintain and project positive thoughts and feelings about yourself and others. The old saying, "if you don't have anything nice to say, don't say it" must include "if you don't have anything nice to think or feel, don't think or feel it." If it is difficult to feel or think something nice about someone, don't think about them at all!

Did you know that when you cross your arms in front of your solar plexus it partially protects you from the emotional influence of others? This is an easy tool to use during an unpleasant conversation with negative or insulting people. Just cross your arms. You will notice how easy it is to become detached, creating a space for you to become calm without being pulled into the drama. On the other hand, when used in the presence of people whose company you enjoy, crossing your arms sends the wrong message; a feeling of disconnection or rejection on some level.

The physical body is a priceless gift and it informs us of things gone awry through its aches and pains. The relation between a negative emotional charge caused by anger, hatred, fear, traumas, etc. and physical health has been scientifically proven.

Hypnotherapy is a great example of a professional practice that resolves stored negative energetic charges and brings about corresponding physical healing. When negative psychoemotional energy tries to pass through our energetic anatomy, it moves as a charge from the astral body, through the chakras and meridians, into the etheric body, then to the physical. It behaves in a similar fashion to muddy water flowing through a kitchen faucet. The water is unable to flow properly or to its full potential. Similarly, the clean vital force of our energy body is restricted or blocked by heavy psychoemotional charges. A lack of vital energy in the energy body consequently results in the devitalization of the physical body when it becomes susceptible to illness in weakened state.

Most physical health problems have a psychoemotional counterpart which cannot be ignored. This is the true reason for illness. Overlooking your emotions usually result in a worsening or reoccurrence of the health challenge. It is not necessarily a bad decision to take prescription medication to alleviate discomfort. The trouble is caused by not realizing that the blockage isn't eliminated by taking the medication. The cause remains and therefore must be dealt with. Here are some examples of suppressed negative charges which may result in corresponding physical health problems; a person holding anger and resentment towards their parents for 35 years; childhood abuse kept secret for many years but often replayed over and over again in the mind of its victim without any resolution; parents who belittle a child repeatedly and enforce the belief that he is bad and worthless. When the child grows up the negative imprint remains in the subconscious mind and creates a constant negative emotional charge. Unexpressed and/or suppressed negative emotions are toxic. Applying healing and transformational methods to release these energetic time bombs dramatically improves not only physical health, but overall well-being.

"The degree of one's emotion varies inversely with one's knowledge of the facts - the less you know the hotter you get."

Bertrand Russell, British philosopher, logician (1872 -1970)

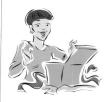

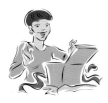

For most, it is a long journey of introspection and healing to address all recent and old emotional issues. During one's lifetime only a little portion may be resolved. That an individual soul is reborn over and over again until all lessons are learned and all issues healed is taught in many religions. They teach that it is easy to observe children, to spot where strong behavioral characteristics or tendencies show up shortly after birth. If everyone was born with a blank slate, why would infants have different personalities, range of abilities and development? As they grow into adolescence, why do some have well developed virtues and others do not, often regardless of parental influence? Wouldn't everyone start out pretty much the same? This concept of re-incarnation states that the start of subsequent lives places an individual in similar conditions, to those they left in their last life. Their life path and social conditions will be a perfect match to resolve and learn what was missed previously. For those who do not believe in other lives or are hoping that a sudden acceptance of religious beliefs or idols at the time of a fast approaching death will spare personal responsibility for an unwholesome life, it may be a good time to consider this possibility.

> "Children's past-life memories are a natural phenomenon. It happens all the time. Very young children, as young as two years of age, make spontaneous statements about past-lives. Their families are convinced that the statements are genuine because the children reveal information they couldn't have possibly learned any other way. And they sometimes exhibit behaviors, such as phobias, that correspond exactly to the past life statements."
>
> *Children's Past Lives*
> by Carol Bowman

> "If the virtuous man who has not done any evil act in this birth suffers, this is due to some wrong act that he may have committed in his previous birth. He will have his compensation in his next birth. If the wicked man who daily does many evil actions apparently enjoys in this birth, this is due to some good Karma he must have done in his previous birth. He will have compensation in his next birth. He will suffer in the next birth. The law of compensation is inexorable and relentless. "
>
> *(Swami Shivananda, Practice of Karma Yoga, Divine Life Society, 1985, p. 102)*

Disease, the physical manifestation of negative psycho-emotional charges is nature's strongest way of informing us that the subtle hints it has sent were already missed and that some imbalance or underlying issue has been ignored to long. There are a many subtle signs that call our attention to underlying negativities in the energy field before the physical manifestation of illness occurs. Daily mishaps and repeated difficulties are a good example. By eliminating the negativity that attracted them in the first place, nature does not have to "reach" for the stronger measure of physical illness to call attention. Psychoemotional negative charges in the energy field that go unheeded begin to attract negative situations. These are usually random negative events one coincidentally runs into, drawn to you by the biophysical Law of Attraction.

> "People deal too much with the negative, with what is wrong. Why not try and see positive things, to just touch those things and make them bloom?"
> -
> Thich Nhat Hanh
> Zen Buddhist monk,
> a teacher, author

The Law of Attraction is an invisible force as are the laws of gravity and magnetism in physics. They cannot be seen but their results can be felt. If an ice-cream cone slips out of your hand it won't fly up towards the sky. It will end up on the sidewalk or sofa. Regardless of where it lands it always falls down, due to the law of gravity, which never fails. If a magnet is put in close proximity of a refrigerator door, by the magnetic law, it will stick to the fridge because the metal corresponds to the magnetic force of the magnet. This is similar in nature to the biophysical Law of Attraction. The psychoemotional field and its emanation or lifeforce field works as a biomagnet. When the field is filled with thoughts and emotions, they begin attracting their equivalent. The circumstances attracted depend on the quality of the psychoemotional charge present. Based on the Law of Attraction, if the energy field vibrates with happiness and health, it will attract its equal as happy and healthy circumstances. On the other hand, an energetic charge of anger and sadness will correspondingly attract situations resonating with anger and sadness.

For example; a young woman wakes up and listens to happy music. She sings in the shower and enjoys her morning cup of tea. Before leaving home she looks in the mirror and realizes how happy she looks and feels. Driving to work, she pops in a CD with her favorite band and does not even register the morning traffic. After arriving at work at a small local law firm, she accidentally runs into a person in the elevator who asks where to find a good lawyer for his case. Inviting him to her office, she gives lots of helpful information. It turns out that he is a very successful businessman who admires her level of expertise so much that he offers her a lucrative legal position with three times the salary she currently earns. Is it a coincidence? She could have just as easily run into an angry person who happened to dislike lawyers. She attracted the opportunity. Not consciously, but by the energy she generated. Her positive energy would not have been a match for an angry bitter person. The Law of Attraction states that like attracts like, therefore her happy energy attracted a happy situation in the form of a stranger in the elevator.

On the other end of the spectrum, a young man awakened by noisy construction workers across the street becomes upset. Walking to the bathroom he accidentally stubs his toe on the edge of his bed frame. In the mixture of pain and anger he realizes that he is running late for work. Quickly jumping into his car, he pulls out of the driveway and overlooks the oncoming car which then hits his minivan. Is this a coincidence? By leaving three seconds later, he would have avoided the oncoming car. He attracted himself to a situation matching his energetic charge of pain and anger. If one realizes that there has been a chain of mishaps and frustrating situations, the first question should be: why was this attracted to me? What do I carry in my field that works as Velcro for these situations? Very often the negative psychoemotional charges originate in the subcon-

Some people believe that emotions are bad. They say, "I am not emotional," but what they actually mean is, "I am disconnected from my emotions." Not being connected to our emotions is like driving and ignoring the traffic lights. For example, anger can be a constructive force to help us change things; fear tells us to be careful! It is fine to feel negative emotions as long as we know how to listen, and after interpreting them, let them go. It becomes dangerous when negative emotions are ignored and remain, lurking inside of us. That is when The Law of Attraction unmercifully strikes. In order to let go of negative emotions, you need to understand what they mean and that requires paying more attention to them.

"Each of us makes his own weather, determines the color of the skies in the emotional universe which he inhabits."

Archbishop Fulton J. Sheen, American television's first preacher (1895 - 1979)

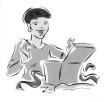

scious mind. Some say, "I am perfectly fine, I feel okay. This still happened to me and seems to be a huge injustice." It is irrelevant whether the negativity is generated consciously or subconsciously. What is important is its presence. And the attraction of a reality to match your feelings.

Imagine your thoughts, feelings, conscious and unconscious sense of well-being corresponding to one of the five men below. Each color represents a particular life event, experience or situation. From the dark circle (miserable) to a pink circle (ecstatic). In life, things tend to be organized by cosmic laws. Our pool of experiences also represents a certain order. By the Law of Attraction, miserable is grouped with miserable, unhappy with unhappy, doing ok with other oks, and so on. Your energetic fields also represent (radiates) a certain level of well-being. Symbolically drawn by the five men below. When jumping in to the pool of experiences (life), where will you be attracted? When you find your place, imagine, that your sense of wellbeing suddenly shifts. What will happen in your pool of experiences? Will you be drawn towards the group on the periphery or toward the center? By understanding this principle and the simple picture below, it should also be clear that when the overall sense of wellbeing shifts, one drifts towards the vibrationally corresponding group. Of course, if one decides to make a major shift from Miserable to Ecstatic, it will take some time to be attracted into the new Ecstatic group. Temporary resistance and friction will occur.

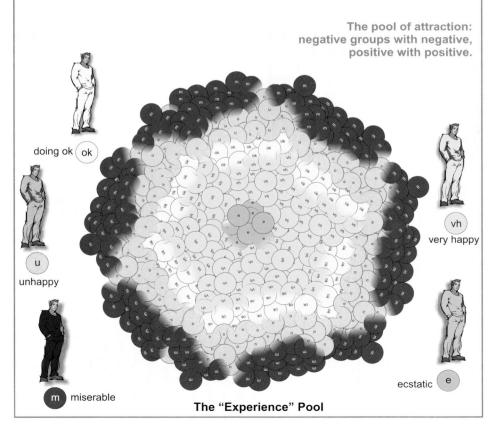

The pool of attraction: negative groups with negative, positive with positive.

doing ok (ok)

very happy (vh)

unhappy (u)

ecstatic (e)

miserable (m)

The "Experience" Pool

It would be foolish to give up when facing the first signs of resistance or friction. Keep going and ultimately your desired destination will be reached. This scheme can be applied to any life aspects - financial conditions, medical conditions, spiritual conditions, etc. Just replace miserable for poor - ecstatic for rich, or miserable for sick, ecstatic for relatively healthy. It gets a little tricky, when you realize, that all aspects of your being are governed by the same law simultaneously. It is not so simple to understand other people's lives because they are a reflection of many experience pools occurring simultaneously (experience pool of health, experience pool of prosperity, etc.) If one could separate all of life's aspects (experience pools), it would be easier to identify which areas need the biggest improvement.

Metaphysical practitioners and healers understand that conscious and subconscious thoughts and emotions create one's reality. Some might say, "Well, I would never create this! I'm not responsible. It's not possible." Most people don't consciously wish for much of what they get, but certain patterns created from the frequency of their current or past psycho-emotional mass attract situations matching that particular frequency, regardless of their will. This is like the magnet wishing that he would never be attracted to the refrigerator door again and he was not responsible for it happening. Implementing this newfound knowledge by choosing thoughts and emotions carefully gives everyone the ability to begin consciously creating a positive, successful, healthy life. Granted, this is not easy to do all the time, but it comes with practice. Often we react emotionally to circumstances based on old habits. Let's say that someone calls you a vulgar name. What makes you react angrily towards that individual? HABIT. That's how I always react. Other's do it. I, the ego, was offended.

> If negative situations occur frequently in your life, try this 3-day exercise. Every time you notice that your thoughts or feelings are negative, say "bingo!" If you discover that bingo has not been said often, and negative situations still persist, you may consider a session with a qualified professional, such as a hypnotherapist or life-coach, to help you uncover the originating cause. Sometimes all it takes is one session to give you a hint as to why this happens.

It is unnecessary to habitually personalize others' actions and then react with a matching negative vibration. Remember in school, parents and teachers would comment on bad behavior "You are no better than the other kid if you act like they do!" Reacting to garbage with garbage pulls you down to a low vibration. What if the next time someone said or did something you didn't like, you simply CHOOSE not to let it affect you? You CHOOSE not to engage in creating destructive negative emotions. It does not mean that you don't take action, but it is not emotionally based. The negative emotions are avoided along with their tendency to attract more of the same.

"Control your emotion or it will control you."

-
Samurai Maxim,
A Seventeenth
Century Samurai

Every disease or illness has its own low frequency or vibration, just as negative thoughts and emotions do. Based on the Law of Attraction, it is typically impossible to attract disease without first having a corresponding low vibration. They may not be easy to recognize in oneself but a good healer or hypnotherapist

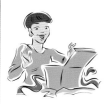

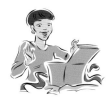

can help uncover where the negative charge is hiding. Almost all manifestations of illness can be traced to negative thoughts and emotions. An example of lowering ones vibration to the point of attracting disease would be the improper care of the physical body. Not eating properly, not exercising, and so on. This is not the emotional root. One would have to look deeper to discover that a poor self-image and its corresponding negative charge was the actual problem which resulted in the outer manifestation of poor physical selfcare. A possible subsequent attraction resulting from poor self-care might be lowered immunity which in turn would attract corresponding viruses or illnesses matching that vibration. Now, on the surface one would not make the connection that he or she attracted a virus or illness, but upon closer investigation it would become obvious. The permanent cure would involve healing the issues surrounding low self-esteem and the related psychoemotional charge.

It is possible to attract the energetic vibration of an illness to one's field, but to have not yet manifested the physical aspect of the disease. This is how clairvoyants are able to identify and therefore predict the future mishaps of an individual. The energetic pattern is already present in the field but it has not yet manifested physically and they can see this pattern as subtle energy. Energy healing is able to remove the psychoemotional counterpart before it has a chance to manifest physically or attract negative situations. It can be considered as a preventative tool and recognized as complementary medicine. Following healing and the removal of the psychoemotional Velcro it will no longer be possible to attract the same pattern of disease as long as it is not recreated consciously or subconsciously. Many herbs and some pharmaceuticals also have similar effects. Their corresponding energetic aspect raises the frequency of the energy field and the disease pattern is released. Homeopathy also works with energy frequencies. It is based on the principle of like attracting like. Homeopaths administer the vibrational essence called a *remedy* and by altering the energetic frequency, the body becomes able to resist the disease.

Negative situations are helpful hints warning that something is out of alignment and must be corrected. If overlooked or misinterpreted, the next, stronger hint could be some form of illness. Natural law preserves the health of the physical body and considers health the number #1 priority. It will attempt to use all kinds of negative experiences before "going after" physical health to get one's attention. It can be likened to caring parents who warn their child over and over not to do something. After several warnings and the child still is not listening, they let the

Henrik Ling (1776-1839) the father of modern Western massage said, "Our negative thoughts are not just in the brain, but also collect in various locations through-out the body and in the aura. The places where negative thoughts and feelings collect is where Ki is restricted in its flow. The physical organs that exist at these locations are restricted in their functioning. If the negative thoughts and feelings are not eliminated quickly, illness results."

child learn through a more severe personal experience (as long as it's not too dangerous). How quickly the child learns. This seemingly cruel act results in a valuable life lesson, preventing them from a possible future tragedy. Forevermore, the child will use the memory of the experience to avoid harmful situations.

Psychoemotional energetic self-care is not common knowledge, but it is easy to learn. It's easy to see if someone is lacking physical hygiene. Imagine if you were able to see the psychoemotional level of hygiene. There are people who can and they will tell you it's not a pretty sight!

It is often incorrectly assumed that all thoughts and feelings belong to oneself. This is not always the case. In fact, thoughts and emotions can easily be picked up or transferred from others. This is referred to as *energetic contamination*. One can take on others' energies of anger as well as their good mood. If someone has fallen into the mud and their clothes are filthy, it would be foolish to think that you could hug them without getting stained. The energy field of a person filled with negative thoughts and emotions can be

> Therapists whose job is to consult their clients on emotional traumas often find themselves in a situation of emotional breakdown without any particular, apparent reason. This is due to the transfer of emotional energy from their clients during therapy. When the client verbalizes their problems - externalizing, the therapist's job is to listen - absorb. The more involved the therapist becomes, the more emotional energy is absorbed. Even though you are not a therapist, learning how to detach from other's emotional baggage is essential for one's psychoemotional health. Being detached does not imply lack of care or assistance!

Summary on the care of the etheric body

Keep your conscious and subconscious thoughts and emotions positive and supportive. This is easier said than done. Here are two main steps:

A) Remove the patterns and origins of negativity - learned in childhood, inherited genetically, or formed as a result of traumas and painful experiences - from your energetic field and body by:

❏ Swimming in the ocean or taking a salt bath as explained in detail in the previous chapter *The Etheric Body*. The energetic aspect of the salt water solution has a cleansing effect on the energetic charge caused by thoughts and emotions in the energy field.

❏ Regular physical exercise. Exercise decreases levels of cortisol - the stress hormone - supports the natural release of endorphines which are the body's 'feel-great' hormones. It also creates the opportunity to interact with other active people. All of these help to improve one's mood while helping to put aside the daily problems or worries, discontinuing the pattern of generating and accumulating negative thoughts and emotions in one's field.

❏ Incorporating a powerful technique called "Emotional Freedom Techniques" (EFT). The manual with instructions can be downloaded for FREE at: " www.learn2heal.com/EFT." EFT is a new discovery that has provided thousands with relief from pain, disease and emotional issues. Simply stated, it is a unique version of acupuncture except needles are not used. Instead, you stimulate main energy meridian points on your body by tapping them with your fingertips. The process is easy to memorize and you can do it anywhere. It can be learned within a few short weekends.

❏ Immediate disconnection from negative people who always complain or bring you down.

"It is well known that panic, despair, depression, hate, rage, exasperation, frustration all produce negative biochemical changes in the body."

Norman Cousins, journalist, author, professor, (1915 - 1990)

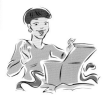

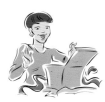

☐ Scheduling regular healing sessions that are designed to remove or dissolve negative thoughts and emotions: Pranic Healing, Reiki, EMCC, Integrated Energy Therapy, Hypnotherapy, Homeopathy, Sound Therapy, etc.

☐ If you continuously experience negative thoughts and emotions for long periods of time, have your doctor test you with a simple blood and hair analysis to rule out chemical and hormonal imbalances and vitamin deficiencies.

B) Replace them with new, supportive patterns in order to attract supportive situations.

☐ Read books from the masters in the field such as:

● **Excuse Me, Your Life is Waiting**: *The Astonishing Power of Feelings* - the nuts and bolts of harnessing the raw power of your feelings. Learn how to turn the negatives into positives and draw good things to you, by Lynn Grabhorn

● **The Truth Will Set You Free, Overcoming Emotional Blindness and Finding Your True Self** - by embracing the truth of our past history, we can heal pain in the present, by Dr. Alice Miller

● **Waking the Tiger, Healing Trauma** - overcome the destructive force of trauma and learn to harness and transform the body's intelligent energies, by Peter Levine

☐ When you are in a "negative thought rut" do something out of the ordinary to break up the destructive pattern. Activities such as running, listening to music, reading and watching funny movies will create a positive shift.

☐ Watch or listen to educational CDs and DVDs and learn to generate positive thoughts and emotions:

● **Enhancing My Self Esteem** - utilizes a specially designed musical composition combined with the technology of binaural audio tones to create a profound and deep state of relaxation. Allowing your unconscious mind to easily and effortlessly accept positive affirmations to improve your self-esteem and transform your life - www.enhancedhealing.com

● **Emotional Freedom and Transformation Technique -** On video or DVD, present a technique you can easily learn. The instruction shows how the tapping sequences are done. With the right attitude, mental and emotional expectations, and a willingness for change, you will be guided to release blockages of negative emotional energy. A fast and easy-to-use technique - www.artofawareness.homestead.com

● **Changing Emotions**, Hypnosis Stress Management Program - is both a healing and peak performance program. For those living a life full of anxiety, low self-esteem, anger or depression, this program offers a light at the end of the tunnel - www.luxevivant.com

☐ Attend free introductory lectures or classes such as:

● **Free Arts Programs for Abused Children** - dance, drama, writing, music, and painting are used to encourage children to channel emotions; release anger; model positive methods of communication; and develop a renewed trust in adults - www.freearts.org

● **Free Introduction to Pranic Healing** - Introductory classes and healing clinics. Learn how your emotions affect your physical health and what you can do to heal them - www.pranichealing.com, www.learn2heal.com

● **Free Reiki Tummo Mini-Workshops** - experience and benefit from the peaceful, calming and spiritually lifting energies of Reiki TUMMO - www.h2amedia.com/la.html#free

"As human beings we all want to be happy and free from misery. We have learned that the key to happiness is inner peace. The greatest obstacles to inner peace are disturbing emotions such as anger and attachment, fear and suspicion, while love and compassion, a sense of universal responsibility are the sources of peace and happiness."

-
His Holiness the 14th the Dalai Lama

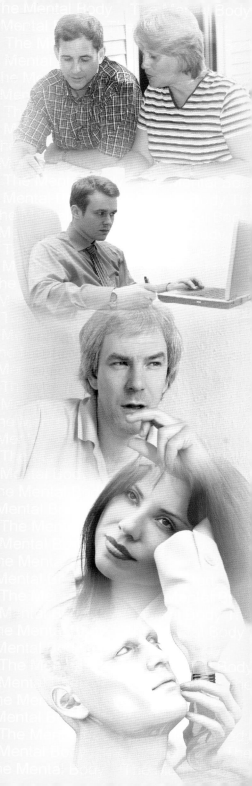

The Mind

Your Mental Body

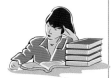

The Mind

Your Mental Body

The mastery of thoughts is undoubtedly the biggest breakthrough in our understanding of human potential. In 1966, educator and scientist, Jose Silva announced an amazing technique. The Silva method is a step-by-step process, that allows an individual to develop their astounding powers of mind, helping to unlock life's endless possibilities. [www.silvamethod.com] Later on, similar systems flooded the market, teaching others how to change their thought and belief habits, promising miraculous results. Clichés such as "Think pink," "Think Positive," or "Be positive," became popular and were easily memorized. Each system referred to the discovery of the profound influence of thoughts on our physical reality. The scientific explanation for why these thought systems worked was not publicly known at that time and such techniques were not widely accepted and practiced.

In 2004, a clearer, scientific view of this subject emerged and was introduced to the general public. The documentary movie, *What the BLEEP Do We Know!?* was released in February, 2004, in Yelm, Washington. The film revealed the uncertain world of quantum fields, hidden behind what we consider to be our normal, waking reality. It was a sneak-peek into the realms of science, and it outlined a possible explanation for how thoughts and emotions affect our physical life. It explains that within the understanding of quantum physics, human thoughts are energy, with limitless power. [www.whatthebleep.com]

In 2006, yet another movie, *The Secret,* enlightened the public with an understanding of the mysteries of our human powers and took another in-depth look at the energy of thoughts. [www.thesecret.tv] It is not a coincidence that our mental powers are the focus of more attention than in the past. As evolution progresses, humanity is becoming more intelligent and our mental strength is increasing. This is evident in the latest generation. Children are achieving mental maturity and deliberation of action much sooner than their parents did.

As society is reintroduced to the Law of Attraction and its corresponding statement: "Wherever the attention goes, the energy

Henrik Ling (1776-1839) the father of modern Western massage said, "It must be understood that the mind exists not only in the brain, but also throughout the body. The nervous system extends to every organ and tissue in the body and so the mind exists here also. It is also known that the mind even extends outside the body in a subtle energy field 2 to 3 feet thick called the aura. Because of this, it is more appropriate to call our mind a mind/body as the mind and body are so closely linked."

"I find, by experience, that the mind and the body are more than married, for they are most intimately united; and when one suffers, the other sympathizes."
-
Philip Dormer Stanhope, 4th Earl of Chesterfield, British statesman (1694 - 1773)

flows," the control of one's thoughts becomes a necessity. Similar to the emotions, thoughts are also energetic in nature, but their energy is much finer than etheric or emotional matter. As a result of our increased power and consciousness of our powers, when someone thinks of someone or something, the flow of energy projected by their focused attention is much stronger. The strength of our thoughts increases our personal power and with this power comes responsibility. The mind can be a powerful tool of mastery, as well as a weapon of social and self-destruction.

The mental body is not only a separate body, as its name suggests, it is also the independent vehicle which carries our consciousness after the physical, and later, astral death, or disintegration of the astral body. The mental body corresponds to concrete intelligence. The mental body, is established in the same manner as the astral body and its nature depends on the quality of the energy of the thoughts that are generated - how refined or coarse they are. Low and selfish thoughts will produce coarse or low vibrating forms, a low mental vibrating building matter; good and altruistic thoughts will produce fine forms, a high vibrating mental building matter.

> ☯
>
> **Due to the increased mental powers and abilities of many, an outburst of negative or destructive thoughts and emotions, directed at someone or something, intentionally or unintentionally, can be powerful enough to cause a negative physical situation for all involved. Use your mental power in a healing way, to control harmful emotions.**

As previously mentioned, some people are aware of their astral existence during sleep and are able to remember fragments of their experiences, upon awakening. The existence of the mental body and mental realms can also be remembered, but unlike the astral, where a strong sense of individuality persists, the mental existence opens one's perception of oneness. Those who remember fragments of time spent in their mental body, describe situations where individuality is maintained, while the knowledge of being one with other people or entire groups takes place. This awareness of oneness does not equate to a loss of personality. This is only a fragment - the beginning stage of what is referred to in spiritual scriptures as "being one with all," or as it is more commonly said, "We are one."

Mental body - mental field

"We are one, after all, you and I. Together we suffer, together exist, and forever will recreate each other."

-
Pierre Teilhard De Chardin,
French paleontologist and a philosopher
(1881 - 1955)

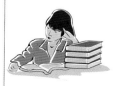

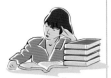

Oneness expressed in world religions:

☐ **Christianity:** "Though we are many, we are one body in Christ!"
(Romans 12 v5)

☐ **Native American :** "Humankind has not woven the web of life. We are but one thread within it. Whatever we do to the web, we do to ourselves. All things are bound together. All things are connected." *(Chief Seattle)*

☐ **Budhism:** "Hurt not others with that which pains yourself."
(From the Udanavarga 5.18)

☐ **Hinduism:** "Do naught to others which if done to thee would cause thee pain." *(From the Mahabharata 5.1517)*

☐ **Sikhism:** "Don't create enmity with anyone as God is within everyone."
(Guru Arjan Devji 259. Guru Granth Sahib)

☐ **Taoism:** "Regard your neighbor's gain as your own gain; and regard your neighbor's loss as your own loss." *(Tai Shang Kan Ying P'ien)*

Oneness has been described in many ways, but to grasp its meaning, one has no other choice than to experience it. One example could be a leafy tree. Every leaf appears to be independent, but they all part of the same tree - all are connected. We cannot say with certainty what each individual leaf is thinking, but we believe that each has a simple choice. To think as a separate leaf, and therefore die in the autumn after separating from the tree - old and yellow; or to realize that it is the tree, a part of the whole. Then it's life will never end. Oneness is the realization that we are not separate from the whole.

"The mind is like an iceberg, it floats with one-seventh of its bulk above water."
-
Sigmund Freud, Austrian neurologist (1856 - 1939)

So, what does all this have to do with healing our physical life? Thoughts can bring happiness, as well as pain. Thought energy combined with emotional energy is the secret ingredient which creates our daily events. Thoughts must be wholesome so that the daily situations we attract to ourselves are pleasant.

No one wants to think unwholesome thoughts, especially after realizing their ability to manifest waking reality. But how many times have you caught yourself by surprise: "Oh my! Did I really think that?" or, "Where did that come from?" or, "I can't believe I just thought about that!" Meditation techniques in which prolonged concentration and awareness is required, bring about the experience of realizing thoughts, previously hidden. A secret room of the subconscious mind opens and a parade of thoughts, accompanied by feelings no one has ever claimed to own, come marching through one's head. In actuality, these thoughts were always there. They were running deep in the background of the mind, but were continuously overshadowed by the momentarily more important daily thoughts. The subconscious mind is described as the deepest level of consciousness that we are not directly aware of which still affects their conscious behavior.

A great example of how the subconscious mind develops is that of someone who has just learned how to drive a car: they sit behind the wheel, watch every curve and road bump, focus on maintaining the suggested distance from the car ahead and try to stay in the center of their lane. Every traffic sign is acknowledged and each driving process - using the turning signal, shifting gears, employing the wipers - is carefully selected. This can be considered "conscious driving." The ideal way of driving suggested by the Department of Motor Vehicles. After a few years, the intense concentration while driving subsides and driving becomes automatic. Some drivers are so immersed in daydreaming or cell-phone conversations, that when they arrive at their destination, they are amazed to find themselves there. This is a dangerous habit, yet offers a great example of subconscious behavior. Similar subconscious acts - thinking negative thoughts and constant daydreaming being the worst offenders - occur regularly and sometimes people arrive forty, sixty and eighty years later, wondering what happened to their life.

You are what you daydream. Those who suffer much injustice, fear or problems in their daydreams, experience the same negativity in their real life. Daydreaming is a hidden tool for success. Many great inventors were notorious daydreamers. At advanced corporations, direct daydreaming is implemented as a deliberate exercise to find the best solutions. Monitor your daydreams and evaluate their nature. If they problem-solve and are positive, you are on the right track, but watch out for those filled with problems and negativity!

There are several ways in which subconscious habits are developed. Our conscious mind serves as a filter to prevent unwanted information from reaching the subconscious levels. During childhood, this filter is not fully developed and any information received may cause a negative subconscious imprint in a child's brain. This is difficult to reverse (heal). A mother, who tells her child repeatedly that he is bad or lazy, even if it is not true and she does not really mean it, has created a situation in which the child's brain may accept this as his internal truth. Later on, this may become the underlying issue for self-esteem problems in adolescence and adulthood. Also, there are emotionally dishonest families, who, instead of being role models for their children, pursue the path of being a talk-model. "Do not look at what I do, follow what I say!" Words end up being unimportant, while behaviors, rather than language, are imprinted on the unguarded subconscious mind. These behaviors later manifest as corresponding behavioral patterns.

Any situation has the potential to be handled incorrectly and cause subconscious damage. For example: A child uses a pen to draw on the wall. If the parents react with, "Look at what you have done! You are a bad boy (or girl)," this sends the message to the child that they are bad. This simple statement has the potential to cause a subconscious imprint. A better parental response would be, "Look at what you have done! Drawing on the wall is bad!" This same scenario can apply to all similar situations - *i.e.*, spilling a glass of orange juice or picking on siblings.

G.A.Bernard, Ph.D.

"Whatever the mind can conceive and believe, it can achieve."

-

Napoleon Hill, American author (1883 - 1970)

The subconscious mind can also be directly influenced during mental or emotional trauma. When the conscious mind becomes overwhelmed with too many informational inputs and its protective "barrier" fails. For example: A driver loses control on an icy road, and is about to cause an accident. The driver in the second car is caught by surprise. Seconds before the impact all of his fear, stress (trauma) and focus is directed on the possible tragic outcome of the oncoming car. He does

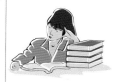

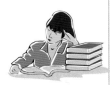

not notice that the soda between the car seats has spilled into his lap. This minor "soda incident," seemingly unimportant, may - in such a state of trauma - be registered by the deeper, subconscious levels of the mind and a negative association between the soda and the accident could be made. This may later manifest as sudden feelings of anxiety and stress each time the same brand of soda is consumed. A common example of this is - being attacked by a dog in childhood. This is frequently experienced as an unexplainable fear of dogs in adulthood. It does not matter if the dog actually caused physical damage, only how the incident was perceived and the trauma it caused.

Repetition of certain habits also programs the subconscious mind. Eating disorders are an example of this, *i.e.,* anorexia and bulimia are often developed from a repetitive thought of being unatracttive and related fear of food consumption. Litle by little, this later manifests as a subconscious negative eating habit that is hard to break. Not all subconscious habits are bad. The efforts of a parent repeating, "Wash your hands after using the bathroom," pays off throughout one's life as hands are washed "automatically" when leaving a restroom.

It is in your best interest to uncover and dissolve as many negative subconscious programs as possible. When Jesus said, "*Go thy way; and as thou hast believed, so be it done unto thee." (Mt. 9: 5-13),* he not only announced the Law of Faith and the Law of Attraction, but he actually explained how it works. One may surmise that a determined conscious will is strong enough to overcome negative subconscious programming. It is possible, but the effects are proven to only be temporary. The subconscious programming always wins. One may decide to stop smoking or run for better health every day, but good intentions often end up falling by the wayside after several weeks. The subconscious mind is a giant intelligence, which by the age of eighteen, makes most of your decisions. Even though it may seem that decision-making is happening consciously, the subconscious mind always has the last word. Many are told what to do from the time they are born and by the time they reach legal age, their thinking processes often remain in the pre-programmed safe, old grooves and patterns. Consciously attempting to overcome the subconscious mind can be compared to sailor on deck attempting to stop the Titanic from sinking by shouting, "Iceberg!" If the boat is already sinking it is too late. To positively reprogram the subconscious mind and avoid life's mishaps created by its destructive patterns, the proper tools must be used. Understanding the influence of the mind on well-being inevitably brings another aspect of hygiene to the forefront.

The latest research suggests that we should only trust our conscious mind with simple decisions. When we use our conscious mind to decide larger, complex issues, the tendency is to over-think, which blocks the important messages coming from our subconscious mind, helping us to make a more wholesome decision. Before making a big decision like buying a house or changing career, it is best to sleep on it - sometimes more than once.

"The mind is a superb instrument if used rightly. Used wrongly, however, it becomes very destructive. To put it more accurately, it is not so much that you use your mind wrongly - you usually don't use it at all. It uses you. This is the disease. You believe that you are your mind. This is the delusion. The instrument has taken you over."

-
Eckhart Tolle, contemporary spiritual teacher and writer on spirituality

Mental Hygiene. This is the process of deliberately removing unsupportive or destructive mental habits.

Changing negative thought processes and replacing them with supportive or neutral ones, minimizes the amount of negative (coarse) psychoemotional mass one generates. The result is a healthy flow of life force and the attraction of positive life situations. This supports one's wellbeing on all levels and manifests as health. It is easier to say: "Be positive!" and "Keep smiling" than to do so,

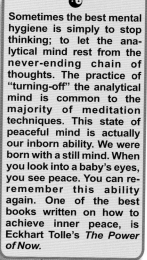

Sometimes the best mental hygiene is simply to stop thinking; to let the analytical mind rest from the never-ending chain of thoughts. The practice of "turning-off" the analytical mind is common to the majority of meditation techniques. This state of peaceful mind is actually our inborn ability. We were born with a still mind. When you look into a baby's eyes, you see peace. You can remember this ability again. One of the best books written on how to achieve inner peace, is Eckhart Tolle's *The Power of Now.*

Methods to address negative mental "programming" or beliefs:

❑ **Hypnosis:** a state of intense relaxation in which the conscious mind temporarily loses its ability to guard access into the subconscious level. This state is induced by a hypnotherapist who uses a form of therapeutic language to resolve or alter the issues and perceptions lodged in the subconscious. This helps to create a new and beneficial reality for the client.

❑ **Subliminal messages:** Communication with words, sounds, smells or images which are below the threshold of waking consciousness. This communication is believed to target and influence (manipulate) the subconscious mind to produce the desired changes in one's personality.

❑ **Binaural beats:** The effect created by the interference between two different sounds (sound waves) was discovered in 1839 by Heinrich Wilhelm Dove, Prussian physicist and meteorologist. This is done via the use of stereo headphones. Each ear is subjected to different sounds, creating an effect of a third, pulsating sound similar to the natural brain frequency. This technology can produce intense states of deep relaxation as well as other health benefits.

❑ **Affirmations:** Our subconscious does not know the difference between actual experience and artificial experience induced by the imagination. Affirmations consist of positive self-talk or self-generated images which produce an imprint on the subconscious mind and results in substantial life-improvement.

❑ **Autosuggestion:** Repetitive, self-affirmations which are deliberately employed during a state of light hypnosis. The hypnosis is self-induced with the help of visualization techniques, autosuggestion tapes or CDs. Autosuggestion differs from hypnosis. The suggestions in hypnosis are given by trained professional, while autosuggestion uses one's own voice.

❑ **Program Authoring the Human Subconscious (P.A.T.H.S.):** A subliminal technology believed to deliver millions of instructions to the subconscious mind in a short period of time (Rapid Data Transfer Protocol). This technology claims to induce various health and other well-being related results. (Editor's note: this reference is presented for our reader's information only. P.A.T.H.S. results have not yet been validated by *Healer's Guide* staff.)

❑ **Eye Movement Desensitization and Reprocessing (E.M.D.R.):** A relatively new therapeutic technique, developed by Francine Shapiro, Ph.D. This method targets a link between negative thoughts or mind images and particular eye movements. When the eye movement is engaged, the negative thoughts or images loose their "charge" and are no longer upsetting to the patient. It can be used for the treatment of traumatic experiences, grief resolution, relief from chronic pain, performance enhancement, addiction cessation and depression among others.

"Our minds can work for us or against us at any given moment. We can learn to accept and live with the natural psychological laws that govern us, understanding how to flow with life rather than struggle against it. We can return to our natural state of contentment."
-
Richard Carlson, American movie actor
(1912 - 1977)

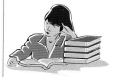

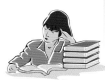

● **Waking Rapid Eye Movement State (W.R.E.M.S.):** This tool claims direct access to the subconscious mind, in particular, the levels where memories are stored. When a particular memory or trauma is accessed it can be "desensitized," which creates a state of calm and resolution. The rapid eye movements (R.E.M.) are a key to the effectiveness of this technique.

● **Neurofeedback, (EEG biofeedback):** The direct training of brain function, based on electrical brain activity, by which the brain learns to function more efficiently. With the help of EEG, individual brainwave activity can be shaped towards a more desirable, better regulated performance. Neurofeedback addresses problems within the spectrum of anxiety-depression, attention deficits, behavior disorders, various sleep disorders, headaches, migraines, PMS, and emotional disturbances. It is also useful for organic brain conditions such as seizures, the autism spectrum, and cerebral palsy.

when under the surface of one's consciousness are twenty-year-old forgotten beliefs such as - "If I am too happy, something bad will happen," or other similar dysfunctional beliefs.

The books and workshops which discuss methods of bringing health, abundance and prosperity into one's life, the secret laws of manifesting success, or "How to become a Trillionaire," are brilliant super-tools of the modern age. However, good results will not be experienced if the old mental trash remains. Take action and eliminate it. Mental Hygiene is an important aspect of Holistic health care. It cannot be ignored when assessing one's state of well-being. Some still carry the tendency to transfer the entire responsibility of their well-being onto a heath professional. In this case, "spill the beans." Mention not only your physical problems and symptoms, but what is happening emotionally and in your mind. Then, your health condition can be treated efficiently, effectively, holistically.

> **☯**
> When a traumatic situation is not processed properly - resolved in the moment when it happens - it is pushed into the subconscious mind where it waits for the right time to resurface to be dealt with. When traumas are suppressed, an enormous psychoemotional energetic charge, released at the time of the trauma, "freezes" in our system. This is how the most severe energetic blockages happen! Falling from a bicycle in severe shock and pain while pretending that nothing happened and that you are fine, is one example. Old traumas must be resolved so that we may heal.

> "Within you right now is the power to do things you never dreamed possible. This power becomes available to you just as you can change your beliefs."
> -
> Maxwell Maltz, cosmetic surgeon, developer of Psycho-Cybernetics
> (1899 - 1975)

Subconscious exercise:
Sit calmly and clear your mind. Think of sliced watermelon on a plate in front of you. Red, sweet, cooling and juicy. Now notice how your mouth is watering just from the thought. You did not tell your body what to do, but it happened anyway. This was your subconscious mind in action. It remembered your past experiences eating watermelon and the reaction of your body, just prior to tasting it. The body and mind work as a team. Whatever is produced by your mind also affects the body.

Mental hygiene can be compared to cleaning up old files in your personal computer. After a certain time, the hard-drive becomes a mess. Full of old, fragmented files, viruses or spyware. Until all this junk is removed, the computer will not perform optimally. Similarly, until the mind is free of unsupportive patterns and programming, the quality of life suffers or may simply be perceived as such. Mental hygiene is essential to the experience of a satisfying life. Refer to one of the techniques listed on page 209 to begin.

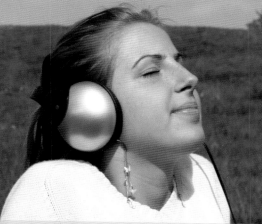

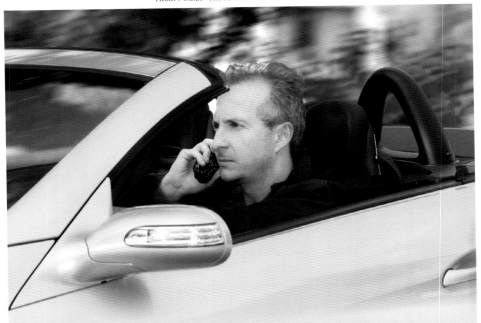

According to the National Highway Traffic Safety Administration (NHTSA),
at any given moment of the day, 500,000 drivers of passenger vehicles
are talking on handheld cell phones.

Conversing on cell phones while driving
can lead to significant decreases
in driving performance

Driving Under the Cell-phone Influence is
DANGEROUS TO EVERYONE

GET OFF YOUR CELL PHONE!

Healer's Guide 2007

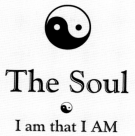

The Soul

I am that I AM

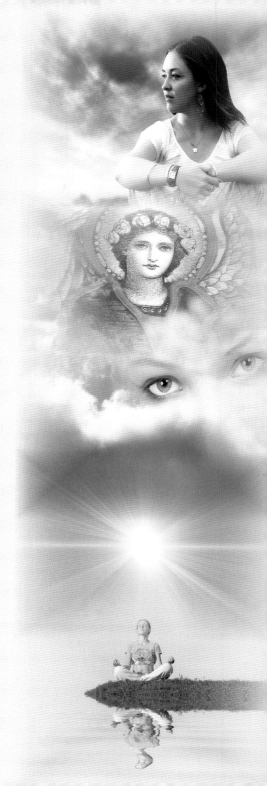

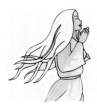

The Soul

I am That I Am

W hen people think of their soul, they usually imagine a vague, sort of ghost like figure, out there, somewhere. And perhaps, this, they think, is a possible answer to what they will be or how they will exist after death. For those who have heard the expression "you are a soul having a human experience" this may be old hat. If this expression presents a new paradigm, then hold on to your hat!

The word reincarnation is usually used to describe subsequent lives. In actuality, it is possible to reincarnate or "re-invent the wheel" several times in one lifetime and this happens quite frequently. Think about the different lives you have lived in your life. Through change and growth we often take on new roles and new identities and discard the old. Evolution is a choice.

Imagine that you are a soul having a human experience. What exactly does it mean to be a soul and how does the experience of this human life operate? The books covering this topic are countless and include the Bible, the Essene Gospel, the Vedas, The Bhagavad Gita, the works of Parmahansa Yogananda, Pantajali, Rumi, the esoteric literature written by authors belonging to the Theosophical Society, as well as the more recent and practical teachings of Master Choa Kok Sui, Barbara Ann Brennan, Lucille Cedarcrans and Mantak Chia. The list goes on. To thoroughly educate yourself will take a little time, but here is a simple overview to wet the whistle, so to speak.

A definition of the Soul:

The unique, immaterial essence of each living being animating its material form; A spark of energy with ego-free consciousness, aware and one with all other sparks and its source. In religious and spiritual teachings the source is referred to as God; The soul consciousness, while in the physical body, does not have to be fully realized by the brain. The brain, when free of thoughts, allows one to experience the consciousness of the soul. The brain with its many thoughts, likes and dislikes, creates a sense of personality or ego that most people identify with. This perception of oneself, considered to be the "I," accompanies the individual, often for an entire lifetime, without the individual realizing their true spiritual soul nature.

"And the Lord God formed man of the dust of the ground, and breathed into his nostrils the breath of life; and man became a living soul."
-
Genesis 2:7

From the common thread of information running through spiritual teachings, we learn that when a human soul is about to be born into a physical body, the soul extends a portion of itself down into the body, at a certain astrologically correct moment, in time and space. The astrological influences help create the complexity of the personality, nature and subtle bodies and serve as a guideline or timetable for one's life events. At the time of birth, you have almost forgotten the experience of being a soul and slowly begin to identify with the physical body, but the soul connection remains. Time goes on and full immersion into the experience of life happens. Little by little the earthly existence becomes the only reality - unless one is fortunate enough to have a spiritual teacher, guru or enlightened parents throughout childhood. The nature of the thoughts, emotions and deeds, wholesome or unwholesome, throughout one's life determines the strength of the soul connection. Choices and actions determine whether the connection grows stronger or weaker. If one becomes so far removed from their soul connection or soul consciousness, they are referred to as a lost soul. This is considered to be a most unfortunate and difficult situation to overcome.

What should you believe or should you believe at all?

"Believe nothing on the faith of traditions, even though they have been held in honor for many generations and in diverse places. Do not believe a thing because many people speak of it. Do not believe on the faith of the sages of the past. Do not believe what you yourself have imagined, persuading yourself that a God inspires you. Believe nothing on the sole authority of your masters and priests. After examination, believe what you yourself have tested and found to be reasonable, and conform your conduct thereto."

~Buddha~

A definition of the Lost Soul:

The aspect of the soul that lives in the physical body is often referred to as the incarnated soul. The originating soul aspect of the incarnated soul is referred to as the overshadowing or higher soul. The connection between the incarnated soul (inhabiting the body), overshadowing soul (higher aspect) and Source (God or Universe), may be distantly compared to the connection of an electrical cord - between the power outlet and an appliance. When plugged in, the electricity (source energy) flows freely and powers the appliance (incarnated soul). The term "lost soul" refers to the situation that occurs when the power cord - connection between overshadowing and incarnated soul - is damaged. After that (at the time of physical death), the appliance (incarnated soul) runs out of internal energies and the game is over! To completely destroy the cord is unlikely, since it is made out of tough material, however it can become damaged and non-functional when one carelessly performs unwholesome actions.

A portion of our sustenance or vital energy comes from the environment and from the food that we eat. This energy is commonly referred to as life force. A larger portion of our vital energy comes from the Universe (God) through the higher soul and vivifies the life of the incarnated soul occupying the physical body. This is usually called Soul Energy or Universal Life Force. Death of the physical body occurs when this vital energy is withdrawn. When the energy becomes partially withdrawn or the flow is impaired by a blockage, it results in a weak soul connection, a reduced amount of vital force for the physical life and accompanying difficulties and illness. The importance of this statement cannot be stressed enough.

"Through our soul is our contact with heaven."

-

Sholem Asch, American novelist, dramatist (1880 - 1957)

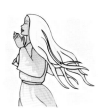

215

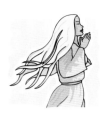

Earlier, it was mentioned that you are the one who makes healing possible. Now we know that "you" does not refer to the body. You, actually refers to you the soul. Your will and desire to heal, in some cases is often enough to invoke or bring down enough soul energy which results in healing. Strengthening the connection with Source through meditation, prayer, faith and wholesome living, enables healing to occur at an accelerated rate. The increased connection with one's guidance (higher soul), leads to increased intuition which allows your waking consciousness to grasp the life lessons of events such as illness. In cases of a weak will or a lack of desire to make the effort to heal, energy healers, are often able to help patients overcome weaknesses by eliminating obstacles and strengthening the obstructed soul connection. The patient often experiences a "rebirth" while in the physical body, discovering a new life path and reason for living.

The virtues universal to all religions are:

● **Loving Kindness and Non-Injury**

● **Generosity and Non-Stealing**

● **Accurate Perception and Correct Expression**

● **Moderation and Non-excessiveness**

● **Constancy of Aim and Effort and Non-Laziness**

Virtues are the basic foundation for one's evolution. Without virtues the soul connection is weak.

A short meditation:

1) Be aware of your right hand. Move it up and down and ask the following question: "Am I this hand or am I moving this hand?"

2) Be aware of your head. Move it side to side and ask the following question: "Am I this head or am I moving this head?"

3) Be aware of your eyes. Close them and move them side to side asking the following question: "Am I those eyes or am I moving them?"

4) Shift your attention from your closed eyes to the inside of your head, into your brain area. Be aware of your brain and ask the following question: "Am I this brain or am I aware of it?"

5) With your eyes still closed, shift the attention from your brain area to the awareness of your whole body. Move it from side to side and ask the following question: "Am I this body or am I just moving and feeling it?"

6) Remember of all your previous answers, "I am not my hand," "I am not my head,", "I am not my eyes," "I am not my brain," " I am not my body." Ask yourself the following question: "Who am I?"

7) Do not answer the question yet. Just hold this question in your mind and with your eyes closed, gently explore your entire body. Take your time, search with your inner awareness into each part of yourself and ask this question: " Where am I?" Look at your legs, your belly, your chest, your head, look everywhere. Then silently affirm " I am not my body. I am the soul."

"The soul is pure when it leaves the body and drags nothing bodily with it, by virtue of having no willing association with the body in life but avoiding it.......Practicing philosophy in the right way is a training to die easily."

-
Socrates,
ancient Greek philosopher
(470 - 399 BCE)

After having enough suffering, trials and tribulations, hardships, illness and the like, one begins to ask. What is life about anyway? Is there a point? Who am I, really? Am I just a bag of bones, flesh and randomly firing neurons in my head? These questions lead to an investigation and eventually to a "remembering" of who you really are. What or who is the power behind this life? Unfortunately, for many, this question is prompted by severe illness, accident, near death experience, fear or

On Meditation
By Elissa Michaud

Meditation has numerous physical, mental, emotional and spiritual benefits. The number one goal of meditation is to connect with Source also known as spiritual energy or life energy. Source is the energy everyone must connect with to renew and heal the body and the emotions. This is the energy that keeps the body from aging, that your mind uses to create your reality, and that your body uses to heal itself. On a daily basis, everything that we do and every choice we make affects our connection to Source and how much lifeforce we are able to access and receive. Our incarnated soul is connected to our higher soul, or higher intelligence by an energy cord, refered to in ancient teachings as the *antakharana*. This cord has the ability to increase or decrease in size and it does so in accordance to our thoughts, emotions and actions. If the thoughts and actions are wholesome, it increases; if they are unwholesome it decreases. When the size of the antakharana gradually increases due to regular meditation, we become more intuitive and make better decisions; our energy increases, therefore maximizing our innate self-healing abilities.

There are several types of meditations and each one brings with it a specific result. Some meditations are designed to increase your energy; some are designed to still the mind; others are designed to develop focus and concentration, strengthening the mental body. Thoughts and emotions are energy. When we are using our available lifeforce to think intensely, generate emotions and for the physical body to run around here and there, the result is less available lifeforce for the body to direct towards healing. By practicing the type of meditation in which we quiet the thoughts and emotions, our connection with Source increases and the increased energy may be used for healing the physical body. It also gives us a chance to relax and go within. By doing so, we are able to clearly see and hear patterns of negative thoughts and emotions which are related

to physical illness. Meditation also increases the connection to our intuition and higher wisdom, enabling us to see circumstances clearly and discover solutions to life situations.

When you begin your meditation, do not have an agenda or expectations. Meditation starts with your personal intention. It may be that you desire healing, or a solution to a problem, or greater intuition. Do not repeat your intentions over and over during the meditation. It has already been set. Meditation is not about psychic or paranormal experiences, such as visions or colorful lights, although these may happen to some individuals, if it is important for their development in some way.

Many meditation teachers and practitioners talk about kundalini energy. This is a powerful life energy which for most people lays dormant in the base of the spine. Kundalini energy is an evolutionary energy. It helps us to evolve and is released gradually when the time is right. In general when a certain amount of purification has been done to the mental, emotional and physical bodies, the spiritual energy which is increased and brought down through meditation, will meet the kundalini energy in the base of the spine, mix with it, and travel back up the spine. This energy in particular, helps to evolve our souls and specifically the human brain. Kundalini meditations should always be learned through special yoga practice. Both Arhatic and Kriya Yoga are time-tested, proven, safe methods of instruction.

Meditation is also a great tool to use in a group setting. When many people come together with a common purpose to meditate as a group, the spiritual energy increases exponentially. It is a valuable service to humanity to participate in groups who come together for the purpose of peace or blessing the earth. The benefits are increased many-fold. Most meditation groups in Los Angeles have free or donation-based teachings and regular meeting groups. If you would like to learn more, find a community or discipline you like and study this excellent practice!

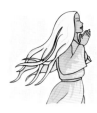

approaching the end of one's life. Why wait? Don't let life dish you a side of misery to get your attention. Meditation is the tool used to embark on a path of introspection and the discovery of one's true self on a deeper level.

After some time is spent searching for answers and studying the various paths of spiritual knowledge, one begins to draw new conclusions regarding their personal truths and reality. As each new piece of information is assimilated, it creates a new level of awareness. Every experience throughout your lifetime is stored in what is referred to as your soul memory. Everyone is familiar with the expression, "You can't take it with you." This only applies to material or earthly things, not to wisdom and spiritual development. This does not apply to the karma generated by service and good deeds and certainly not to the development of your energy body. As mentioned in previous chapters, every wholesome experience, thought or action creates refined psychoemotional matter and generates good karma. Unwholesome actions create gross psychoemotional matter and the retribution of the law of cause and effect.

For those interested in developing and evolving their spirit and energy body, or who desire rapid spiritual growth during this physical life, the science of yoga, including meditation, is the fast track program. Kriya Yoga taught by Self-Realization Fellowship Center and Arhatic Yoga, taught by Master Choa Kok Sui are examples of practical yoga teachings and are tailored for easy assimilation by our western society. For eons, science and spirituality have been considered to be worlds apart, while in fact, they go hand in hand. The exercises and meditations taught to spiritual seekers are largely based on a scientific foundation. We are now re-discovering that ancient spiritual teachings are, in fact, in-line with natural laws and scientific breakthroughs, but are called by different names, due to differences in cultural backgrounds.

Consider the things that provide nourishment for your soul. High on the list will be a spiritual practice and prayer; learning something new; experiencing joy through family and friends; the satisfaction of using your gifts to build, create or play; helping someone in need or serving others; solitude and moments of introspection; taking care of your body to provide a healthy vehicle for the soul's expression; and, doing what you are truly passionate about. What about the things that take away nourishment with negative emotions such as hatred, guilt, being moody, laziness, working without passion, not making time for spiritual practice, dishonesty, being unkind, greediness, jealousy, wasting time. And the list could go on.

Planetary Meditation for Peace and illumination is being practiced in more than 58 countries throughout the world. It is a form of world service because the earth is blessed with loving kindness during the meditation. Divine energy flows through you, cleansing your aura and thus, has a healing effect. It is a safe practice that can be done daily.

www.meditatepeace.com

"You don't have to be religious to have a soul; everybody has one. You don't have to be religious to perfect your soul; I have found saintliness in avowed atheists."

-
Rabbi Harold Kushner,
The Lord Is My Shepherd: Healing Wisdom of the Twenty-Third Psalm

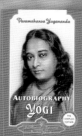
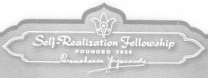

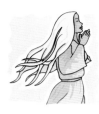

From time to time, it is a normal part of the human experience to feel lost; fearful; abandoned; out of touch with one's guidance and God; and, that there is no clear indication for direction or purpose. More than ever, these are the times to meditate, pray and and to be introspective. Do things that employ the heart aspect and that bring joy. Attempt to reconnect with the divine aspect of your soul and develop intuition. This is also the time that a spiritual psychologist or life coach, counselor, guru and spiritual/energy healer have much to offer. This is not usually the best time to be pushing hard in the world of affairs, immersed in work, distracted through television and other popular pacifiers. Study the art of meditation and yoga or take a workshop to learn how to connect with your guidance. Be introspective. This may be the appropriate time to shift some outer aspect of your earth experience, be it career, lifestyle or relationship. Be aware and rediscover that you are, in fact, a soul in a human body.

> **Everyone has free-will. We come into our lives with certain circumstances and events predestined. By our choices we may either improve or ruin our opportunities. A strong soul connection developed through meditation, enables us to be more connected with our guidance and therefore, make better choices, improving our lives.**

Bringing Our Lives Into Balance
By Brother Achalananda

In the following article (courtesy of Self-Realization Fellowship, Los Angeles), condensed from a talk given in Los Angeles, Brother Achalananda – a senior member of the Self-Realization Fellowship monastic communities – shares Paramahansa Yogananda's wisdom on how we can achieve balance and well-being in our lives amid the complexities of the modern world.

> "We do not destroy religion by destroying superstition."
> -
> Marcus Tullius Cicero, philosopher of Ancient Rome (106 BC - 43 BC)

What does balance consist of? The great yoga master Paramahansa Yogananda taught an ideal that encompasses the material, psychological and emotional, and spiritual aspects of our lives - an ideal that is tremendously motivating and inspiring. We all want to have a healthy body, free of problems and weaknesses; we don't want it to be a hindrance. We want our mind to be alert and our emotions and feelings to be working for us and not against us; we want them to contribute to harmonious and fulfilling relationships with those around us. And above all, we very much want and need to connect with the spiritual side of our being - with that most natural and all-satisfying part of ourselves, our soul; and with God.

However, to achieve that balance we have to invest some energy and time and attention. Balance doesn't come just by our hoping it will somehow happen; we have to make it happen through a definite plan and effort.

To balance all the aspects of our life we need something to balance them on, some point of equilibrium. The more complex our lives become, the more we need to realize that there is only one reliable point of balance - and that is God. Only God pervades everything, underlies all the material and spiritual activities of life. We have to learn to make Him our balance point. There is no other answer.

When you look at life with clear understanding, it all boils down to this: Balance means finding God; and finding God means meditation.

Balanced living - real spiritual living - said Paramahansaji, "consists in seeking the comfort of meditation first and then making material life very simple....Why spend all your valuable time in seeking perishable things? Why not spend your time seeking God first through deep meditation until you actually contact Him? When you commune with Him you will receive the imperishable treasures of heaven and all you need of the perishable material benefits of this life."

All of us have a lot of demands on our time. To find time to seek God we have to simplify our lives. Find ways to bring God into your life every day as much as possible. Take a moment to let the mind go within, become aware of the spiritual eye, and even though you may be very busy with work, repeat, "For You, God, for You." Then go on with your duties. That constant reminder, that bringing the mind back to the focus point, helps us keep our inner balance.

During the 20th century, Asian spiritual practices were introduced in the West. The second Industrial Revolution brought great spiritual teachers overseas. Until then people who were interested in having a direct spiritual experience had little access to these teachings in the local Western religions. It seemed strange at first due to cultural differences, but the message is one of God-communion, love, unity and integration - harmonious with all world religions. Growth requires you to rise above cultural and religious differences.

Making time for recreation and wholesome activities you enjoy is a necessary component of spiritual and psychological balance. In the long run you will get much more accomplished in your work and in your spiritual life - and you will be healthier physically - if you remember this. Ideally, the week should consist of five days working at your regular job; the sixth given to relaxing, recreation, doing things around the home; and the seventh day should be for deepening your relationship with God.

Ultimately, the secret of balance is to put first things first - and that means seeking God. Schedule your life; plan a balanced routine of meditation so that you're getting a certain amount every day, and then follow it.

"Our intellect has achieved the most tremendous things, but in the meantime our spiritual dwelling has fallen into disrepair."
-
Carl Gustav Jung, Swiss psychiatrist, founder of analytical psychology, *The Archetypes and the Collective Unconscious*

The whole secret of spiritual success: Never give up! You are a divine soul; and the pressures and stresses you feel can never dim that radiant spark of divinity within you. They are simply challenges to be faced and overcome, joyously! You already have within you everything you need to do so. All you have to do is uncover it.

Brother Achalananda has been a monk of the Self-Realization Fellowship monastic communities for more than 50 years. Presently, he serves as senior minister at Self-Realization Fellowship's Lake Shrine Temple in Pacific Palisades, California and as a member of the SRF Board of Directors. He has lectured extensively on the science and philosophy of Yoga and the universal teachings of Paramahansa Yogananda (who founded SRF in 1920. For more information about SRF, visit www.yogananda-srf.org.

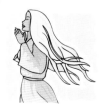

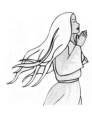

Free or donation-based meditation resources:

◻ **Sahaja Yoga** - choose from several daily introductory classes, meditation workshops, walk-in meditations - www.sahajayogala.org/

◻ **Shambala Meditation Center of Los Angeles** - Free meditation instruction is available, as well as a wide variety of classes and programs in meditation - http://la.shambhala.org

◻ **Sant Mat Meditation Center** - All programs are free of charge and open to the public; information about Sant Mat is given by authorized initiates of Sant Baljit Singh - www.knowthyselfassoul.org

◻ **Sivananda Yoga Vendanta Center** - open houses, open class and free satsang (Meditation, Chanting & Discourse) - www.sivananda.org/la/free.htm

◻ **Urban Dharma Los Angeles** - free meditation, workshops and classes - www.urbandharma.org/buddhala.html

◻ **Krs Edstrom's Retreat Experience** - free online guided meditations for stress, pain, relaxation and spiritual growth - www.askkrs.com/serenity.htm

◻ **Vijja - 18 -Body** - instruction and meditation class on line or in person - www.18body.com

◻ **Los Angeles Meditation Center** - free weekly classes on meditation and spiritual development to the public - www.lameditioncenter.org

◻ **Agape International Spiritual Center** - New Thought-Ancient Wisdom tradition of spirituality, services and meditation - www.agapelive.com

◻ **Self Realization Fellowship Center** - universal teachings of Paramahansa Yogananda, services and meditation - www.selfrealizationfellowship.com

◻ **US Pranic Healing Center** - Planetary Meditation for World Peace full moon meditation - www.pranichealing.com

◻ **Guru Singh** - listen to audio files of lectures and yoga classes online - www.gurusingh.com

Books:

◻ *Autobiography of a Yogi* - comprehensive introduction to the whole science and philosophy of Yoga, revealing the underlying unity of the great religions of East and West, by Paramahansa Yogananda

◻ *Initiation* - an autobiographical novel unveiling mystical truths communicated in modern terms, by Elisabeth Haich

◻ *Journey of Souls: Case Studies of Life Between Lives* - uncovers the mystery of life in the spirit world after death, on earth, by Michael Newton, Ph.D.

◻ *Meditation on the Soul* - discusses the meaning of Soul Realization and includes two advanced meditations - Meditation on Twin Hearts; Meditation on the Soul, by Master Choa Kok Sui

◻ *Teachings of Rumi* - a collection of mystical poetry written by Jelallundin Rumi, illuminating the heart and mind, conveying an experience of Divine Love, by Andrew Harvey

◻ *The Seat of the Soul* - discusses the values of the soul and the alignment of the personality with the soul, by Gary Zukav

◻ *The Causal Body and the Ego* - discusses the vehicle which survives the death and disintegration of the physical, mental and emotional bodies, by Col. Arthur Powell

◻ *The Nature of the Soul* - A course of instruction in The Wisdom. It is designed to facilitate step-by-step unfoldment from individuality to group awareness and conscious service to the One Life, by Lucille Cedarcrans

"Whether one believes in a religion or not, and whether one believes in rebirth or not, there isn't anyone who doesn't appreciate kindness and compassion."
-
His Holiness,
14th the Dalai Lama

The Healing Modalities

The Modality and Practitioner Guide

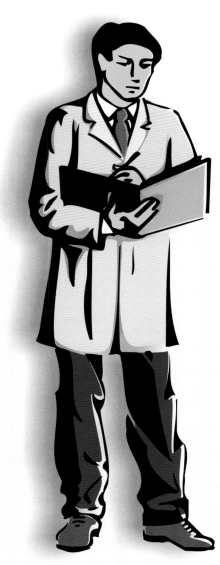

- Acupuncture
- Ayurveda
- Biofeedback
- Chinese Medicine
- Chiropractic
- Colon Therapy
- Cranial Sacral Therapy
- Doula
- Energetic Balancing
- Feng Shui
- Holistic Dentistry
- Holistic/Integrative MD
- Holistic Senior Care
- Homeopathy
- Hypnotherapy
- Integrated Energy Therapy^{AE}
- Life Coaching
- Massage Therapy
- Naturopathy
- Neurofeedback
- Neuro Linguistic Prog.
- Nutritional Counseling
- Osteopathy
- Physical Therapy
- Pranic Healing^{SM}
- Reiki
- Rolfing®
- Spiritual Psychology
- Transitional Healing

Acupuncture

~

What is Acupuncture? Acupuncture is a complete Chinese medical system. Acupuncture needles are inserted into specific body points (acupuncture points) for therapeutic purposes, to relieve pain, correct the flow of chi, or produce regional anesthesia. Acupuncture works by influencing the Chi (life energy) which circulates throughout the energy channels or meridians in the body. Acupuncture points are where the chi is most accessible. There are 12 main meridians and each is related to an organ: lung, kidney, gallbladder, stomach, spleen, heart, small and large intestine, urinary bladder, san jiao (triple burner) and pericardium. In addition there are 8 extraordinary channels which supply chi to the other 12 channels.

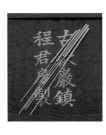

When the ultra-thin, flexible needles are properly placed on the acupuncture points the imbalances are corrected by increasing, or decreasing the flow or amount of chi through the meridian. Most patients feel no pain during treatment. Some feel energized, while others feel relaxed. Improper needle placement or movement of the patient may cause slight soreness during treatment.

Licenced Acupuncturists diagnose by asking the patient questions and by observing their pulse and tongue. They also look for signs of imbalance as indicated by the relationship of Yin and Yang. Yin diseases demonstrate signs of deficiency, while Yang diseases demonstrate signs of excess. An example of yin imbalance would be fatigue; an example of yang excessive imbalance would be high blood pressure. Health can often be restored by diet and lifestyle suggestions designed to balance the yin and yang.

It is widely practiced in the United States. There are thousands of licensed practitioners. Acupuncture is recommended by physicians and dentists, for pain relief or other health conditions.

The 2002 National Health Interview Survey stated that an estimated 8.2 million U.S. adults had used acupuncture.

Origin and History: Acupuncture has been a major part of primary healthcare in Asia for thousands of years and originated in China. The earliest recordings of acupuncture are found in the Nei Jing (The Yellow Emperor's Classic of Internal Medicine), a medical text book, believed to be as old as 200 BC.

Applications: Acupuncture is effective for managing pain. It effectively treats disorders related to the following body systems: respiratory, gastrointestinal, neurological, hormonal and musculoskeletal. It is effective in treating migraines, headaches, sciatica, menopausal and PMS symptoms, infertility, ulcers, diarrhea, constipation, gingivitis, allergies, certain vision problems, asthma, anxiety, chronic fatigue, fibromyalgia, osteoarthritis, irritable bowel syndrome, hypertension, insomnia, depression, chronic pain conditions such as arthritis and bursitis, injuries, post traumatic and post-surgical pain, stroke rehabilitation, and addictions such as alcoholism, smoking, and eating disorders.

Research: Acupuncture is one of the most thoroughly researched and documented of the alternative medical practices. Many research and controlled studies have shown success evidence of treating the above-mentioned health conditions. Studies have shown that there is a correlation between the electromagnetic fields in the body and the channels or meridians.

Cautions: Few complications have been reported. Those reported were a result of inadequate sterilization of needles or improper delivery of treatments. Practitioners must use a new set of disposable needles for each patient/visit. Proper licensing indicates that the practitioner has met certain standards.

Insurance: Frequently covers treatment.

Practitioner quick reference:

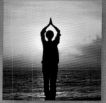 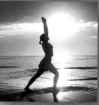 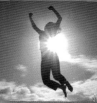 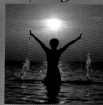

Use of Chinese Medicine for Fertility, Pregnancy and Childbirth
By Azita Moallef, L.Ac.

Acupuncture can be applied in the early and late stages of pregnancy as well as during labor for pain relief. Various pathological conditions can be treated effectively during pregnancy and labor, without the side effects of more common therapies.

In the late stages of pregnancy, acupuncture can promote the maturity of the cervix and birth channel therefore reducing the duration of labor significantly. During the process of labor Acupuncture Analgesia is the key method for reducing most of the labor pain and can be very effective for inducing labor. Moxabustion is effective for turning a breached baby. Acupuncture Analgesia for labor utilizes a mild application of electrical stimulation.

Evidence of treatment of infertility with Acupuncture dates back to 11AD. It can help reduce stress, increase blood flow to the reproductive organs, and normalize ovulation and the menstrual cycle.

Chinese Medicine uses a Whole Person Fertility program, which offers a revolutionary, mind-body-spirit process to help women conceive. it works with women and men to increase their opportunity to get pregnant and carry to term. This work recognizes that fertility difficulties are not necessarily only a medical problem, but are often related to issues in one's personal history and current life. This process helps couples reclaim their reproductive rights and offers tremendous potential for transformation and healing.

Some of the conditions treated with Chinese medicine:

Breached Position, Promoting Labor, Childbirth Facilitation, Insufficient Lactation

Digestive:
morning sickness, nausea, vomiting, stomachache, diarrhea, constipation, hemorrhoids, indigestion, gastric reflux

Musculo-skeletal:
muscle, tendon, and ligament pain and discomfort, groin spasms, leg cramps, sciatica

Immune System and Other:
fatigue, gestational Diabetes, side effects of western medication

Respiratory:
cold and flu, sore throat, bronchitis, asthma, smoking

Gynecological/Genito-urinary:
menstrual pain, hot flashes, infertility, endometriosis, mastitis, vaginal and UTI, difficult urination, incontinence, sexual dysfunction, prevention of miscarriage, uterine hemorrhaging

Cardiovascular:
high blood pressure, palpitations, varicose vein, eclampsia and pre-eclampsia, nose bleeds

Emotional and stress related:
depression, adjustment to parenthood, confusing emotions, fatigue, insomnia, anxiety, irritability, stress

www.4wellbeing.com
See Ad on page 227

Acupuncture & Herbs
for Pregnancy, Birth & Beyond...

Azita Moallef, L.Ac.

Acupuncture ❧ Acupressure ❧ Herbal Medicine ❧ Energy Medicine

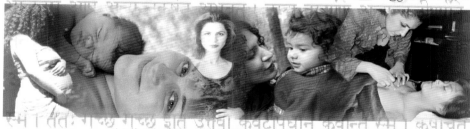

❧ Whole Person Fertility Program ❧

❧ Childbirth Preparation Sessions ❧

❧ Breached Position and Labor Induction ❧

❧ Postpartum Holistic Weight Loss Program ❧

❧ Placenta Preparation and Nutritional Counseling ❧

❧ Pregnancy, Postpartum, Infantile Tui Na Massage ❧

Azita is an Oriental Medicine practitioner with expertise in women's & children's holistic health in private practice. She has facilitated many births using acupuncture and herbs working in hospitals as well as home birth setting. Her own experience of childbirth - first by cesarean and second naturally - was a priceless experience of personal growth, where she understood the pain process in a new empowering way, radically different from the usual. She regards pregnancy and birth as a rite of passage integral to a woman's evolution into mothering and believes that healthy pregnancy and natural birth are processes which have lifelong impact on a woman's self esteem, her health, her ability to nurture, and her personal growth.

Azita Moallef, B.A., L.Ac., M.T.O.M. - Santa Monica, CA. 90403

310 - 453 - 5717

www.4wellbeing.com

What is the AcuFitness Technique?
by Suzan Brudow

Just as we see many solo practitioners "merging" to offer a variety of alternative services within one location, so too we find innovative holistic professionals combining their healing talents to develop new treatment techniques.

One such treatment, developed over the last six years right here in Southern California, is The AcuFitness Technique™, a fusion of Pilates, weight training and acupuncture. Co-created by long time fitness expert, Javier Jacobo, and Master Acupuncturist, Nicole Bradshaw, AFT has evolved into an authentic treatment program with a track record of results, testimonials and protocols. Until now, AFT treatments have been offered only at Javier's Studio City fitness practice (HottieBodies, Pilates & Wellness), but that's about to change. The partners expect to launch an AFT training program in 2007, offering certification for AcuFitness Technique™ practitioners.

The process: Javier Jacobo's studies and experience of anatomy, kinesiology and nutrition were combined with Nicole Bradshaw's experience in acupuncture and traditional oriental medicine in an integrative fashion. This fusion was the foundation that created The AcuFitness Technique. The Aha! moment came when Nicole revealed to Javier how conditions could be treated via the ear using auricular therapy - a system of diagnosis and treatment based on the knowledge that many acupuncture points of the ear correspond to a different part of the body. Her expertise in auricular point activation was the key to being able to support and improve vital organ functions, while encouraging the body's natural ability to heal while in motion. They began offering this service to their respective clients, personalizing the placement of the needles and the exercise regimen to the client's specific needs.

When fitness is combined with acupuncture it helps to accelerate health and wellness and promotes weight loss. It does this by reducing cravings, improving digestive functions, and balancing hormone levels. These are all key factors in being able to loose weight and achieve health. Some conditions addressed quite effectively by this technique include severe back pain, shoulder pain, knee pain, addictive food cravings, stress/anxiety and low energy.

The technique provides the benefits of a full body acupuncture treatment and an unrestricted physical workout simultaneously. The results were immediately evident. Following are some case studies.

Case Studies:

#1 - 75 year old female regularly went to the hospital for mysterious episodes of dizziness and frequent sciatica. AFT treatments commenced once a week, focusing on strengthening the structural region and general nourishment to the internal organs, She has continued a once-weekly maintenance routine for the past two years with no trips to the hospital.

#2 - Male; age 54 with neck, shoulder, left knee pain and chronic low back pain due to a near-fatal auto accident. Patient had surgically replaced muscular regions in the foot and chronic structural misalignments. Pain generally dominated the left side of his body. AFT treatment resulted in relief of pain with noticeably improved circulation. Client maintains very active lifestyle, has had periodic flare-ups but overall relief. He credits the AFT treatments with his ability to pursue advanced physical performance.

#3 - Female; age 41 scheduled for back surgery and in a brace to minimize pain. During her menstrual cycle, hormonal spikes manifested unusual bloating that completely altered her physical appearance. She began AFT treatment 2-3 times per week. Within two months she canceled her surgery and to this day she has no back problems and her hormonal changes have completely normalized.

Javier and Nicole are just two of many examples of an emerging new breed of multi-faceted medical professionals making the future of healthcare look very bright indeed.

See Ad on page 165

Ayurveda

The Vedic System of Health Care

What is Ayurveda?: Ayurvedic Medicine is a complete Indian medical system, which recognizes the importance of the relationship of body, mind, and spirit. Two people may have the same symptoms, but their energetic constitutions may be completely different, therefore treatment is individually tailored. Ayurvedic philosophy states that disease is a result of misuse of the senses, misuse of the will, simple-wear and tear or trauma to the physical body. Good health is a direct result of one's positive and wholesome relations with their environment.

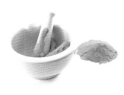

The clinical subspecialties of Ayurveda as traditionally practiced are as follows: Internal medicine, general surgery, Otorhinolaryngology, pediatrics and Obstetric/Gynecology, psychiatry, toxicology, nutrition, detoxification and rejuvenation, fertility and virility. Constitutional assessment is done via questions and observation. Practitioners ask their patients about their diet, digestion, behavior, personal habits, lifestyle practices. At each visit practitioner checks the patient's urine, pulse, stool, tongue, teeth, eyes, skin, weight and overall appearance. Treatments may include the following:

• Enemas, fasting and special diets to eliminate impurities in the digestive tract; and the use of medicated oils administered through nasal sprays to eliminate impurities in the respiratory system.

• Reduce symptoms and stress through careful recommendation of herbs, small amounts of metal and mineral preparations, lifestyle modifications, yoga, exercises, meditation, stretching, breathing and meditation techniques and sun.

• Bodywork similar to acupressure and/or massage with medicinal oils are recommended for physical and psychological problems and to reduce pain, lessen fatigue and improve circulation.

Origin and History: Ayurveda is a holistic system of healing which evolved among the Brahmin sages of ancient India 3000-5000 years ago. Two-thirds of the Indian population use Ayurvedic Medicine. Ayurvedic practices were handed down by word of mouth before there were written records. Two ancient books, written in Sanskrit 2,000 years ago - the Caraka Samhita and the Susruta Samhita - are thought to be the first texts on Ayurveda. They cover many topics including pathology, diagnosis, treatment and philosophy.

Applications: Ayurveda is effective for most health related problems and treats in accordance to the balance of the three "Doshas" or constitutions:

• *The Vata Dosha:* Space and air. The most influential and the moving force behind the other two. Controls the flow of blood, nutrients and cell division, the heart, breathing, and the mind, Vata is disrupted by staying up late, eating dry fruit, or eating too often. Diseases indicating imbalance are neurological, and mental disorders, insomnia and loss of joy for life.

• *The Pitta Dosha:* Fire and water. Controls the hormones and digestive system, chemical and metabolic processes. Imbalance is created by eating too much spicy or sour food, excessive sun, and anger or fear. Diseases of imbalance include arthritis, heart disease and heartburn.

• *The Kapha Dosha*: Water and earth. Promoting love, compassion, understanding, forgiveness, loyalty, patience. Kapha controls strength, growth, immunity & self-healing. Imbalance is created by too many sweet foods, overeating, and excess salt. Resulting illnesses are diabetes, gallbladder and respiratory problems, stomach ulcers and impotency.

Cautions: Caution for treatment outside of the U.S. In 2004 a study revealed that 1/5 of the 70 Ayurvedic remedies purchased over-the-counter, manufactured in South Asia contained lead, mercury or arsenic at harmful levels. For safe use it is advisable to use remedies under the supervision of an Ayurvedic practitioner.

Practitioner quick reference:
Ione Linker - page 238

Biphone Biofeedback

A Science of Mind-Body Interactions

What is Biofeedback? Biofeedback is a system which evaluates the biological signals produced by the body. It is based on the body's innate ability and potential to influence automatic functions through the exertion of will and mind resulting in self-regulation of the body.

It is a relatively new modality since it was only during the

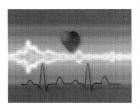

late 1960's that scientists discovered that normally unconscious, autonomic biological body functions could be controlled voluntarily. Biofeedback involves measuring a individual's bodily processes such as blood pressure, heart rate, skin temperature, galvanic skin response, breathing rate and muscle tension. Bio-signals are collected through special sensors attached to the skin of the individual and information is presented to the client in real-time. It is then transported through the "interface" into the computer where the information becomes analyzed and presented in the form of moving graphs or audio tones interpreted by a Biofeedback specialist.

During the treatment sensors are attached to the surface of the skin at various locations on the body (usually the shoulders, fingers, back, and head) to collect the reading of the patient's vital signs as indicators of their health issue. The result helps the individual by bringing awareness and the ability to control biological responses in order to improve certain health issues.

Origin and History: The origins of biofeedback are based on studies completed in the late 1960s by neuroscientist, Neal Miller, Ph.D. of Rockefeller University. His experimentation showed that laboratory animals (rats) could be trained to increase or decrease their heart rates by stimulating the pleasure center of their brain with electricity or simply by being rewarded for producing the desired physiological responses. In 1969-1970, research psychologist Barbara B. Brown Ph.D. created and popularized the word biofeedback

and co-founded the Biofeedback Research Society, which later evolved into the Association for Applied Psychophysiology and Biofeedback [www.aapb.org].

Applications: Clinical biofeedback techniques are used to help with stress-related conditions such as: headache, cardiac arrhythmia, asthma, muscle injury, pain relief, insomnia, TMJ, high blood pressure, digestive disorders, attention deficit disorder, incontinence, poor posture, tennis elbow, golfer's elbow, epilepsy paralysis, irritable bowel syndrome, hyperactivity, Raynaud's disease, ringing of the ears, constipation, esophageal dysfunction, and others. The American Association for the Study of Headaches endorses biofeedback as a valid form of treatment.

Research: Several successful research studies have been conducted. The research of Elmer Green, Ph.D., director of the Menninger Foundation's Psychophysiology Laboratory related to testing biofeedback as a possible method of treatment of mental and physical conditions with an emphasis on migraine headaches.

The research of Thomas Budzynskl, Ph.D., Johann Stoyva, Ph.D., and Charles Adler, M.D., at the University of Colorado investigated the influence of biofeedback on muscle tension and the resulting pain.

A pilot study by Joseph Sargeant, M.D., director of the Department of Internal Medicine at Menninger, used headache patients as subjects. The research proved that the technique was successful in reducing and even eliminating headaches in the vast majority of the subjects.

Cautions: Individuals with the following issues should avoid biofeedback therapy. Persons with severe psychosis, depression, or obsessional neurosis, debilitated patients or those with psychopathic personalities. It is recommended for diabetics and those with endocrine disorders to check with a doctor, to see whether this is an appropriate treatment, as it can change the need for insulin and other medications.

Insurance: Insurance coverage for biofeedback is often available but it may vary based on the insurance coverage plan. Contact your local biofeedback provider to discuss coverage issues.

Quick practitioner reference:
Synergy Holistic SkinCare - page 167
My Bio Body - page 246
(Quantum-Biofeedback)

Chinese Medicine

Traditional

What is Traditional Chinese Medicine? Traditional Chinese Medicine consists of several components - acupuncture therapy, herbal/diet therapy, tui na - a therapeutic massage composed of over 20 manipulations and techniques for relaxation or rehabilitation, and chi gong - exercise. Therapies such as moxibustion (applying heat to an area of the body or to the acupuncture needles; useful for pain relief, weakness and fatigue) and cupping (the application of glass cups to acupuncture points or the affected part of the body which creates a vacuum suction created and helps stimulate blood circulation, improve the energy flow and removes toxins; the technique is used for muscle injuries, joint pain and bronchial congestion) are applied. Lifestyle management through diet, tai chi, chi gong and meditation are recommended.

The source of disease is said to be related to one or more of the following three causes:

- Internal - emotional factors,

- External - climatic conditions, and miscellaneous

- Injury, diet, fatigue, exercise, and our constitution.

The goal of all practitioners of Chinese Medicine is to improve the patient's overall wellbeing – body, mind and spirit, rather than merely treating symptoms. Treatments are designed to balance a patient's chi.

A patient's overall health is evaluated to find the cause of illness. The initial visit is usually about an hour and a half. Your practitioner will take your vital signs and examine your pulse and tongue, and perhaps do an abdominal palpation and facial diagnosis. Generally the acupuncture treatment takes about 20 minutes and then the practitioner may prescribe some Chinese herbs.

Origin and History: The exact origins of Chinese Medicine are rather vague as most of its developments took place before the appearance of written text. The Emperor, Shen Nung, is said to be the forefather of Chinese Medicine and he was born over 5400 years ago. He is stated to have written the great herbal, "Shen Nung Pan Tsao." and taught people how to raise crops, animals and to identify therapeutic herbs. His knowledge was handed down verbally through generations. The oldest medical book, the Huang Di Nei Jing - The Yellow Emperor's Classic of Internal Medicine - is attributed to the Yellow Emperor who is thought to have lived 4700 BC. Differing opinions date the book between 800 BC. and 200 BC.

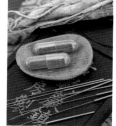

Applications:
Chinese medicine effectively treats addictions, allergies, arthritis, asthma, anxiety, chronic fatigue, cardiovascular, paralysis, gastrointestinal, gynecological and neuromuscular disorders, depression, headaches, immune system deficiency, migraines and stress.

Cautions: The herbal formulas usually consist of two or more herbs which target the symptoms as well as the underlying cause of the illness. The formulas may be taken as a tea, tincture, or in a capsule. Chinese herbs are quite potent and therefore should only be prescribed by a licensed practitioner. Even though the side effects are minimal while taking them, you should be monitored during the course of treatment. Special caution for herbs manufactured outside of the U.S. They may contain heavy metals.

Quick practitioner reference:

3000 Years Health Center

Acupuncture   Chiropractic   Chinese Herbal Medicine

Aternative Health Care for Maintaining A Balance And Healthy Life

We heal people everyday... that's what we do best.

We provide comprehensive natural health care with the following therapy:

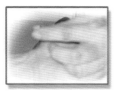

Herbal Medicine

*Acupuncture
*Moxibustion
*Cupping
*Facial Rejuvenation
*Therapeutic Massage
*Nutritional Supplements

*Herbal Medicine
*Nutritional Counseling
*Chiropractic
*Physio-therapy
*Exercise Programs

Acupuncture

For more information,
please contact us:

3000 Years Health Center
823 N. Broadway
Los Angeles, CA. 90012
Phone: 213-680-8754
Fax: 213-680-9385

www.3kyears.com

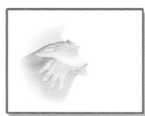

Chiropractic

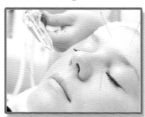

Facial Rejuvenation

Restore your MIND, BODY and SOUL.

Chiropractic

Body Alignment

What is Chiropractic? Chiropractic is a health care discipline which emphasizes the innate power of the body to heal itself without the use of drugs or surgery. The practice of chiropractic focuses on the relationship between the spine and the nervous system. The chiropractic adjustment removes any energetic disruptions or distortions which are caused by vertebral misalignments, referred to as subluxations. This restores the normal flow of nerve energy. The premise of chiropractic is that if the nervous system is healthy and functions well, then the other systems under its control will also be able to function optimally. The nervous system controls the respiratory, digestive, muscular and immune functions and includes the brain, spinal cord; the spinal nerves that exit the vertebral column through openings on the sides of each vertebra; and all the peripheral nerves that branch off to the organs, tissues, blood vessels and muscles. The foundation of chiropractic care involves: an emphasis on prevention through diet, exercise and lifestyle and the administering of nutritional products such as vitamins, minerals and herbs where necessary, manual adjustments, physical therapy and rehabilitation. Chiropractors are trained to diagnose all conditions and prescribe laboratory tests, MRIs and X-rays. They are required to refer patients to a specialist or other healthcare provider if the condition requires further treatment not in the scope of their practice.

The first visit lasts about one hour while subsequent visits are usually no more than twenty minutes. The patient is interviewed and a complete health history is given: past injuries and illnesses; current conditions, medications, lifestyle, stress levels, diet, exercise and sleep habits. During the physical exam, the chiropractor tests for flexibility and range of motion. If necessary, they may perform diagnostic tests, such as blood pressure and X-rays. Patients lie down on a low table on which the chiropractor performs the spinal manipulations. The spinal column is aligned by several low force thrusting motions. The chiropractor also may use or recommend massage or similar soft-tissue therapies. Some people experience some stiffness for a few days after the adjustment. Each condition is different and therefore the chiropractor will recommend the suggested frequency and number of visits.

Origin and History: The first recorded chiropractic adjustment was performed on September 18, 1895, by Dr. Daniel David Palmer, a Canadian-born magnetic healer. He "stumbled" across the technique when he cured a man suffering from deafness and acute back pain by realigning a displaced vertebra in his back. Palmer opened his chiropractic school-Palmer Infirmary and Chiropractic Institute - in 1897. However, some of the earliest healers in the history of the world understood the importance of having a healthy spine. "Get knowledge

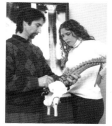

of the spine, for this is the requisite for many diseases," said Hippocrates. Chiropractic today, is second only to medicine as the largest primary healthcare modality in the western world.

Applications: Chiropractic is effective for acute and chronic low back pain, neck pain, headaches including migraines relating to sublaxations, sports injuries such as frozen shoulder, tennis elbow, carpal tunnel syndrome, digestive problems and menstrual and premenstrual pain which are frequently a result of impeded nerve functions, asthma and most musculoskeletal disorders.

Cautions: Individuals with bone fractures or infections, advanced osteoporosis, acute arthritis, and tumors should avoid chiropractic therapy in areas affected. Patients should have caution with chiropractic if they are experiencing numbness, tingling, or other neurological problems. In these cases be sure to ask the doctor if it is alright for you to be treated.

Insurance: Many plans cover treatment.

Quick practitioner reference:

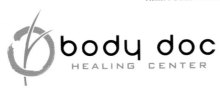

Dr. Paul D'Alfonso joined the holistic facility of Body Doc Healing Center to expand the level of services and to share the Body Doc vision to treat patients with love & service.

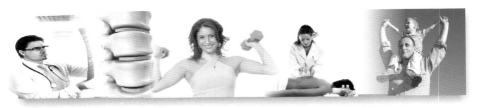

Dr. Paul offers the perfect blend of Eastern and Western medical philosophy. "Organic Healing" is achieved in this 10.000 sq. foot state-of-the-art facility by combining his services with the best Chiropractors, Medical Doctors, Massage Therapists, Physical Therapists, Acupuncturists and Estheticians.

Dr. Paul D'Alfonso
serves patients with a Holistc Approach

- Chiropractic techniques for infants to seniors.
- Massage Therapy & Physical Therapy
- Stress Management & Pain Management
- Anti-aging & Hormone replacement
- Hyperbaric Oxygen Therapy & Laser Therapy
- Clinic for special needs children
- Detoxification & Ionic Cleansing Footbaths
- 2,000 square foot Gym & Personal Trainers
- Natural whole food anti-oxidant supplements
- 2,600 square foot Training Conference Center

1924 B East Maple Avenue, El Segundo, CA 90245

(310) 546-6863

chiropractic - www.BodyDocChiropractic.com

supplements - www.Myviaoffice.com/DoctorPaul

One time use! **50%Off** Expiration 12/31/07

Receive 50% off of your first Hyperbaric Treatment + COMPLIMENTARY Neurological Scan

---

One time use! **$99.00** Expiration 12/31/07

Receive the package of 3 Ionic Detoxification footbath (regularly is $169) for $99 + COMPLIMENTARY Neurological Scan

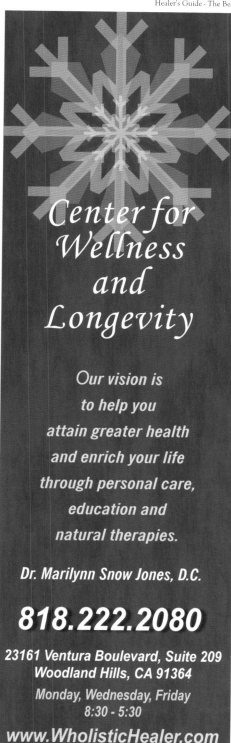

Center for Wellness and Longevity

Our vision is to help you attain greater health and enrich your life through personal care, education and natural therapies.

Dr. Marilynn Snow Jones, D.C.

818.222.2080

**23161 Ventura Boulevard, Suite 209
Woodland Hills, CA 91364**

Monday, Wednesday, Friday
8:30 - 5:30

www.WholisticHealer.com

Non-Force Chiropractic

Manipulation and Applied Kinesiology
With the understanding that the structures of your body influence its function, we have a wide variety of gentle, safe techniques to restore balance in your spine, musculature, and even your visceral (abdominal) organs.

NAET

(Nambudripad's Allergy Elimination Techniques)
NAET is a successful, drug free, natural treatment which allows your brain to reinterpret what is used to think was a poison, seeing it now as a harmless, acceptable substance, leaving you allergy-free. NAET elimination is achieved by a combination of acupressure, spinal manipulation, kinesiology and energy medicine.

EFT

(Emotional Freedom Techniques)
EFT is an easy, powerful technique that provides freedom from pain and the limitations caused by emotional, mental and physical stressors. You can receive help with variety of issues such as: phobias, pain, insomnia, smoking, weight loss, depression, panic, PTSD/abuse and headaches, to name a few.

"My 6-year old daughter had many ear infections and nothing helped. I worked with Dr. Jones, who not only stopped the pain, but eliminated the allergy through NAET."
-Diane N.

"I was diagnosed with Fibromyalgia, and the pain decreased through EFT. I am so pleased. I even have more freedom of movement."
-Judi L.

- Chiropractic
- Acupuncture
- Massage Therapy
- Clinical Nutrition
- Nature's Pharmacy
- Metabolic Screening
- Amino Acid Therapy
- Bio Cranial

Dr. Marilynn Snow Jones is a top holistic health practitioner who has specialized in Non-Force Chiropractic for over 20 years. Other areas of expertise include over 15 years of NAET experience, weight loss, clinical nutrition, detoxification, kinesiology, EFT and energetic healing.

Allergy Relief
By Marilynn Snow Jones, D.C.

How many of us live our lives with the following symptoms: fatigue, sleeplessness, depression, irritability, digestive disturbances, headaches, migraines, skin disorders, sinus congestion, and pain? Many of these symptoms may be due to allergies. Some of the main symptoms are due to inhalants, things we come in contact with, or the food we eat. There are environmental factors such as chemicals, pollutants, pesticides, heavy metals, household products, fertilizers, and sprays as well as dust, molds, pollens, and animals. Another cause of allergies are the things we ingest, these are generally the foods, vitamins, and minerals we consume on a daily basis. When you find yourself with any of these symptoms or exposures, there is something you can do to help lessen the reaction.

The most sensible change in your life would be to start a nutritional, anti-inflammatory diet and to address your allergy symptoms with a health care professional. One of the biggest problems we have is that the majority of us structure our diets around convenience or fast foods. They contain the most inflammatory nutrients available, unhealthy vegetable oils, trans fats, and high ratios of omega 6 oils. This standard American diet deprives you of the anti-inflammatory and anti-oxidants benefits you receive from fruits and vegetables.

What you are trying to do is create an environment in your body that is very alkaline. There are two types of food, acidic and alkaline. You will get the most anti-inflammatory reactions by staying in the 70% alkaline range of foods you eat. What are the acidic foods? They are mainly sugars, grains and proteins. Because we need protein to sustain life, we must eat healthy meats. That means the basic foods we should stay away from are all sugars and most grains. You need to consume fresh fruits, vegetables, and seeds. Another important nutrient we

need is omega 3 oils. You need a good balanced oil supplement and if you consume wild caught fish and grass fed beef, you will round out a balanced diet. When you consume this type of food source, you allow your body to have building blocks of anti-inflammatory compounds. Your immune system will calm down, and the things you come in contact with or items you ingest will have a lesser reaction and your symptoms will decrease.

Allergies on the other hand, must be addressed by a health care professional who is trained in allergy elimination. There are new, natural alternative ways to reduce and eliminate a majority of allergy symptoms.

Case Study:
A female patient came into my office complaining of headaches, classic allergy symptoms, joint pain, fatigue, sciatica and excessive weight. She had many absences from work and had difficulty completing simple tasks because of her condition. She was an avid yoga enthusiast, but her performance was limited by her pain. We started by addressing her allergy symptoms with a natural, proven technique. During this time, we also eliminated sugars and grains in her diet. This forced her into eating vegetables, fruits, proteins, plus a balance of beneficial oils. She found she was losing weight, she had more energy and her headaches disappeared. When she went to her yoga class, she noticed her joint pain and sciatica were greatly relieved. This is not an exceptional case. The majority of people find themselves feeling better by following these simple dietary rules and by eliminating allergic pollutants.

Sometimes taking good care of our bodies can be confusing. It is important to consult with a healthcare professional and learn the optimum way to healthy diets, proper exercise, and allergy prevention.

www.wholistichealer.com
See Ad on page 235

Colon Therapy

Hydrotherapy

What is Colon Hydrotherapy? Also known as colon therapy, colonics or colon irrigation, is a gentle and safe infusion of water into the colon for thorough cleansing. There are a variety of symptoms which indicate an unhealthy colon, including constipation, diarrhea, abdominal pain, bad breath, body odor, abdominal gas, confusion, bloating, irritability, skin blemishes, frequent headaches, backaches and fatigue. The average adult is said to possibly have between 10-25 pounds of dried fecal matter in his/her colon.

After completing a health history form and consulting with the colon hydrotherapist, the client is draped, lies on a colon therapy table and a small disposable speculum about ½ inch in diameter, is inserted into the anus. Then, approximately 20 gallons of warm, clean water is slowly released, in a continuous flushing process, in and out of the colon, freeing the toxic waste. During the treatment the therapist may apply a light massage to the abdominal area to facilitate the process. The client may feel some discomfort in the abdomen area or cramping if there is impacted fecal matter or gas pockets.

The water causes the muscles of the colon to contract repeatedly, called peristalsis, which pushes the feces out through the hose into a closed waste system. Colon therapy prevents toxic absorption through the intestinal wall and strengthens the peristaltic action of the colon assisting the colon to return to its natural shape and functional ability. The session takes about one hour.

Origin and History: Colon Hydrotherapy is said to have been used as early as 1500 BC. Colon irrigation became popular in the late 1800s and early 1900s as a treatment for autointoxication. John Harvey Kellogg, M.D., founder of the Kellogg cereal company, was one of the earliest known advocates of colonics. By the 1930s, most physicians no longer believed in autointoxication. As laxatives grew in popularity, colonics became less popular. Many holistic healthcare professionals recommend colonics. Colonics have regained their popularity as of late.

Applications: Colon Hydrotherapy is used primarily for relief of constipation. Constipation caused by poor diet and lack of fiber and water, can lead to many health problems, prevent the absorption of nutrients and create an environment where harmful bacteria, yeasts and parasites can thrive. The toxins and waste may be reabsorbed through the colon wall and enter the bloodstream causing autointoxication. Fecal matter often accumulates and hardens in the colon and may increase the risk of colon cancer. Colon Hydrotherapy removes accumulated waste from the colon, preventing constipation and improving health.

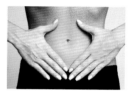

Research: The brain is profoundly influenced by impulses coming from a distended bowel. There are reflexes from the colon that affect the entire nervous system. There is a vast overlap of neuropeptide activity in the gut and the brain (Pert et al., 1985). As early as 1907, B. Robinson documented the vast and complex nervous system of the abdominal viscera. The enteric nervous system has become an active area in physiological research with over 600 articles listed on Medline since 1985. Modern medicine recognizes the involvement of the abdominal nervous system in several neurological disorders, including migraine, epilepsy, and autism (McMillin et al., 1999). *www.meridianinstitute.com/reports/colonic1.html*

Cautions: The following conditions are contraindicated - pregnancy during the first and third trimester, severe hemorrhoids, Crohn's disease, ulcerative colitis, heart disease, abdominal hernia, gastrointestinal cancer, recent colon surgery, and intestinal tumors. Nausea may be present following a treatment. After colonics it is very important to replenish the healthy colon bacteria, with food supplements called probiotics.

Quick practitioner reference:
Holistic Medical Center - page 28
Ione Linker - page 238

Linker
Elemental Healing
Unlimited

Ayurveda

Yoga

Massage

Colon Hydrotherapy

Rebirthing Breathwork

Flower of Life Workshops

Ione Linker, Clinical Ayurvedic Specialist, Intern

(310) 951-5138
ionelink@netzero.com

Cranial Sacral

~

What is Cranial Sacral Therapy?

Cranial Sacral Therapy is a gentle method of enhancing and balancing the functioning of the craniosacral system which is comprised of the membranes and cerebrospinal fluid that mobilizes, surrounds and protects the brain and spinal cord. Its reach extends from the bones of the skull, face and mouth all the way down to the sacrum. The role of the cranial sacral system relates to the development and performance of the brain and spinal cord. Any imbalance in it can cause sensory, motor and/or neurological disabilities.

Cranial sacral therapy is practiced by practitioners trained in the healing art. Many massage therapists and body workers also add this modality to their repertoire of skills. The technique restores the natural movement between the twenty-two bones of the skull and aids the circulation of the cerebrospinal fluid throughout the central nervous system and dissipates the stress, thereby healing the nervous system. This dissipates the body's stress. The cranial sacral system assists the body with its natural healing ability.

The vital energy coming into the human body produces distinct subtle rhythms. The cerebrospinal fluid has a particular rhythm of expansion and contraction. These cranial rhythmic impulses move at a cycle between 8 and 14 times a minute. The rhythm and restrictions are easily felt by the trained practitioner who lightly touches areas or key body points on the head, spine and sacrum. The practitioner is then able to evaluate the flow and apply slight movements and pressure to release restrictions, balancing the flow and thus improving the functioning of the central nervous system.

Origin and History: The presence of the subtle rhythms of the body on which cranial sacral therapy is based was discovered by osteopath Dr. William Sutherland over 100 years ago. He discovered that cranial

sutures have small degrees of motion. He concluded that the movements were produced by the body's inherent life force, which he referred to as the "Breath of Life." and that the motion of cranial bones is closely connected to the subtle movements involving a network of tissues, cerebrospinal fluid, central nervous system, the membranes surrounding the central nervous system and the sacrum. The healing art was further pioneered and popularized by osteopathic physician, John Upledger, D.O., following extensive scientific research from 1975 to 1983 at Michigan State University, which confirmed Dr. Sutherland's theory. The technique is based on Cranial Osteopathy.

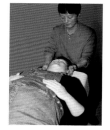

Applications:

Patients with soft tissue injuries, chronic pain, sinusitis, asthma, ear-nose-throat problems as well as muscle tension, migraine headaches, chronic back and neck pain, scoliosis, sciatica, vertigo, TMJ, dyslexia, autism, central nervous system disorders, stress related disorders, neuro-vascular disorders, brain and spinal cord injuries, autism, learning disabilities, fibromyalgia, benefit from therapeutic sessions. It is highly recommended for those with head or spinal injuries resulting from an accident. It is ideal for infants and newborns with birth trauma, due to the light touch used (the weight of a coin).

Cautions: Acute aneurysm and cerebral hemorrhage are contraindicated.

Insurance: May cover treatment if combined with other medical practices. Check with your provider.

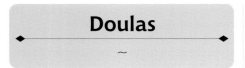

Doulas

~

What is a Doula: A birth doula is a healthcare practitioner and supportive companion professionally trained to provide labor support to the mother. Doulas are present during births in hospitals, birthing centers and at home. They work in cooperation with the Ob-Gyn physicians, nurses and mid-wives. They provide education in the prenatal period, during labor and birth and are familiar with all alternatives and options to help parents make informed decisions. Doulas provide physical, emotional, educational and practical support to the mother-to-be and her partner during labor and birth. Their role and acceptance is rapidly growing. Doulas do not provide clinical duties or diagnose. A doula's knowledge and experience covers the areas of recovery, breast feeding and infant care and does not extend into the area of physical exams or fetal assessment. Doulas attend both medicated and unmedicated births. A doula's support begins at the start of labor until two hours following the birth.

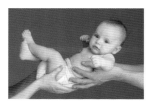

Doulas understand the physiology of the birth process and the emotional needs of women. While medical staff comes in and out of the birthing room during labor, and the doctor comes in just prior to the birth, doulas remain by the side of the mother-to-be throughout the entire labor, helping with breathing, relaxation, positioning and massage. Some doulas are trained in special massage techniques, acupuncture, visualization techniques and more. They also facilitate communication between the laboring woman, her partner and the clinical care providers. Faced with the fears and uncertainty of labor, many women find reassurance in having a doula by their side. Having a Doula boosts confidence and takes the pressure off of the husband or partner. The chances of having a healthier and more empowering birth are improved.

After delivery, a *postpartum doula* will provide in-home support. Their care focuses on the well-being of the mother and they provide advice, support and assistance with baby care, household chores and other light duties. They are hired on an hourly basis and will support, listen, and answer any questions the new mother may have.

Origin and History: The word, "doula," comes from ancient Greek meaning "woman's servant." Throughout history and in much of the world today, women have supported women through labor and birth, giving massage and providing continuous emotional support.

Applications: Women with high-risk pregnancies, teenager mothers, women with a history of abuse or psychiatric problems and single women all benefit greatly from a doula's service.

Research: Research has found that women who have one-on-one professional labor assistance tend to have shorter labors, fewer complications, and healthier newborns. It has been demonstrated that mothers who have this support produce lower levels of stress hormones during labor than women in strictly clinical situations. The risk of having a cesarean section, forceps delivery, or episiotomy drops. The ability to cope with the pain improves, decreasing the possibility of needing pain medication. The relationship with a partner is likely to grow stronger. Women are more likely to be confident in their mothering skills and be more successful with breast-feeding. Statistics include: 50% reduction in cesarean rates; 25% shorter labor; 60% reduction in epidural requests; 40% reduction in oxytocin (pitocin) use; 30% reduction in analgesia use; 40% reduction in forceps delivery.

Insurance: Some insurance plans may cover care. Check with your provider.

Quick practitioner reference:

Childbirth
at home...

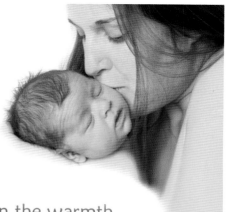

Give birth to your baby in the warmth, love and comfort of your own home.

it's safe,
it's natural,
it's empowering!

We provide homebirth and womens health care services to the greater Los Angeles area.

Call today for more information:

310.278.6333

TLC *Tender Loving Childbirth*
Midwidery Care and Womans Health Center

www.tenderlovingchildbirth.com

Energetic Balancing

~

What is Energetic Balancing? Energetic balancing is the scientific application of energy healing. According to Einstein's physics, all of the "stuff" in the universe is energy - energy moving, or vibrating, at different frequencies. Quantum physics presents the theory that all that energy comes in small packages called quanta, and that each quanta has a distinct frequency, and that those frequencies can be read and affected. Energetic balancing includes a number of different techniques and technologies including quantum biofeedback. Energetic balancing often works in conjunction with homeopathy to support the healing process. Sound, color, light and energy of varying frequencies may be transmitted through a practitioner's hands to the client or via cutting-edge scientific equipment. This rebalances the physical and subtle energetic bodies. These technologies also operate in the realms of the subtle and spiritual worlds. Humans are energetic beings living in a world of subtle energies, within gravitational and magnetic fields. Every function of our body is affected by outer stimuli. The goal of energetic balancing is to realign the individual to restore harmony with the universal lifeforce.

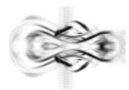

Quantum technology (Quantum Biofeedback) evaluates energy, blockages and dysfunction in the energy field and supplies safe, accurate, subtle and powerful healing frequencies which positively affect the subtle energy field and raise the lifeforce of the human body. Quantum technology identifies imbalances through their frequency by measuring electrical conductivity at responsive points (meridian points) on the skin - typically on the hands and feet. Twenty of these meridians end on the hands or the feet. Everything - every thought, emotion, disease, pathogen, parasite or toxic chemical has its own frequency which can be "read" by quantum field scientific equipment. The client assumes a co-creative role with the practitioner. Some people notice the changes during the session, but many changes occur within the next several days.

Origin and History: Royal Raymond Rife was a scientist born in 1888 and died in 1971. After studying at Johns Hopkins, Rife developed technology which is still commonly used today in the fields of optics, electronics, radiochemistry, biochemistry, ballistics, and aviation. He developed the world's first virus microscope and the Universal microscope. Rife invented a technology which was able to measure specific frequencies. He also discovered the frequencies which specifically destroyed herpes, polio, spinal meningitis, tetanus, influenza, cancer and other dangerous disease organisms. Similar technology has been invented and developed since then by several manufacturers.

Applications: Works on the subtle levels to effectively address many problems on the physical, mental, emotional and spiritual levels. The results are reported to be enhanced balance, greater circulation of lifeforce energy, pain relief, increased rate of healing, reduced stress and anxiety, relaxation, improved sense of wellbeing, increased mental clarity and emotional stability. Distance-healing and healing for pets.

Research: In 1934, the University of Southern California appointed a Special Medical Research Committee to bring terminal cancer patients from Pasadena County Hospital to Rife's San Diego Laboratory and clinic for treatment. The team included doctors and pathologists assigned to examine the patients - if still alive - in 90 days. After the 90 days of treatment, the Committee concluded that 86.5% of the patients had been completely cured. The treatment was then adjusted and the remaining 13.5% of the patients also responded within the next four weeks. The total recovery rate using Rife's technology was 100%. Unfortunately, the original Rife technology has been destroyed and the machines that are available now are only an approximation, with some probably more efficacious than others.

Quick practitioner reference:

EMC2 - page 243
My Bio Body - page 246

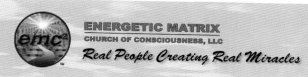

ENERGETIC MATRIX
CHURCH OF CONSCIOUSNESS, LLC
Real People Creating Real Miracles

AIM PROGRAM OF ENERGETIC BALANCING

■ EMC²'s AIM Program of Energetic Balancing provides balancing energies to help you remove your subtle energy imbalances. More than 40,000 people worldwide have participated in the AIM program. AIM stands for All Inclusive Method, a comprehensive spiritual technology for delivering focused healing prayer which specifically addresses your imbalances. Twenty-four hours a day, seven days a week, you receive all the balancing energies that have been revealed to EMC². This spiritual process is performed by making subtle energy balancing frequencies available to your photograph. Based on the holographic principle, your photograph acts as an energetic surrogate for your energy pattern.

■ Scholarships for the AIM Program are available for individuals with the frequency of autism or Down Syndrome.

■ EMC² (Energetic Matrix Church of Consciousness, LLC) believes that imbalances in subtle energy impede the flow of lifeforce and that you can heal yourself by removing these imbalances. This allows free-flowing life force to manifest wholeness, creativity and wellness in all areas of your life, including spiritual, emotional, mental and physical. Stephen Lewis, Evan Slawson and Roberta Hladek formed EMC² in 1998 to assist in healing the planet, one energetic being at a time.

● *My prostate had been enlarged for at least 20 years. I just returned from having a physical and the doctor told me that my prostate was small, like the prostate of a 20 year old. I believe the AIM Program is wonderful.*

● *Depression runs in my family and I used to get depressed for seemingly no reason at all. Now, I don't get depressed about anything. AIM's been a life-changing phenomenon for me mentally, spiritually and physically.*

● *I just wanted to pass something on to you that I think is a result of my self-healing through the AIM Program. I have a family history of high cholesterol and in December 2003, my total cholesterol was 198. After 8 months on the program, my cholesterol was 163.*

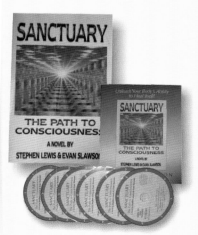

WOULD YOU LIKE TO...
HAVE MORE ENERGY?
HAVE BETTER HEALTH AND WELL-BEING?
HAVE BETTER RELATIONSHIPS?
BE MORE SUCCESSFUL?
FULFILL THE PURPOSE OF YOUR LIFE?

Learn more about the AIM program of Energetic Balancing and discover your self healing powers...

Order your FREE Information Kit !

1-877-500-3622
EnergeticMatrix.com

The Technology of Healing
An Interview With Stephen Lewis

*I*n *May of 2003, Stephen Lewis, co-founder of Energetic Matrix Church of Consciousness, LLC (EMC²) was interviewed by Vermont-based economist and ecologist Susan Meeker-Lowry, author of "Economics As If the Earth Really Mattered" and "Invested in the Common Good."*

Susan Meeker-Lowry: I'd like to start with some basic questions about the AIM Program and the process of energetic balancing. What are they and how do they work?

Stephen Lewis: AIM stands for "All-Inclusive Method." It is a spiritual technology, the purpose of which is to remove energetic imbalances which impede the flow of the life force. These imbalances exist in what we call the Energetic Matrix, or the higher self or true self. Participants' photographs are placed on the QID (the computerized Quantum-Consciousness Imprinting Device), which is referred to as being "on the tray." Subtle energy balancing frequencies are applied to the person's photo which are transmitted via the photo directly to the participant. The balancing energies are used by the participant's higher self to neutralize energetic imbalances.

Tell me more about these frequencies.

Everything is energy. You, me, trees, emotions, illnesses, everything. And everything vibrates at a unique frequency, including diseases. For every imbalance there is a frequency that will neutralize it. AIM delivers thousands of balancing frequencies for both physical and karmic (hereditary) energetic imbalances. It also delivers special activating frequencies that enable your higher self to select those frequencies you need, and ignore those you don't need. That is also

true for enhancing frequencies that help increase your lifeforce and your ability to respond to energetic crises.

You give the frequencies the names of illnesses, yet you don't actually cure illnesses?

I have never been given so much opportunity for so many disclaimers in one sentence. I am truly blessed. First of all everything does have a frequency, including diseases; however, there is no acceptable proof that the frequency of the disease is actually the disease. In this country there are very specific laws about how diseases may be diagnosed. We use no acceptable diagnostic technique. We make no claims as to disease nor are we permitted to do so. On the other hand, I believe we are the authority on energetic imbalances. If we find an energetic imbalance associated with a disease in units of consciousness, we say just that, you have that imbalance in your consciousness. As to your next politically incorrect statement,

Susan, EMC² does not cure anything. In fact we don't heal anything either. What we do very simply is help YOU heal yourself. Of course, no one else can heal you but you. Our holographic technology simply forces you to focus on your healing without cessation.

Why do you use a photo?

Photos are easier to identify, and easier to store than blood, spit or hair. Are you familiar with holograms?

They're three dimensional pictures and any piece of the hologram contains the whole?

Right. The holographic principle is a concept in physics. Thus anything that is unique to you, including your photograph, contains all existing information about you at any level. I could use hair or spit or blood or a tooth, but photos are easier to work with, and less invasive.

So it seems that the indigenous people who won't let their picture be taken because they believe it will steal their soul were on to something.

These so-called primitive people understand the holographic principle. And, most importantly, they live it. They can't do the math but so what? I think it is worth noting that the holographic principle is a contemporary name given to a spiritual reality that is fundamental and basic to human consciousness. As such, it provides an indestructible link between science and spirituality. To me, the hologram is our path to the God particle.

EMC² stands for The Energetic Matrix Church of Consciousness. Why do you consider it a religion?

Because what we do is in the realm of healing, as opposed to the realm of curing, it must have a designation that indicates that distinction. Treating and curing proceed from the outside, in. Healing begins at that deep, dark, dense mass that is within us and brings it to the outside, to the light...of consciousness.

You said you were guided to discover AIM. How?

I've been fascinated by energy all my life. I've studied Oriental medicine, philosophy, and religion which are based entirely on energy. In fact, among my degrees, are those in acupuncture and homeopathy and I knew, intuitively, that if everything is energy, then anything can be changed. I also understood that consciousness creates the way we live, our well-being, our ill-being, etc. So, I realized that to implement and use this knowledge, I'd have to find a method of measuring life in units of consciousness. That was my goal, that was my vision, and eventually it was my revelation. And the revelation came to me, I believe, because of that prolonged, sustained vision. I think that's the link between vision and revelation.

Was this a process of many years?

Oh absolutely. It still is. The book, Sanctuary, is just a coalescence of things, "thus far." The vision was the basis, the revelation is the continuing fruition. I take no credit for this revelation of how to measure life in units of consciousness. It came from a higher source. I understood that consciousness creates your ill-being or well-being.

The best examples are the studies of people with multiple personality disorders (MPD). Take something as concrete as diabetes. It's sugar in the blood. It's material stuff. Now when these people who have MPD shift personalities, in an instant, not in the 120 days it takes to make red blood cells, they are no longer diabetic. This has been documented countless times. The diabetes was created by a particular consciousness, and once that was no longer present the manifestation of diabetes disappeared. Then when they went back to the first personality, immediately, the blood was diabetic again. The second personality may have had hemorrhoids, but that's a different personality's problem. Think about that for a second.

How would you define healing?

Healing is the process of using your consciousness and elevating it to remove imbalances that are created by a lower level of consciousness. That lower level of consciousness was inevitably created by the manifestation of a failure, a failure of the courage required to feel something emotionally painful. That's the basis of why only you can heal yourself. No healer can heal you. That doesn't change the fact that healers are the most important people in our lives. But, they don't heal anyone. Only you can heal you.

For more information about energetic balancing, contact EMC² at
1-877-500-3622
www.energeticmatrix.com

See Ad on page 243

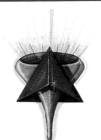

'Energy is Life'
Stress = Disease
De-Stress, Feel Better!

Balance & Wellbeing Can Happen by Choice... What will you Choose?

- Preventative Aging
- Identify & Clear Toxins
- Trauma & Anxiety Reduction
- Menopause Alleviation
- Pain Management
- Address Electro Environment
- Increase Cellular Vitality
- Healthier Organs
- Quality Energy & Better Sleep
- Improve Circulation & Brain Function
- Feel Centered & Balanced

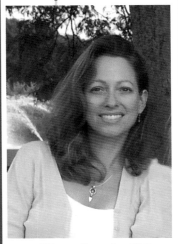

Diana Carsola, CBT

Located on
Sepulveda at National

what we resist persists...

Book a Session Today
310-202-0295

"Practitioner of Quantum Biofeedback Technology"
www.mybiobody.com   info@mybiobody.com

Quantum Physics... Ancient Healing... Modern Technology...

1) Did You Know? Children are more vulnerable to CELL PHONES and 'EMF' radiation due to their scull-thickness still growing and maturing?

2) Did you Know? Today's Processed Foods are Toxic. The 7 Principles of Health: Fresh Air & Sunshine, Water, **Whole Foods**, Walking, Relationships, Passion, a Good Night's Sleep.   **Learn What You Can Do for Protection.

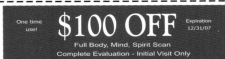
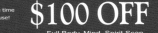

"Hook Me Up" - Quantum Biofeedback and Electrophysiological Reactivity
by Diana Carsola, CBT

Stress is linked to six of the leading causes of death: heart disease, cancer, lung ailments, accidents, cirrhosis of the liver, and suicide. Learning about stressors and the management of them by alleviating the cumulative factors associated with today's electronic environment is the most positive action toward preventative health care you will ever make. Our autonomic nervous system containing the sympathetic (fight or flight) and parasympathetic (regenerative) branches are in desperate need of balance, especially when we live in cities. Understanding how our nervous system functions, gives us clear clues on how to nurture our health, state of mind, and inspirations.

After having seemingly unrelated ailments and hospital visits for 15 years, (at the age of 40) I was diagnosed with Lupus and discovered cysts on my ovaries and cervix. Realizing that traumatic experiences, some lifestyle choices and care giving for years may have contributed to my disease. This was my wake up call to create the possibility of a life, that I love, and truer wellbeing. In order to achieve this, I had to regain my personal responsibility for my thoughts, words, actions and preventative care.

I had studied The Healing Tao, Ayurveda and herbal remedies for many, many years. These experiences and the passion for Quantum Physics have played a key role in my choice not to have taken any steroids or medication for Lupus, to date. Needless to say, when I discovered Quantum Biofeedback, I realized the possibilities, "Got Hooked Up" and have since shrunk my cysts and further balanced stressors that induce Lupus flair ups before the physical signs manifest - by 88% so far. I let go of a business I'd had for 20 years and became a qualified practitioner, certified in Quantum Biofeedback Technology and have dedicated my life to further education, while serving and encouraging others in their discoveries of preventative care and truer wellbeing.

The premises of Quantum Biofeedback Therapy are that the body is electrical in nature, innately intelligent, and has the ability to heal itself if the right conditions or stimuli are provided. The testing capabilities of today's energetic devices such as the EPFX/SCIO system can be invaluable in detecting deep levels of stress, not only physical, but also mental, emotional, nutritional, metabolic and electro-pollution stressors. Imagine an ultra-sophisticated devise that combines biofeedback procedures with the most advanced, up-to-date technology for scanning the human body, in much the same way as computer anti-virus scanning software.

Quantum Biofeedback is non-invasive, requiring five comfortable sensor straps for the wrists, ankles and forehead. The speed of Electrophysiological Reactivity lies at around the speed of ionic exchange (1/100 per second), and thanks to the speed of modern computers, this system is currently testing over 9,700 reactions in a 3-minute test. As neither the patient nor the operator is aware of which item is being tested, this is a truly comprehensive double-blind test. Once general patterns of stress have been verified, a qualified practitioner can readily observe which remedies, nutrients or therapies produce the most beneficial response. Therapists can thereby address the biological, psychological and etiological uniqueness of the individual in designing a therapeutic protocol.

Perhaps the greatest value, in this quantum leap of energetic technology, is in its ability to detect dis-ease or deficiency states before they manifest symptomatically. True 'Health Care' is preventative, and the role of a health practitioner is educative. Today's healthcare crisis presents an unprecedented opportunity for regaining responsibility. What a client is able to learn about their areas of risk, weakness or deficiency, can empower them to make informed decisions as to their own future health.

See Ad on page 246

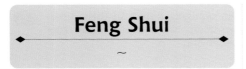

Feng Shui

~

What is Feng Shui? Feng Shui is the Art and Science of Environmental Energy Mastery. Feng Shui is rapidly becoming a standard healing practice for creating the ideal and balanced environment in which to live and work. Professional Feng Shui practitioners utilize and apply the laws of

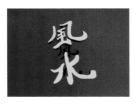

nature in order heal our homes and office environments.Feng Shui helps us to create balance and harmony in our personal space by promoting the flow of positive energy and neutralizing or minimizing negative or destructive energy. Feng Shui practitioners believe that taking care of our physical bodies is a good place to begin, but is not enough. It is extremely important to clear, cleanse and energize our surroundings. Our homes and offices have their own energetic pattern or energy flow which directly affect our lives on all levels.

In a typical Feng Shui assessment the practitioner will do a detailed interview and examination of the environment; she will have you fill out a questionnaire and provide a rough sketch of or plans; examine the seen and unseen influences; explain how they affect the client and others living or working in the environment; thoroughly assess both the supportive and obstructive influences on a physical and energetic level and share with you how to enhance or correct/minimize them; provide a detailed assessment of each room and the proper positioning of sleeping and working areas; provide a detailed explanation of all changes and make corrections if necessary.

Additionally, most feng shui practitioners will conduct a space clearing ceremony prior to making any adjustments. Space clearing is the removal

of all unhealthy energetic patterns or residues from an environment. This is achieved by utilizing a variety of powerful cleansing and energy techniques.

We all have a feeling nature which some people call it intuition or a "gut feeling." If you don't feel quite right in your home, or if you feel that since you have lived in a certain environment, you are not as happy, or if things are not going well, this is a good sign that the environment may not be supportive for you and that it needs to be corrected through Feng Shui. Another indicator is long lasting or chronic health problems, often for more that one person in the environment.

Origin and History: Feng Shui is a natural science and it's history goes back more than 2000 years. Feng Shui literally means Wind and Water. The oldest know writing on the subject of Feng Shui appeared in 25 A.D. during the East Han Dynasty. Feng Shui theory is primarily based on Yin/Yang theory. The Yin/Yang theory became very popular during the period from 770 BC to 475 BC, which indicates that Feng Shui originated from this same period.

Applications: When you move into a new home, apartment or office; annually or periodically - as a yearly cleansing and adjustment; during financial difficulty, before building a new home, in conjunction with interior design changes; during relationship difficulties; after a death in the family; when there is severe or chronic illness; before becoming pregnant/before childbirth; before embarking on a new career; when things are not manifesting in your life as you desire; to help the sale of a property.

Consider Feng Shui and environmental testing when experiencing fatigue and/or lowered immunity, blurred thinking, lack of focus, frequent colds, headaches, chronic cough, depression, irritability and anxiety. Some other indicators that feng shui may be required are: repeated negative thoughts and emotions; children having difficulty academically or socially; difficulties with relationships, creativity or finances.

Quick practitioner reference:

True Feng Shui - page 100

Holistic Dentistry

~

What is Holistic Dentistry? Holistic dentistry is also referred to as Environmental dentistry, Biological dentistry or Biocompatible dentistry. Holistic Dentists perform all traditional dental procedures in addition to holistic applications. The mouth is an integrated part of the entire body and an important indicator of overall health and many diseases can first be detected from the health of the gums and teeth. The goal is to remedy dental problems holistically, with as little impact on the rest of the patient's system. Curing the ills of the body often requires repairing teeth, removing mercury fillings, or treating gum disease. The health of the gums and teeth often require nutritional supplementation or dietary modifications.

Holistic dentists understand that each tooth is related to an acupuncture meridian and that each meridian is connected to an organ, vertebrae, gland, and a cranial nerve. When a tooth decays or contains toxic dental material the associated meridian may develop signs of dysfunction and if this state continues for some time, the meridian-related organ, nerves and vertebrae are affected and will show signs of distress.

Holistic dentists use biocompatible materials that will not adversely impact their patient's immune systems. Most holistic dentists test for bio-compatibility (how a material interacts with your body) for allergies and possible toxic reactions, prior to performing dental work.

Some common complications and their influence on the whole body system include: infected root canal-treated teeth have strong connection to the development of cancer and heart disease; pockets of gangrene in the jawbone are often found at the sites of previous extractions by conventional dentists; implants done without biocompatibility testing are related to auto-immune problems; periodontal-disease related infections affect health and may be related to heart disease.

Materials, ranging from most biocompatible to the least, include: Pure Gold is used for very small cavities; gold alloy is used on crowns and inlays. Gold or platinum are the most durable of filling materials lasting 20 years or more; Non-gold alloy is used for crowns and is less durable, expensive and biocompatible; Silver or Mercury Amalgam: a combination of silver, tin, copper, or zinc dissolved by elemental mercury which makes up 50% of the amalgam mass. Elemental mercury is a poisonous heavy metal and accumulates in body tissues affecting the central nervous system. Composites include a variety of materials and last about 6.5 years, some are biocompatible.

Applications:

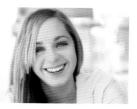

Consider holistic dentistry for all dental work. If your system is sensitive, or especially suceptible to stressors; or if you have symptoms of allergy or immune stress, then testing is recommended. Holistic dentistry offers alternatives such as acupuncture instead of anesthesia and is often used in conjunction with Osteopathy. Problems with the jaw joint such as TMJ, may involve the head bones, the neck, and spinal column; and spinal structural problems can effect the jaw, therefore holistic orthodontic dentistry is supported with orthopedic orthodontics, aligning the muscles and bones.

Research: Research demonstrates a connection between mercury and Alzheimer's and Lou Gehrig's Disease. Mercury vapor is released from the fillings and is absorbed very rapidly in the body, primarily by inhalation and swallowing. Direct correlations in autopsies have been found between the amount of mercury found in the brain and the number of mercury fillings. Mercury is able to pass through the placenta to an unborn baby and is more toxic than lead, cadmium, and even arsenic and small amounts can damage the brain, heart, lungs, organs and glands and suppress immunity

Cautions: Some dentists claim to be holistic but they are only mercury-free dentists. Holistic dentists follow safe mercury removal procedures.

Insurance: Most dental plans cover treatment.

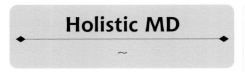

Holistic MD

~

What is a Holistic M.D.? Holistic medical doctors are physicians that have completed their post-graduate degree as either a medical doctor (M.D.), or a doctor of osteopathic medicine (D.O.) and their three-year residency. In addition, holistic medical doctors have several years of study and clinical training in one or more alternative therapies such as naturopathy, homeopathy, neurofeedback or biofeedback, nutrition, herbal medicine, chiropractic, and acupuncture. Additional alternative techniques such as Emotional Freedom Therapy, Kinesiology, Total Body Modification, and N.A.E.T are often used.

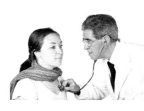

The services offered by a holistic medical doctor include a blend of conventional Western medicine and alternative medicine. Therefore the patient benefits from the technology and wisdom of both. Holistic medical doctors realize that no single healthcare modality has all the answers. The practitioner is devoted to treating the health of the whole person; their body, mind, emotions and spirit. Holistic medical doctors will continually upgrade their skills during their years of their practice, in the newest and most effective alternative methods of treatment for their patients.

During the first appointment with your holistic medical doctor you will have an in-depth discussion of your medical history and the appropriate diagnostic tests will be performed or scheduled. A first visit with a holistic medical doctor lasts approximately 1 – 1 1/2 hours. During the follow up visit the results are discussed and the most effective treatment methods based on your health problem and unique physiology are outlined. The doctor communicates openly with the patient regarding their options of treatment, both

alternative and western, outlines the pros and cons of each, and involves them with the decision-making process. Most holistic medical doctors gravitate towards using alternative methods as their primary treatment mode and use western medicine as long as it is not accompanied by harmful side effects, and often as a last resort. Treatment plans are tailored to each patient. A one-size-fits-all approach is not the signature of a holistic medical doctor. They educate patients thoroughly and discuss prevention and lifestyle, empowering them to take responsibility for the care of their health.

Applications: This approach is very effective at treating virtually any health problem. The more severe the disease, the more the services of a holistic medical doctor are invaluable. This type of care is suitable for anyone that believes in the healing power of the body and prefers a preventative and natural approach, using surgery and medication as a last resort; and for those who would like to heal chronic conditions for which western medicine offers only medication. Good examples of conditions which fall in the later category are cancer, HIV, high blood pressure, depression, PMS, diabetes, infertility, heart disease, chronic fatigue syndrome, fibromyalgia, lupus and digestive diseases.

Insurance: Covered by most insurance. Certain treatments and nutritional products are usually not covered.

Quick practitioner reference:

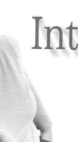

Integrative Medicine

WAEL ALOMAR, M.D.

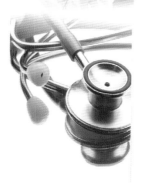

- The goal is not to give you more medication, but to reduce your medication through diet and natural remedies, and to treat the cause of your disease not the symptoms.

- Our patients are healthier, have fewer side effects to medication, and are less likely to be hospitalized or go to the emergency room.

- While you cannot put a price tag on health, we find that in addition to the tremendous health improvement, our patients save money when we reduce or eradicate their need for medications, or supplements.

Our practice includes but is not limited to:

- allergy
- heart disease
- asthma
- digestive diseases
- high blood pressure
- high cholesterol
- diabetes
- arthritis
- cancer
- lung disease
- kidney disease
- weight loss
- fibromyalgia
- fatigue
- headache
- sinusitis

Wael Alomar, M.D.
1752 Ocean Park Blvd.
Santa Monica, CA 90405
(310) 433-5249

For more information, please visit our website

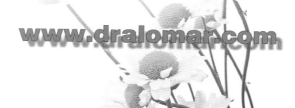

www.dralomar.com

Holistic Senior Care

~

What is Holistic Senior Care? Holistic Senior Care provides lifestyle enhancements for the elderly that enable them to live better by helping them to be physically healthier, mentally agile and more mobile at any age.

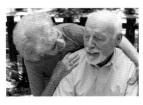

Holistic services which are beneficial to seniors for age-related difficulties include:

• Physical therapy, acupuncture, chiropractic and massage. These modalities are highly beneficial for rehabilitation, pain management and strengthening unused muscles. Practitioners will recommend appropriate exercise, stretching and balance training, following an assessment and treatment to keep the body active and limber. Physical therapy is especially effective for regaining functional abilities such as walking and for help to those who use assistive devices for physical movement.

• Neurofeedback treatments are excellent for maintaining, restoring and even increasing mental focus and agility. This is a great solution for seniors with a lack of interest in preparing and eating meals - a common problem.

• Nutritional practitioners will demonstrate how to prepare quick, easy and nutritious meals. They will also be able to address particular nutritional deficiencies and advise on proper dietary changes and supplementation.

• Naturopathic Doctors will assess and recommend herbs which are supportive for specific health issues. They will also advise particular lifestyle and management techniques.

• Holistic Medical Doctors will run the appropriate tests and be able to determine if there is an alternative treatment to support any existing health issues.

They will also determine if there are suitable alternatives that can be used in place of, or to reduce the amount of prescription medications.

• Energy healing therapies are effective and an important part of keeping the energetic components of the subtle body cleansed and functioning properly. As the physical body ages, the chakras tend to slow down and are not able to draw in as much prana or lifeforce. As the number of health conditions increases, there are more obstructions or diseased energies in the centers. This decreases the amount of prana absorbed, leading to overall weakness.

It is highly beneficial for seniors to have access to quality holistic care. Senior assisted living care is quite a new concept and holistic senior care is a rare service to come by. Senior assisted living offers medical and alternative services, proactively and reactively, combined with education and lifestyle management to retain and improve independence. Typically, there is a medical doctor or nurse on duty twenty-four hours a day. All of the staff are trained and experienced in working with the elderly and understand the complications that are associated with diseases specifically associated with aging such as heart conditions, post-stroke, alzheimers, parkinson's, diabetes, and impaired physical and mental functioning.

Fitness is emphasized and it is a necessary part of the daily routine, important for longevity, and is a critical factor in maintaining independence and activities. Lack of exercise leads to muscle mass loss, loss of range of motion and flexibility, cardiovascular endurance, and neuromuscular coordination The residents are encouraged to participate in walking, yoga, chi gong, tai chi and meditation, all of which are excellent for keeping the body, mind and spirit young and supple.

Insurance: Most private insurance plans cover care.

Quick practitioner reference:
Olympia Happy Home Care - page 253

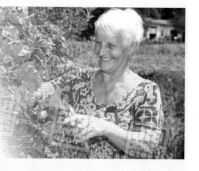

Olympia Happy Home Care

At Olympia Happy Home Care we not only understand the importance of individualized service but we also enforce quality training for our caretakers to ensure the best possible care for our elderly residents.

Our Integrative quality services include:

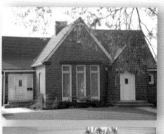

- **Programs for social & recreational activity**
- **Three nutritious meals, snacks, & special diets**
- **Supervision of medication & medical routines by RN**
- **Linen and personal laundry service**
- **24-hour quality care & supervision**
- **Ambulatory & non-ambulatory care**
- **Assistance with activities of daily living** (bathing, hygiene, etc)
- **Holistic Approach**

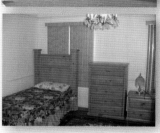

Specialized Services:

- **Dementia waiver for specialized care**

CPR Training/Program: As Red Cross Certified instructors, we also provide training seminars for caregivers (We also help the caregivers to increase their effectiveness by teaching them meditation, emotional freedom technique(EFT) and other helpful practices)

- **In-service training for staff to ensure up-to-date and quality care**

6446 San Vicente Blvd Los Angeles , CA 90048
Phone: (323) 273-8676 Fax: (323) 932-6508
www.olympiahappyhome.com

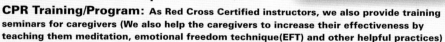

Homeopathy

~

What is Homeopathy? Homeopathy is an alternative medical system with its own approach for diagnosing, classifying, and treating. It is based on the premise that every person has a vital lifeforce, which when disrupted causes illness. Homeopathy stimulates the body's healing responses by ad-

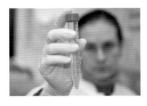

ministering small doses of substances called remedies, which if given to healthy individuals in large doses would produce the same symptoms of the disease. This is referred to as the "similia principle" or "like cures like." Remedies are derived from plants, minerals, or animals and prepared by diluting the substance. Vigorous shaking of the diluted substances makes the remedy more effective by extracting its vital essence. When the dilution is such that the substance's molecules are gone, the "memory" is held in the surrounding water molecules.

Treatment is tailored to each patient after evaluating symptoms, emotional and mental states, nutrition and lifestyle. During follow-up visits the patient's progress is assessed to determine further treatment.

According to a 1999 survey of Americans and their health, over six million Americans had used homeopathy in the preceding 12 months. Homeopathy is an integral part of the national health care systems Germany, the United Kingdom, India, Pakistan, Sri Lanka, and Mexico. In Europe, training in homeopathy is considered a primary professional degree with three years of study.

In the US, practitioners obtain their knowledge through diploma programs, certificate programs, and correspondence. Homeopathic training is part of the medical education of naturopathy. Homeopathy is generally practiced alongside other modalities in which the practitioner is licensed, such as conventional medicine, naturopathy, or acupuncture.

Applications: Homeopathy is used to treat the most acute and chronic problems. Practitioners experience good results with homeopathic remedies when treating yeast, bladder, sinus and ear infections, skin problems, allergies, headaches, asthma, eczema, anxiety, depression, chronic fatigue and autoimmune issues, autism, women's health issues such as PMS, menopausal symptoms and dysmenorrhea.

Origin and History: The term homeopathy comes from the Greek words homeo, meaning similar, and pathos, meaning suffering or disease. The concept and system of homeopathy was first developed in the 1700's in Germany by Samuel Hahnemann, a physician and chemist. He found that by eating cinchona bark used to cure malaria, he developed malaria-like symptoms. Homeopathy was introduced to the United States in 1825 by Hans Burch Gram and in 1835, the first homeopathic medical college was established. By the 20th century, eight percent of all medical practitioners in the US were homeopaths, with 20 homeopathic medical colleges and over 100 homeopathic hospitals.

Research: A Nuclear Magnetic Resonance (NMR) study showed that all twenty-three different homeopathic remedies and potencies tested had distinctive readings of submolecular activity, while the placebos did not. This demonstrates that homeopathy's function is not so much chemical but energetic. Published in the *Journal of Holistic Medicine*, 5 (Fall-Winter 1983).

Cautions: It is recommended that homeopathic remedies be recommended by a trained professional. Homeopathic remedies are regulated by the FDA.

Insurance: Insurance companies are more likely to cover homeopathy when the person providing the service is a licensed healthcare professional, such as an M.D. or D.O.

Quick practitioner reference:
Holistic Medical Center - page 28
Tender Loving Childbirth - page 241
Dr. Randy Martin - page 255

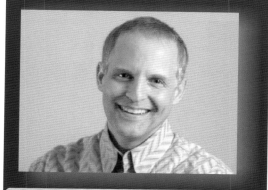
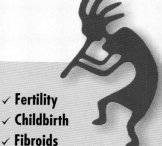

Premenstrual Syndrome
By: Dr. Randy Martin, O.M.D

What Is PMS? Premenstrual Syndrome is one of the most common health problems facing women. About one third of women experience some sort of PMS. This translates into a lot of missed days at school or work, severe stress on relationships, needless breakups and divorce, and suffering. I can't tell you how many times women have thanked me for literally saving their marriage. Symptoms of PMS begin as early as ten to fourteen days prior to the start of menstruation and end the first few days after the onset. There are more than 150 symptoms associated with PMS. Listed below are some of the most typical: irritability, anxiety, moodiness, anger, headaches, skin problems, vertigo, weight gain, chocolate craving, joint pain, back pain, cramps, constipation, diarrhea, sugar craving, sore throat, vision problems and bloating.

What Is The Cause of PMS? PMS is caused by both psychological and physiological imbalances. Psychologically, the primary cause is stress. Physiologically, the primary cause is an imbalance of estrogen and progesterone. Other secondary causes include poor diet, heredity, and lack of exercise. From the point of view of Oriental medicine, the primary meridian and energy systems involved with PMS in most women are the liver, spleen and kidneys.

General Treatments for PMS. Diet is the first and foremost factor that is within your control. Foods known to increase symptoms of PMS, which should be reduced or eliminated include: caffeine, milk, hard cheese, salt, chocolate, sugar, alcohol, beef, pork, lamb, and pickled foods. Foods helpful in reducing the symptoms of PMS which should be added to the diet are: whole grains, brown rice, oatmeal, millet, Pritikin-type breads with no added oils, salt or sugar; all vegetables, but especially beets, carrots, collard greens, mustard greens, and beet tops; fish, and all kinds of beans are your best sources of protein. Certain vitamin supple-ments are also helpful depending on your particular needs. The two most important are vitamin B6 for bloating and water retention; and magnesium for cramps and uterine pain. Vitamin C combats stress, as do all the B vitamins. A quality, well-rounded multiple high in vitamin B is a good preventative. If you suffer from cramps, be sure to take twice as much magnesium, as you do calcium. Also take evening primrose oil or black currant seed oil.

Can Homeopathy Help With PMS? For menstrual cramps there are a number of different remedies. *Colocynth* type of cramps are relieved by doubling up, bending forward, applying pressure or warmth, as are *Magnesium phosphoricum* cramps. Always stop taking the remedy if you feel worse or if the symptoms stop. When the symptoms decrease, also stop taking the remedy. If you keep taking the remedy after the symptoms stop, they will come back again. Note: often only one dose of the correct remedy, in the correct potency is all you need. Be sure to follow all the other rules listed. They can be found in the homeopathy section of my book, *Optimum Health.*

● For symptoms of fatigue or weakness, try *Calcium (carbonate).* This remedy will be particularly helpful if you also experience headaches, sweating and are cold in general. Also good for fatigue is *Sepia.* For Sepia to be indicated usually you will also have low back pains, lower abdomen cramping, loss of interest in sex, an increase in anger and intolerance for others. Depression and moodiness is common.

● For excessive weeping, sadness, or over sensitiveness, the primary remedy is *Pulsatilla.* Other indications for Pulsatilla are a desire for company, a desire to be outside or to have windows open, nausea, giddiness, fainting, and unpredictable or changeable moods. *Chamomile* is another remedy for excessive moodiness, with fault-finding and snapping over little things. It will also show symptoms of cramps that feel like labor pains. The *Lachesis* personality may be angry and moody with ovarian pains that are worse on the left side. Dizziness and diarrhea, a dislike for tight clothing, or anything tight around the neck, are characteristic of Lachesis.

See Ad on page 255

Hypnotherapy

~

What is Hypnotherapy? Hypnotherapy is a complementary therapy and a psychological healing tool, which facilitates change on the subconscious mental levels, by using the therapeutic application of hypnosis, as the primary technique. Hypnotherapy is used to treat somatic, psychological and behavioral illness by altering unwanted behavioral patterns and creating new ones. During the session, you are in a hypnotic state where you become physically, mentally and emotionally, relaxed. In this increased state of awareness you and your therapist are able to access your subconscious mind which is much more responsive to new ideas. When the subconscious is spoken to directly, it may be possible to reprogram old behavior patterns and introduce new ideas and positive suggestions. These positive suggestions may then help you to make the changes you desire. Hypnosis is gaining credibility as a valuable mental and psychological tool. Holistic doctors and dentists often refer their patients to hypnotherapists. Hypnotherapy has been approved as a method of therapy since 1958 by the American Medical Association.

A hypnotherapy session begins with a medical history and discussion of your treatment goals. The hypnotherapist acts as a guide, helping you to make the desired changes. To induce the state of deep relation, the hypnotherapist uses a variety of techniques such as deep breathing, muscle relaxation, imagery, or counting techniques. Contrary to misconceptions, you do not go into a deep sleep; the hypnotherapist cannot control your mind, and you will not say or do anything against your will.

The hypnotherapist then instructs new ideas and beliefs via visualization, suggestions and guided imagery, to your subconscious mind. During this time the part of your brain that is always analyzing is inert and will not be able prevent the new information from being received. At times you will be listening - especially while receiving these suggestions - and at other times you will be answering questions asked by the hypnotherapist.

When the session is complete, you will return to your fully conscious state and may feel very relaxed.

Origin and History: Franz Anton Mesmer (1734-1815), Austrian physician, is acknowledged as the 'Father of Hypnosis'. James Esdaile, a surgeon, operated on his patients using 'mesmeric sleep' as anesthetic in the 1840s. In 1843, the terms 'hypnotism' and 'hypnosis' were coined by James Braid (1795-1860), a Scottish surgeon. He found that subjects could go into a trance if they fixated their eyes on a bright object. His theory was that a sort of neurophysiological process was involved and he found that hypnosis was very useful in disorders where no 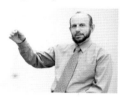 organic origin could be identified.

Applications: Hypnotherapy has been used effectively for a wide variety of problems including: stress management, smoking cessation, insomnia, addictions, phobias, fears, weight control, headaches, pain management, teeth grinding, dental procedures, and anxiety. Hypnotherapy is used to enhance self-improvement goals such as public speaking, self-confidence and to improve sports and academic performance.

Research: Hypnotherapy may decrease the pain and anxiety associated with invasive or uncomfortable medical procedures; this may allow for reduced use of medication(s) as was seen in a group of subjects undergoing interventional radiological procedures (Lang et al. 2000). Hypnotherapy can also improve recovery time, enhance intraoperative patient comfort by reducing anxiety and pain, and may help create optimal surgical conditions (Faymonville et al. 1998)

Cautions: Contraindications include personality disorders, psychosis (Vickers and Zollman 1999), and paranoia (Saichek 2000).

Quick practitioner reference:

Hypnotherapy

WHEN YOU ARE READY

to shift limiting beliefs and make rapid, powerful
and lasting core changes that can dramatically improve your life.
Increase your **confidence** in any situation
Enhance your **relationships**
Heal your past and create your future
Get over your **fears**
Change your body and your habits
and much more

Find out about **HYPNO*SPA**
body sculpting and breast enlargement using the power of your mind!

For a free phone consultation call

Regina Bardo, R.N., C.Ht., C.Mt.
Clinical Hypnotherapist, Certified Master Practitioner of NLP
Certified Master Practitioner of Time Line Therapy™
Certified Therapeutic Imagery Facilitator

(818) 633-4462
Regina.Bardo@hypnosis.edu • www.ReginaBardo.com

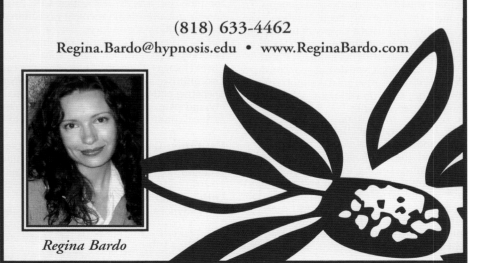

Regina Bardo

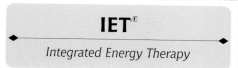

IET^Æ

Integrated Energy Therapy

What is Integrated Energy Therapy®? Integrated Energy Therapy is a powerful, hands-on, gentle energy therapy that focuses on personal empowerment. Integrated Energy Therapy is often referred to as Healing with the Energy of Angels. The philosophy of Integrated Energy Therapy is embodied in the word 'integrated' which was chosen because it conveys the healing vision of integrating the pain of the past, into the power of the present, to bring about the joy of the future. This healing modality is reported to use a divine angelic energy ray and works directly with one's 12-Strand Spiritual DNA. Working with the spiritual DNA clears ancient patterns and helps to facilitate one's evolution. This therapy can be used singularly or in conjunction with other healing arts modalities.

The objective of Integrated Energy Therapy is to provide safe, yet powerful, energetic support to release suppressed feelings, and their corresponding energy blocks and limited energy patterns from cellular memory which facilitates healing on all levels. Each session begins with a short discussion regarding the areas you would like to focus on during the healing. You then lie down, fully clothed, and relax on a massage table. The practitioner may or may not play relaxing music. Using gentle touch, the practitioner will allow and direct angelic healing forces to dissolve negative energy blocks. Some people may feel a slight sensation or warmth from the hands of the practitioner. At the end of the session, most clients feel relaxed and peaceful.

Integrated Energy Therapy® is an attunement-based energy therapy system. Clients may choose to become trained in it as it is easy to learn and practice. Then they are able to work on themselves, their family and their friends. The attunements are done in person by a certified Integrated Energy Therapy Master Instructor.

Origin and History: Steven Thayer is the creator of Integrated Energy Therapy®. He is also the founding director of the Center of Being, Inc. He is an ordained Interfaith Minister, an engineer, a certified Reiki Master and author of the book, *Interview with an Angel.* IET is currently being taught and practiced in over 25 countries around the world including the United States, Belgium, Canada, and Ireland.

Applications:

Complementary to western medical care to support rapid healing for all acute or chronic illness. The benefits of IET include: releasing

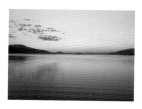

of deeply suppressed feelings; clearing of energy blocks that limit your health, abundance, relationships and creativity; understanding of your soul purpose; healing on physical, emotional, mental and spiritual level; increasing of intuitive abilities and connecting with guidance.

Insurance: Does not cover this form of therapy.

Quick practitioner reference:

Vicki Frederiksen - page 260

Integrated Energy Therapy™

Everything that we see, touch, hear, feel, and think is made up of energy

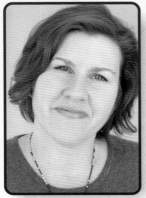

Vicki Frederiksen
Master Instructor

- *As a Certified IET Master Instructor,* Vicki Frederiksen uses powerful techniques to rebalance your energy system back to its natural state of health, ease, and joy.

- *Integrated Energy Therapy™ (IET) is* a safe, gentle, effective way to balance and empower your human energy field and your life. IET helps you release dysfunctional behaviors, thoughts and emotions rooted in the past, while reconnecting you with the possibility of living without fear or limiting beliefs now. Working beyond symptoms, IET always directs healing to the very deepest level of cause.

- *How IET Works:* Your physical body, thoughts and emotions are all comprised of energy. Everything exists in energy systems having vibrational qualities or patterns which can be changed. Blocks occur when your naturally balanced energy field contains negativity, trauma, distress, or fear. This restrictive quality creates dysfunctions limiting your experience of life, resulting in a lack of spontaneity, energy depletion, unrest, agitation or dis-ease. By systematically directing the Integrated Energy, blocks are released and the energy body is restored to its natural state of health and harmony.

Rebalance and Restore Well-Being, Health, Happiness, Purpose, Creativity, & Freedom

818.913.9692

www.energywellbeing.com

Integrated Energy Therapy
by Vicki Frederiksen, Certified IET
Master Instructor

I have been facilitating private Integrated Energy Therapy® sessions at weSpark, a local cancer support center, for three years. This has been a wonderful opportunity to work as a bridge: offering an alternative healing modality to support individuals in the midst of a medical challenge. There is cancer, and there is the person who is experiencing cancer. My purpose at weSpark is to offer healing to the person who is experiencing the challenge of cancer as a patient, survivor, or caregiver.

When a person is diagnosed with cancer, their entire life can change very suddenly. Often, their lives become a blur of doctor's appointments, opinions, medical reports, lab tests, insurance papers, life altering decisions, and questions. Schedules change; priorities change; relationships change; and life rhythms change. Cancer can easily move to the center of someone's life as all activities, resources and conversations begin revolving around the focus on a cure.

As an Integrated Energy Therapy® (IET) practitioner, I can never promise a cure. What I can do is offer healing to the individual who is seeking a cure. While doctors and medical establishments work with medications and procedures that target the cancer, I am able to effectively work with powerful energy balancing techniques that focus on the individual and their personal experience of stress, fear, pain, disharmony, frustration, disappointment and depression (to name a few). When I first began working at weSpark, it was remarkable to me that most clients were seeking support and healing around family dynamics, finances, creative blocks, and life purpose—really no different than clients in my private practice. The fact that few sessions at a cancer support center were actually focused on cancer, told me that the needs of a person with cancer are no different than what we all need to thrive: to feel safe, loved, and

necessary. Healing deep emotional trauma or fearful mis-perceptions that can create a fearful world, IET gently brings us into wholeness.

Using cancer as a metaphor for any personal crisis, we can seek healing at the level of symptoms or we can move deeper to the level of cause. Many of us have personal stories that explain why our "symptoms" exist and behaviors or habits that effectively manage these "symptoms." These stories and behaviors can begin to lull us into a false perception of who we are. True healing occurs when we look beneath the surface and stop identifying with our experiences: we are not our experiences. We are not our thoughts or emotions. Our experiences, thoughts and emotions are essential and rich, but they can not and do not define the truth of who and what we are. They can, however, lead us to the truth.

Healing is an inward journey of discovery. Every experience is here to lead us deeper into the truth of the power of love. We are given countless opportunities to realize that we are the very creation and inspiration of love itself. This love is not passive or conditional. This love is powerful - the very life force that flows through us and around us. This love is the source of fearlessness and wholeness. This love is intelligent and wise, beyond our understanding. The power of this love will facilitate healing by helping us to feel safe in our bodies, have an experience of belonging in the world, and embrace our inherent goodness. This love encourages each of us to delight and prosper in the magnificent, soulful expression of our lives.

When we know ourselves as love, we can begin to expect love to show up in our lives everywhere. Trusting the power of love, we can begin to expect positive, harmonious outcomes in all matters. As love becomes the center of our lives, we can be grateful for the life that we have—just as it is. We are empowered in the presence of love that is boundless, non-judgmental, forgiving, and compassionate. When we move away from fear, anything is possible!

See Ad on page 260

Life Coaching

~

What is a Life Coach? Life coaches are personal guides that work one-on-one with their clients to create life improvements and changes. Most life coaches take extensive courses, sometimes in the areas of their chosen speciality and others prefer to cover a broad range of topics and situations. Changes or life improvements are often desired in the areas of career and business, relationships, family, finances, spiritual or personal growth.

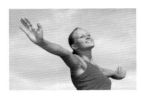

Life coaching is quite different than counseling. Rather than discussing old issues, failures and digging up the past, coaching is pro-active and assists in getting the client to the actions that will change his or her life. A coach will help you eliminate your obstacles and encourage your growth. A life-coach is there to remind you that regardless of the past, you are a powerful being and can change or recreate your life by taking control and making new decisions. It is a personal growth healing service which helps you to take the necessary steps towards creating the life you desire. Coaches will help you to identify and overcome limiting beliefs. They remain objective and therefore can often see the bigger picture with a new perspective.

Your first session with a coach is similar to an interview. They will find out where you are now in your life and where you would like to be. They then formulate your plan, supporting personal growth, including goal setting, life-improvement strategies and behavior modification. It is standard practice for a life coach to assign homework each time you meet. They strive to help their clients achieve balance and success and act as their mentor and cheerleader. Their goal is to help you bring out the very best in you by discovering your untapped resources and helping you put them into action. Life coaches usually meet with their clients weekly to maintain focus and steady growth They will hold you accountable for your actions or lack of them.

Origin and History: Life coaching gained it's popularity in the 1960's. Laura Whitworth and Thomas Leonard founded The Coaches Training Institute and Coaching University and developed a coaching system which is considered to be the core of the profession today. Since then, a variety of coaching systems have evolved based on behavioral sciences and education.

Applications: Subcategories and specialty areas of coaches include: sports, singing, acting, career, relationships, finances, and business. Coaching is effective for implementing goals such as: getting in shape, losing weight, eliminating old unsupportive patterns, developing new attitudes required for success, eliminating obstacles to prosperity, getting out of your comfort zone, when you are considering a career change, growing a new business, building a new practice or starting a new job, specialty professions and for students who need to develop study skills and habits.

Cautions: Some life coaches have training, credentials or degrees, while others do not. It is important for you to choose a coach who is a right match for you and who you feel comfortable with. Take the time to do your research and ask for references from a few prospective life coaches before making your decision. There are training programs for life coaching, but no official regulations or standards exist.

Insurance: Does not cover life coaching. It may be possible if the coach is also a licensed therapist.

Quick practitioner reference:

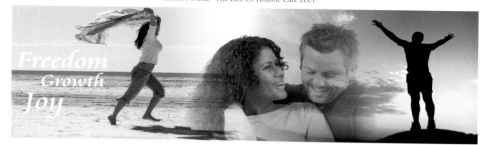

Remove Life Obstacles!

Relationship and Life Coach

• Fran provides a safe haven with non-judgmental support through life transitions, helping you navigate toward your goals. She uses a serious, yet warm and light-hearted approach to coaching and hypnotherapy, making your progress the ultimate priority.

Intuitive Counselor

• Very often those moments in our lives that present themselves as the most difficult and challenging become our greatest opportunity to change for the better, especially with proper guidance and support.

Clinical Hypnotherapist

• Learn grounding, self protection and meditation techniques right for you. Find your own path, follow your heart and soul, and embrace the real you. Fran specializes in self empowerment and coaching through "spiritual awakening."

- *"Thanks to Fran, I am no longer a doormat and now believe I truly deserve to be happy. With Fran's coaching, I got my power back. My career and relationships have completely turned around." - Aileen A. -*

- *"I learned through Fran, that telling the truth and accepting the consequences truly sets me free. I have grown significantly with her help" - Gil S.-*

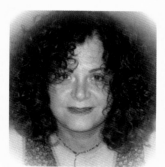

For a FREE consultation,
Take the FIRST STEP and call:
Fran Coleman, CCH
(213) 923-7655

francoleman@sbcglobal.net
Certified Clinical Hypnotherapist
Certified Master of Life Metaphysical Counselor
Pax Graduate

What Do You Want To Be Different?
by Elaine McBroom, C.Ht.

We're all looking for something. Something that will make us feel...some way. Maybe we want to feel happy, content, lovable, good enough, connected, loved or some other feeling. Some of us don't even know we're looking for something to help us feel something different than we feel. The entire television commercial industry is built around the knowledge that we're looking for something.

Some of us try shopping, drinking, eating, watching television, other escapes or even addictions. Some of us try self help workshops, gym memberships, diets, facelifts or other cosmetic surgery. We believe that if we just do something, get something, experience something, understand some-thing, look a certain way, have a certain thing, try a certain thing, we'll feel it, whatever it is. Don't get me wrong, there is absolutely nothing wrong with any of these. That's not my point. While the intent of looking for something to make us feel different is positive, it usually doesn't work. Not because we don't try, but because we're looking in the wrong place. We're looking for the wrong thing. It doesn't come from anything we do or have, change or acquire. It only comes from one place. It comes from in here.

Let me explain, the Theory Of Mind, or affectionately called T.O.M. by Dr. John Kappas, the founder of Hypnosis Motivation Institute will help. As humans, we are all born with only two fears: The fear of falling and the fear of loud noises. We are also born with the limbic system hard wired, that part of the brain that is inherited from those ancestors that had to fight lions and tigers and bears, oh my! This is the portion of the brain that carries the reflex of fight, flight or, I add freeze. We no longer have to fight lions and tigers and bears, so this portion of our brain has converted fight, flight or freeze to stress, anxiety or depression. Other than that, we are born with what one could term a blank slate. Then life starts to happen. Things happen to us and around us. People tell us what they think, show us ways of being, react to things that happen and teach us by example. It's not what happens that creates our beliefs, it's how we interpret what happens. For example, if something happens that makes us sad and mom or grandma,

who wants us to feel better, says "don't feel bad, dear, have a cookie," some of us may decide that a cookie will make us feel better. Some of us may decide that food is love. Some of us may decide that feeling our sadness is not acceptable. It's all in the interpretation.

From the beginning, we start creating our beliefs by interpreting life. We decide what is positive and what is negative. We look for evidence to prove our interpretation and often completely ignore evidence to the contrary. Furthermore, we live life as if our interpretations and decisions are absolutely true. Many of us decided we weren't lovable or good enough. Then we go about looking for what will make us feel lovable or good enough. We look out there. Nothing seems to work, so we keep looking. We probably don't even know we've made these decisions, but they are running our life. And, most of them were made before we were eight or nine years old, when we developed the critical mind. So, basically, our kid is running our life.

In my experience with working with clients over the past five plus years, the thing that works is looking inside, discovering what it is we are looking for, and then giving it to ourselves. I've found that most people are looking for love or protection as a bottom line. They think, "If I have (do, be, know) this (fill in the blank), then I'll feel love (or protection).

So how do we give love or protection to ourselves? We notice when we are not feeling our current age. Yes, believe it or not, we often feel much younger than we currently are. We notice when the feelings that we're feeling are much bigger than the situation that is happening right now. Then we notice what we need in that moment. Do we need love or protection or something else? Many of us have something we want to hear in that moment, like "I love you," or "you're safe." We can tell ourselves that thing we need to hear. We can hear it from ourselves more effectively than from someone else. We may not believe it the first time, but as we continue to practice being there for ourselves and loving ourselves, we start to believe it and the anger, sadness, fear, shame or guilt starts to dissolve. We start to believe we're lovable, good enough or pretty enough. Then we start to feel happy, content, lovable, connected and loved. There are skills that help, like hypnosis, where the adult comes into team with the kid and updates incorrect decisions. Even with help, in life it takes practice loving ourselves, and we're worth it.

Massage Therapy

~

What is Massage Therapy? Massage therapy includes a wide variety of therapeutic approaches which involve using hands-on manipulation of muscles and soft tissue. Therapeutic massage increases the rate at which the body recovers from injury and illness. It is used to prevent and alleviate pain, discomfort and muscle tightness.

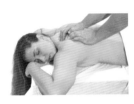

Massage therapy improves blood and lymphatic circulation; relieves muscle tension and pain; increases flexibility by stretching and loosening the muscles which improves mobility; helps clear lactic acid and metabolic waste stored in the tissues; reduces pain and stiffness in muscles and joints; brings oxygen and nutrients to the tissues and this results in an increased rate of healing and stimulates the release of endorphins. On a mental and emotional level, massage therapy reduces stress and anxiety, increases one's ability to think calmly; promotes a relaxed state of alertness and an overall feeling of well-being; and provides compassionate touch.

There are many different kinds of massage therapy: Swedish, Deep Tissue, Sports Lymphatic, Pregnancy Massage, Thai Yoga Massage, TuiNa (Chinese Massage), Reflexology and others. It is a good idea to experiment to find the ones you like.

A massage therapy session begins with a short consultation with the therapist. They will review your symptoms, medical history, stress level and lifestyle. The areas concentrated on during the session are determined by the length of the session scheduled (between 30 min and 1 ½ hours), and your preferences. The therapist then leaves the room and you undress to the level of your comfort. You then will lie face down or up, depending on the therapists instructions, under a sheet on the massage table. The sheet covers your body at being treated. The massage therapist will return and check on your level of comfort. If you have skin allergies, you may want to bring your own lotion. Massage therapy is not painful but you may experience soreness when the therapist works on knots and areas holding tension. Let your therapist know if the pressure is too strong or not strong enough for you.

Origin and History: Massage dates back to the roots of Western medicine in ancient Greece. In the 5th century B.C. in Greece, Hippocrates stated, "A physician must be experienced in many things but assuredly also in rubbing." He said that massage, along with fresh air, good food, baths, music, rest, and visits to friends, is key to treating disease. Sweden's Henrik Ling (1776-1839) is considered the father of modern Western massage.

Applications: Massage therapy is effective in treating back pain, arthritis, tendinitis, headaches, migraines, strains, sprains, stress, circulatory and respiratory problems, post-injury and surgical rehabilitation and helps to boost the immune system. Massage therapy is preventively beneficial for everyone - especially performers, athletes and those with sedentary jobs. It is used with great success for the elderly, the bedridden, those in nursing homes or hospitals and for those with a chronic illness or a sedentary job.

Cautions: Do not have a massage on an area where there is an open wound, inflamed or infected tissue, rash, bruise, tumor, hernia, fracture, or immediately after surgery, radiation or chemotherapy. If you are pregnant, have cancer, heart disease or blood clots, check with your doctor first.

Insurance: Many insurance providers are beginning to extend coverage to include massage. Check with your provider.

Quick practitioner-reference:

OM Holistic Health Center

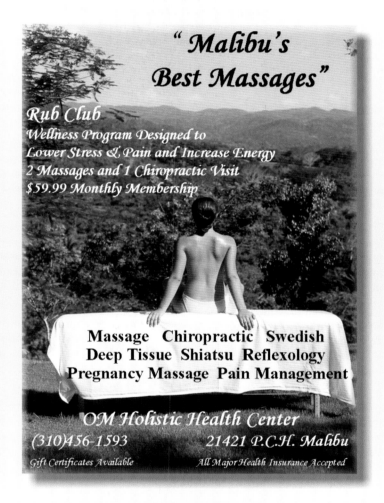

" Malibu's Best Massages"

Rub Club
Wellness Program Designed to
Lower Stress & Pain and Increase Energy
2 Massages and 1 Chiropractic Visit
$59.99 Monthly Membership

**Massage Chiropractic Swedish
Deep Tissue Shiatsu Reflexology
Pregnancy Massage Pain Management**

OM Holistic Health Center
(310)456-1593   21421 P.C.H. Malibu
Gift Certificates Available   All Major Health Insurance Accepted

Massage & Chiropractic

(310) 456-1593

The Gift of Education
by Val Guin

I've always enjoyed helping others, and it seemed that, through touch, I was able to make people feel better. As a child, I would rub my parents' shoulders and feet when they came home from work. When I was 16, my grandfather was recovering from a stroke and my grandmother from mishaps with doctors. The Physical Therapist (PT) would come to the house and teach me what to do to help them heal. I loved seeing the daily improvement that a little loving touch and exercise made possible. I decided to become a Physical Therapist.

I began training as a restorative nurse, assisting a PT at the Spastic Foundation in Sylmar. I also began my training as a PT at the local colleges. On Christmas Eve, I was driving to school early when a drunk driver ran a red light and hit my car. I could not move; my hands and legs were numb. It was not until later that we realized the full extent of my injuries. Due to breaks in the spine and spinal compression, I no longer had complete control of my limbs, nor could I lift anything. This ended my career as a PT.

Soon after the accident, I got married and, against all odds, got pregnant. The doctors had said it would be hard to get pregnant and almost impossible to have a natural childbirth, due to the twisting and compression in my spine and pelvis. The birth of my daughter was several days long, with no medication. The long, slow process actually helped both my spine and pelvis. The doctors were in shock at the difference. I still suffered with pain, but had less intermittent paralysis because I had more space between my vertebrae after giving birth. It was like having internal bodywork. Thank you to my daughter, Natiya!

My career as a PT was over, so I took a job in the health and fitness department of the YWCA, handing out uniforms and towels. My Mom had always said, "If you are going to do something, do it 110%. You never know where it will lead, but you will always be proud of yourself along the way." I did just that, learning everyone's names and encouraging them as we became a supportive family.

There was a massage therapist on staff whom I greatly respected. I shared my story and she offered to train me. After working with me, she suggested I go to school for formal training, telling me, "You're a natural!" We came to an Institute of PsychoStructural Balancing (IPSB) open house and I watched and listened to the teachers speak and do Tai Qi. I loved it! This was the school for me. The problem was my husband was not supportive. I had no idea how I would pay for school. A few weeks later I came to work and I was handed an envelope. My co-workers had collected enough money to send me to massage school. My life has never been the same. At IPSB, I gained the tools to stay out of physical and mental pain, and learned new ways to approach my daily life. Ever since, I have continued learning and growing.

Val Guin is an internationally known, Certified Massage Therapist who has been doing bodywork since 1981. She is a founding member of the Santa Monica Center of Healing Arts, where she has her full time practice. She teaches all levels of massage, including Forearm Dance, the revolutionary massage modality she created. She co-owns, with her daughter, Ohana Productions, which produces educational videos on healing bodywork. She acquired Co-Ownership of IPSB in 2006.

See Ad on page 64

Naturopathy

~

What is Naturopathic Medicine?

Naturopathic medicine is a holistic system of primary health care, based on the healing power of nature. Naturopathic doctors ("N.Ds") are trained to prevent, diagnose and treat disease and are trained in minor surgery and pharmacology. N.Ds utilize a wide variety of non-invasive therapies and techniques such as nutrition, herbal medicine, homeopathy, Chinese medicine/ acupuncture, hypnotherapy, psychology and counseling, detoxification via fasting, enemas and colonics, hydrotherapy and physical medicine. Some NDs have training and certification in natural child birth. Naturopathic doctors are licensed professionals in 14 US states and have four years of post-graduate doctoral education in medical diagnosis and treatment.

NOTE: Naturopaths are healthcare practitioners who also practice in a similar fashion to NDs, but are not licensed medical doctors and do not diagnose disease. They attend vocational schools and are trained in physiology, anatomy and to use the same natural treatments as does an ND.

The first visit will include a thorough examination of all valid factors which contribute to the patient's health problems. The ND ask questions about diet, lifestyle, stress, and other factors. Then the ND performs a physical examination and conventional and alternative laboratory tests such as the comprehensive stool analysis or hair/mineral analysis, if required.

N.Ds treat the whole person, which means they investigate the physical, mental, genetic or hereditary risk factors and environmental, social and spiritual factors. They seek to identify and remove the causes of illness, rather than suppress symptoms. They use the least invasive and least harmful methods to diagnose and treat patients, emphasizing prevention and education. Treatments are designed to support health.

N.Ds and Naturopaths encourage patients to attain optimum health through lifestyle changes and to take responsibility for their own self-care.

Origin and History: Naturopathic medicine dates back to the 18th century European natural healing systems. Benjamin Lust, a German healthcare practitioner, founded the American School of Naturopathy in the US in 1902. Beginning in the mid-1920s, the popularity of naturopathic medicine declined while allopathic medical training, pharmaceuticals and medical technologies became mainstream. Today naturopathic medicine is a synthesis of the best eastern and western methods of natural care.

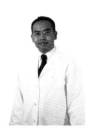

Applications: There is not one single chronic or acute illness that naturopathic medicine is not recommended or effective at treating.

Cautions: Tell your medical doctor (M.D.) about your natural care and tell your naturopath about your conventional care. Some treatments can negatively interact with each other. Therapeutic doses of nutrients or herbs should be administered by a licensed practitioner.

Insurance: State licensing for N.Ds is new in California. The first Californian N.D. became licensed in January, 2005. At this time, most insurance companies have not yet recognized the profession for insurance coverage; however, some patients are able to submit bills and have their visits covered.

Quick practitioner reference:
Holistic Medical Center - page 28
Paramount Herbs - page 270

Naturopathy and You
by John Buratti, ND, Ph.D.

Just what is Naturopathy? It is a system of therapy utilizing physical forces, such as air, light, water, heat, massage and herbs. Notice, I did not mention radiation and chemicals in this definition. Naturopathy is a comprehensive approach which emphasizes supporting the body's physical attempts to eliminate disease and maintain optimum health. Naturopathic methods follow from the central idea that a major cause of dis-ease is an excessive buildup of toxic materials (often due to improper eating, infections and lack of exercise) which clog the avenues of waste disposal (colon, liver, kidneys, skin). A founder of naturopathy stated that disease is, in fact, the result of our individual or collective violation of nature's laws either through ignorance or willfulness and it is in our power to rid ourselves of disease. And it follows that disease which appears to be entirely physical is due to something being wrong in the mental, emotional or spiritual sphere of which the symptom is merely the reflection.

The following six principles of healing form the foundation for naturopathy:

● The healing process is structured within our body's inherent nature (ability) to heal itself and restore health.

● Treat the whole person for an interaction of physical, mental, emotional, genetic, spiritual, and environmental factors disrupting the harmonious functioning of an individual.

● Do no harm. The more gentle and non-invasive the therapy, the less disruptive it will be to the patient's integral whole.

● Identify and treat the cause of the illness by uncovering the underlying reason. When only the symptoms are treated, the underlying causes remain and the patient may develop a more serious, chronic condition.

● Prevention is the best "cure." Naturopaths help patients to recognize their choices and how those choices affect their health.

● Doctor as Teacher - the original meaning of the word. A naturopath is a facilitator for a patient's healing process. As such, a principal responsibility is to educate the patient and encourage self-responsibility. They take the time listen during the consultation.

Americans need to be educated on how their bodies work. If one organ starts to fail then the human body will start to assist the failing organ with another organ. This is called the toxic stress cycle. This cycle can be broken. When digestion begins to fail our colons get backed up. This leads to liver and gallbladder problems. Then the kidneys and bladder work harder and then require the lungs in this cycle. The heart, lymph and circulation are then over hampered and this leads to the spleen for supplementary help. Muscle aches may appear and then lead to spinal problems. And to finish this cycle the brain and nervous system then require help from the endocrine glands which then leads to the beginning of the Toxic Stress Cycle: digestion (what you eat and what you assimilate).

● Do you realize that digestion begins with proper food combining, mastication (chewing) and enzyme availability?

● Do you realize the colon functions for the intestinal assimilation of nutrients and elimination of waste products?

● Do you know what is in your daily multivitamin/mineral supplement?

High levels of inorganic vitamin supplements can tax a weak liver even more, as well as create biochemical imbalances.

"Naturopaths are Holistic Health Practitioners that incorporate a variety of "wholistic" disciplines during their consultations and are a viable alternative to regain and maintain your health by using safe and effective herbal remedies."

Health is often a reflection of how we choose to live.

See Ad on page 271

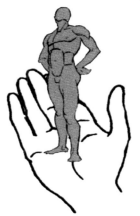
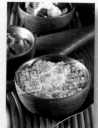

Neurofeedback

~

What is Neurofeedback? Neurofeedback (NFB), also called neurotherapy, neurobiofeedback or EEG biofeedback, is the direct training of brain function, by which the brain learns to function more efficiently. Neurofeedback influences the brain directly by impacting the frequencies and patterns of brain cell activity. When the brain is not functioning well, it usually shows up on an Electoencphalogram test (EEG). When a brain cell is functioning, it produces a change in the electrical field within and around the brain cell. This change in the electrical field can be observed by placing electrodes on the scalp to detect the activity. To treat specific conditions, the practitioner uses targeted frequencies corresponding to the area of the brain which is experiencing problems. The condition dictates the location on the scalp where the practitioner places the probes. In addition, basic neuro-diagnostic and neuro-psychological tests are used to assess brain function. Signals are processed by a computer and reflected back to the client. This information is presented in the form of a video game. The client then plays the video game in order to shape the brainwave activity towards a more desirable and regulated performance. Specific brain training protocols have been developed for each brain-related problem. The brain is trained and challenged to help improve its ability to regulate all bodily functions. Any brain, regardless of its level of function, can be trained to function better.

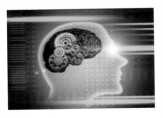

Origin and History: In the late 1960's Dr. Barry Sterman of UCLA was conducting sleep research using EEG to evaluate neurological activity associated with sleep and sleep onset. Dr. Joel Lubar of the University of Tennessee who had studied hyperactivity and attention issues, joined Sterman's research team and decided to research the benefits of neurofeedback in this area. The recent increase in public awareness and clinical use of neurofeedback is attributed to Siegfried and Sue Othmer of EEG Institute. They spent four years developing computerized instrumentation and now offer training courses to mental health practitioners.

Applications: Neurofeedback is highly effective with certain cases of seizures, traumatic brain injury, stroke and autism. In these instances the training does not so much get rid of the problem as it organizes the brain to function better. It is also effective for migraines, birth trauma, autism, cerebral palsy, attention deficit disorder, suicidal behavior, anxiety, depression, bipolar disorder, behavior and sleep disorders, headaches, migraines, PMS, emotional disturbances, bed-wetting, nightmares, sleep walking, and teeth grinding. This modality is ideal for professional athletes, corporate executives, and performing artists to enhance brain performance - a type of 'peak performance training' to achieve levels of excellence. Preventatively, neurofeedback can be used to maintain good brain function as one gets older. The severity of the symptom presentation and the treatment response determines the number of sessions.

Research: The majority of the research has evaluated the use of neurofeedback as it pertains to symptoms of attention deficit disorder and epilepsy. For further research read the following: A Symphony in the Brain by Jim Robbins, The ADD Book, by Sears & Thompson Getting Rid of Ritalin, by Castro & Hill.

Insurance: Insurance plans that cover mental health may cover the cost of neurofeedback.

Quick practitioner reference:
EEG Info - page 69
EEG Institute - page 273

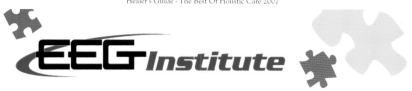

EEG Institute

The Technique is **Neurofeedback**
The Results are **Extraordinary**

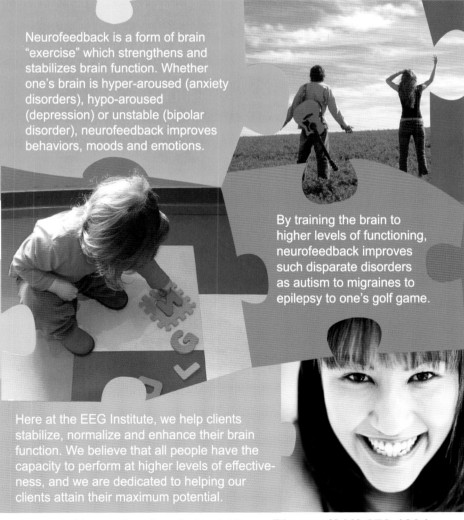

Neurofeedback is a form of brain "exercise" which strengthens and stabilizes brain function. Whether one's brain is hyper-aroused (anxiety disorders), hypo-aroused (depression) or unstable (bipolar disorder), neurofeedback improves behaviors, moods and emotions.

By training the brain to higher levels of functioning, neurofeedback improves such disparate disorders as autism to migraines to epilepsy to one's golf game.

Here at the EEG Institute, we help clients stabilize, normalize and enhance their brain function. We believe that all people have the capacity to perform at higher levels of effectiveness, and we are dedicated to helping our clients attain their maximum potential.

22020 Clarendon St., Suite 305
Woodland Hills, CA 91367

Phone: (818) 373-1334
Fax: (818) 373-1331

NLP
Neuro-Linguistic Progamming

What is NLP? Neuro-Linguistic Programming can best be described as a school of thought, and an offshoot of Hypnotherapy and Psychotherapy. It is a powerful technology that helps to create healthy interpersonal and intrapersonal relationships. NLP combines neurology, language and programming to determine how our bodies function and how we communicate or interact with others. The combination of neurology, language and programming also determine what kind of life experiences we create for ourselves on a daily basis. With NLP principles, we can literally re-create our reality and make better, more rewarding choices. There are two main background beliefs:

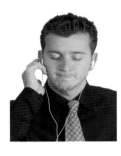

● The Map is Not the Territory. Human beings perceive reality by a unique inner perception or "map" which is based on our sensory systems. By associating a certain meaning to sensory input, we create our inner reality. Our personal reality is often mistakenly perceived as the ultimate reality of all.

● The Universe, nature and the human mind are connected by *Systemic Processes*. Interconnectedness exists between the processes taking place within oneself and all of nature's systems or subsystems. These systems cannot be isolated from each other. They directly and indirectly influence each other and are subject to natural laws or principles which seek to create optimum balance.

When one's inner perception "map" of the individual - consisting of internal and mental and emotional "programs" - are indentified, the self-destructive, unsupportive and stagnating patterns can be eliminated and then replaced with supportive ones. This is achieved by identifying the primary sensory filters (auditory,

linguistic and kinesthetic). Success is achieved when the unsupportive filters are found and then changed or altered. The new established filters help individuals to achieve what they desire, even in highly stressful situations.

Origin and History: NLP originated in 1973 at U.C. Santa Cruz as a result of a research project of two students - Richard Bandler, a mathematician, and John Grinder, a linguist. Their research led to them to analyze the way individuals store and process their thoughts, which lead to a better understanding of how we communicate with others. They published the book *"The Structure of Magic, I" Vol. I & II* (1975, 1976) and *"Patterns of the Hypnotic Techniques" Vol. I & II (1975, 1976)* by Milton H. Erickson, M.D.

Applications: NLP is a proven tool for achieving results and creating success. The use of NLP is effective for, but not limited to: enhancing relationships, addressing learning challenges, achieving relaxation, reducing stress, removing phobias (*i.e.,* fear of public speaking, fear of heights, fear of small places, fears of snakes, spiders, etc.), reducing allergic responses (*i.e.,* food and pollen allergies), asthma, and stopping harmful habits (*i.e.,* smoking, overeating, drinking, and drug abuse).

Research: A one year research study 1993 -1994 into the treatment of asthmatics, using NLP, was done in Denmark by General Practitioner Jorgen Lund and NLP Master Practitioner Hanne Lund. The intervention group received 3-36 hours (average 13) of NLP intervention techniques. The NLP focus was not exclusively on the asthma; it was on how the people lived their daily lives. The NLP group increased their lung capacity by an average of 200ml - the equivalent of reversing four years of damage in a year. Sleep disorders in the NLP group began at 50% and dropped to zero. Use of asthma inhalers and acute medication in the NLP group fell to near zero.

Quick practitioner reference:

Nutritional Counseling
~

What is Nutritional Counseling?

Nutritional Practitioners include dietitians, nutritionists and nutritional therapists. They are educated and trained in the science of food and the body's systems. As a result they are able to recommend the appropriate dietary changes, based on an individual's nutritional needs and health-related goals. They understand that we are biochemical beings. Science has provided the tools to measure the chemical composition and physiological benefits of food and nutrients. The physical body is made of water, chemicals and electricity. When any one of these components becomes out of balance, illness may result. Each body is a uniquely different system and responds to food and supplements in its own way.

Nutritional consultants help to support one's dietary and health-related goals based on their clients personal eating habits and when necessary, supplements are recommend. A survey of a client's diet, lifestyle and general state of health helps nutritional consultants analyze what each body needs and design the best nutritional plan for them. A client's in-depth evaluation consists of a questionnaire and any combination of the following diagnostic techniques: blood panel, hair analysis, kinesiology, biofeedback, physical symptoms, etc.

Nutritional healing works with nature's ability to heal and provides the body with natural substances. Practitioners can address a vast range of medical conditions. Research is constantly providing us with new information as to the effects of food and nutrients on the body; it's direct influence on disease and how one can obtain optimal mental and physical performance and excellent health when one uses the nutritional approach in a preventative manner.

Applications: Practitioners are able to help heal a variety of illnesses including:

anorexia, bulimia, fatigue, arthritis, cancer, digestive problems, stress, allergies, skin disorders, hormonal problems and improve cardiovascular and mental health. In addition they can provide the specialized nutritional support necessary for children; for athletes to achieve peak performance; for prenatal and postnatal needs; to increase energy and stamina. Practitioners often will specialize in particular areas of nutrition.

Research:

In recent years, findings from scientific studies have begun to corroborate the conventional wisdom that fish food is good for the brain. New research from the Framingham Heart Study has shown that eating three or more servings of fish per week may significantly decrease one's risk of dementia and Alzheimer's disease. The protective ingredient in fish is an essential fatty acid known as DHA (docosa-hexaenoic acid) which appears to be important in affecting the risk of dementia.

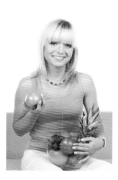

Cautions: It is important to have a medical diagnosis before obtaining detailed nutritional advice for specific health problems. These include high blood pressure, high cholesterol, diabetes, severe food allergies, high blood pressure, certain chronic digestive problems, osteoporosis, kidney disease, cancer, and obesity.

Insurance: may cover treatment

Quick practitioner reference:

Osteopathy

~

What is Osteopathy? Osteopathy is branch of western medicine that follows a philosophy of medical care that centers on the patient, not the disease. It is based on the theory that disturbances in the musculoskeletal system - bones, muscles, tendons, tissues, nerves and spinal column

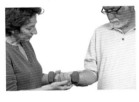

- affect other bodily parts, causing many disorders that can be corrected by various manipulative techniques in conjunction with conventional medical, surgical, pharmacological, and other therapeutic procedures. Mechanical problems which affect the tension of the spine may result in nervous and circulatory problems leading to pain, disability and dysfunction.

Diseases of specific organs can produce pain in other parts of the body. Stomach ulcers consistently cause area of spinal pain and irritation just below the shoulders in the back. The radiation of pain to the loin is the reflection of pain and disability of the left shoulder following heart disease. Reoccurring headaches are often related to problems affecting the cervical portion of the spinal column. By addressing the spine, osteopathic treatment can often relieve headache symptoms.

Doctors of Osteopathic Medicine (D.O.) are fully licensed medical doctors and surgeons and therefore are able to treat and diagnose. They utilize all of the recognized procedures and modern technologies for prevention, diagnosis and treatment of disease, including drugs, radiation and surgery, but their holistic approach offers an alternative and helps patients avoid extreme or unnecessary procedures.

The integrity of the body's musculoskeletal system is crucial to the patient's wellbeing. Osteopaths emphasize proper nutrition and environmental factors. The technique they use is called Osteopathic Manipulative Treatment. Osteopaths use a variety of treatment methods including massage, stretching, cranial osteopathy, low-force manipulations, and traction, among other specialized techniques. The methods used are determined by the patient's age, physique, history and their particular problem.

Osteopathic doctors focus on prevention and make their patients aware of the causes behind their problems. Patients are educated and instructed; givien tailored exercise programs, relaxation techniques for stress, proper body mechanics, and encouraged to take responsibility for their own health.

Origin and History: Osteopathy was developed in America in the 1870's by Dr. Andrew Taylor Still, and is now recognized worldwide as one of the most scientifically validated and effective complementary therapies.

Applications: Osteopathy accelerates the rate of recovery and treats back and neck problems, headaches, back pain related to childbirth, helping to prepare the body for childbirth, sciatica, joint problems including arthritic pain, and ligament strains, sports injuries, tendinitis, work-related and repetitive strain injuries, whiplash, sinus problems and menstrual cramps.

Insurance: Most medical insurance covers treatment.

Physical Therapy

~

What is Physical Therapy? Physical therapy - also referred to as physiotherapy - is the treatment of injury and disease by physical means. It is considered within the realm of conventional medicine. Physical therapy restores wellbeing following injury, pain or disability and improves mobility, relieves pain, and restores function to the impaired areas of the physical body.

During the first appointment, which takes between ½ to a full hour, the physical therapist will discuss your medical history, perform a physical evaluation and assessment, and then discuss your treatment. In the physical evaluation the physical therapist will test for range of motion, strength, posture, balance, motor skills and a cardiopulmonary assessment before your treatment.

Any of the following therapies may be used: ultrasound, electrical stimulation, manual therapies such as massage or myofascial release to mobilize and manipulate the joints, acupuncture, hydrotherapy, traction and provision of aids or appliances such as walking devices. Treatment is applied to the musculoskeletal, cardiopulmonary or integumentary systems.

Patient education is a very important aspect of this practice and the therapist will recommend exercise programs and lifestyle considerations, to prevent further injury.

Here is a brief explanation of some common techniques used by physical therapists.

● Muscle Effect Therapy (MET). A light touch that brings awareness to muscle tension. This often brings old trauma - emotions, memories - to the surface to be released.

● Soft Tissue Mobilization (STM). A hands-on therapy designed to restore the joint mobility.

● Myofascial Release (MFR). A specialized stretching technique to treat patients who have a variety of soft tissue problems.

Fascia is the connective tissue which covers all organs and muscles.

Origin and History: Physical Therapy has its roots as a traditional healing art and history traces its practice back to as early as 3000 BC in China.

Applications: Musculoskeletal physical therapy is proven to successfully treat and improve conditions of back and neck pain, injuries, joint problems such as arthritis , cerebral palsy, spina bifida and bio-mechanical problems. Cardiopulmonary physical therapy treats acute asthma, chest infections, post-myocardial infaction, chronic obstructive pulmonary disease, pneumonia, and problems associated with cystic fibrosis. Neurological physical therapy works with conditions, such as stroke and multiple sclerosis to restore or improve motor function. Physical therapy is used preventatively in treatments that include fitness and wellness programs, movement, reducing pain and therefore preventing disability. Physical therapy is used in private practice, hospitals, sports facilities, elderly and home care clinics.

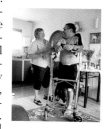

Insurance: California law requires that a patient obtain a referral from a medical doctor or chiropractor before physical therapy treatment. Medical insurance, medicare and workers compensation generally cover treatment. Check with your insurance carrier to determine your coverage.

Quick practitioner reference:

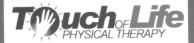
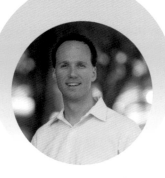
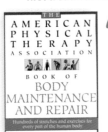

Pranic Healing℠

Ancient Art, Modern Science

What is Pranic Healing? Pranic Healing is a form of energy healing which systematically utilizes the "prana" or life force readily available from the sun, air and ground to heal physical and emotional imbalances. It requires no drugs, gadgets not even physical contact with the subject. The practitioner works directly on the bioplasmic or energy body of the client. The bioplasmic body is commonly referred to as the *aura*. Pranic Healing's effectiveness relies on the fact that there is an intimate connection between these two bodies. As we heal the bioplasmic body it creates a new and perfect pattern for the physical counterpart to follow, resulting in a healing.

Pranic Healing acts as a powerful catalyst to spark the body's inborn ability to heal itself. However, it is not meant to replace orthodox medicine but rather to complement it. Pranic Healing can be easily learned in one or two weekends and follows a step-by-step cookbook approach to healing. Pranic Healing utilizes the following principles:

● Principle of Cleansing - It is by removing the diseased energies from the affected energy centers/diseased organs and then energizing them with sufficient life force/prana that healing is accomplished. Energizing without first cleansing is like pouring fresh coffee into a cup that is already filled with stale coffee. This approach is slow and quite wasteful. A healing crisis may occur if the diseased energy is pushed further into the body by a willful healer. A healing crisis is a process whereby the body attempts to expel stale or diseased energies. Some of symptoms are vomiting, fever, diarrhea, fatigue and heavy sweating.

● Principle of Energizing - When affected areas are thoroughly energetically cleansed, the fresh healthy life-force/prana has to be supplied in order to boost rapid recovery. The Pranic Healing "water pump" approach prevents the healer from becoming drained following a healing or counseling session. By knowing how to properly flow the healing energies through their system and then direct them to the affected area of the client, the healer is able to sufficiently energize the affected areas without draining his/hers own supply of lifeforce.

Origin and History: The founder or Pranic Healing, Master Choa Kok Sui, is the author of more than 14 books including: *Miracles Through Pranic Healing (1987), Pranic Psychotherapy (1990), Advanced Pranic Healing (1992), Pranic Crystal Healing (1996), Psychic Self Defense for Home and Office (1999), Meditations for Soul Realization (2000), Universal and Kabbalistic Meditation on the Lord's Prayer (2001).* Master Choa's style in presenting esoteric concepts and in unveiling inner spiritual teachings, is simple, straight forward, and practical. He managed to conceptualize a fresh and far deeper understanding of energy healing, using the readily available source of all life - Prana, called Pranic Energy or Vital Life Force.

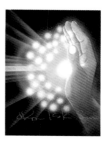

Applications: Complementary to western medical care. Supports rapid healing for all acute or chronic illnesses *i.e.*: asthma, heart ailments, irritable bowel syndrome, arthritis and back pain and other severe ailments as tumorous or infectious diseases. Great results are reported daily for psychological and emotional imbalances. Can be applied distantly and for pets.

Research:
- An investigation of the effect of Pranic Healing on the survival rates of HeLa cells subjected to radiation. The results of this preliminary study are summarized in on page 17.
- A scientific experiment conducted by Dr. Masaru Emoto, a Japanese researcher, on the effects of subtle energy on water, in July 2003. Pranic healers directed pranic energy to a tap water sample in his Tokyo laboratory. The research methodology can be accessed from the website www.hado.net

Quick practitioner reference:

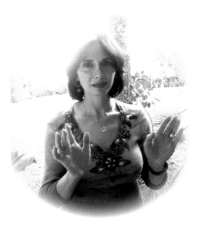

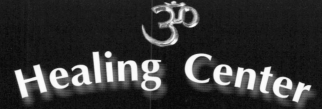

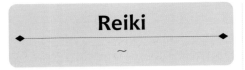

Reiki

~

What is Reiki? Reiki is a Japanese energy technique for stress reduction and relaxation that promotes healing. Rei, in Japanese, means "God's Wisdom or the Higher Power" and Ki means, "lifeforce energy." Reiki is a safe, easy method of spiritual healing. Everyone can use and benefit from it. The ability to practice Reiki is transferred from the instructor who is called a Reiki Master, to the practitioner. This is referred to as an attunement and allows the student to tap into the unlimited supply of universal lifeforce - energy. It is based on the concept that lifeforce flows through us and if one's lifeforce is low, there is a tendency to become sick. If the lifeforce is high, there is a tendency to be healthy. Reiki addresses the whole person - body, emotions, mind and spirit. Although Reiki is spiritual in nature, it is not religious.

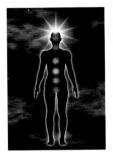

It works with the understanding that the lifeforce flows though the chakras, meridians and nadis, providing nourishment to the physical body. When this flow is disrupted or diminished, it results in the impaired function of the organs and cells of the body. The Reiki practitioner allows the Universal energy to flow from their hands to the energetic system of the client. This raises the frequency of their energy field (where the negative thoughts and emotions are stored), causing them to break apart or disintegrate. Then the lifeforce is able to flow, unimpeded. In Reiki, the practitioner does not decide what to work on. Reiki energy is guided by the Higher Intelligence; it knows exactly where to go and what to do.

During the session the client lays on a massage table, fully clothed.

The practitioner places her hands in a series of positions, held for several minutes on or near the clients' body. A typical session lasts between 45 and 90 minutes. Clients become relaxed and may fall asleep, feeling refreshed and "lighter" afterwards.

Origin and History: Mikao Usui, a Buddhist, who studied Christianity, founded the technique and concept of Reiki after having a mystical experience. In 1914, Usui's personal and business life was failing and he decided to travel to the holy mountain, Mt. Kurama to study Isyu Guo, a spiritual training course. Reiki was brought to the U.S. by Hawaiian born, Mrs. Takata. She received her Reiki training in Japan in 1936, and returned to Hawaii in 1937 and proceeded to establish Reiki in Hawaii. Reiki is not exclusive to the system of healing based on Usui's method. There have been several styles and schools of thought which followed, based on similar principles, although all are called Reiki.

Applications: Reiki is effective in helping virtually every known illness and malady and is used as complementary medicine. It helps to reduces stress, decreases the need for pain medication, improves sleep and appetite; reduces the side effects following regular medical treatments such as chemotherapy, post operative pain and depression and speeds recovery. Complete healings have been reported and confirmed by medical tests before and after treatment. Medical professionals are beginning to recognize its value and have begun adding it to services provided by hospitals, medical clinics, and hospice programs. Reiki can be used for self-healing and distance-healing and on animals and plants.

Insurance: Some insurance plans cover Reiki, Ask your provider.

Quick practitioner reference:
Touch of Life Physical Therapy - page 278
Chani Nicholas - page 283

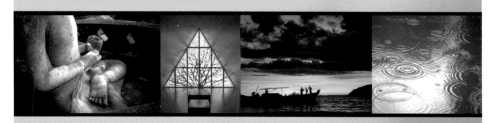

⌘ CHANI NICHOLAS ⌘

CHANIBRIE@HOTMAIL.COM
818.406.8548

REIKI IS A SUBTLE YET POWERFUL HEALING MODALITY THAT WORKS ON THE EMOTIONAL, PHYSICAL AND SPIRITUAL BODIES/PLANES. REIKI IS A HANDS ON HEALING MODALITY THAT ALWAYS GIVES YOU WHAT YOU NEED SO THAT **EVERY SESSION IS COMPLETELY UNIQUE** TO THE PERSON RECIEVING IT.

IN PRACTICING REIKI FOR THE PAST **16 YEARS** I HAVE WITNESSED MIRACULOUS TRANSFORMATIONS IN PEOPLE DEALING WITH EMOTIONAL ISSUES, PHYSICAL DISABILITIES AND TERMINAL ILLNESSES. REIKI TRANSLATED MEANS **"UNIVERSAL LIFE FORCE ENERGY"**, SIMPLY PUT IT MEANS LOVE.

WHEN PEOPLE RECEIVE REIKI TREATMENTS THEY ARE COMMITING TO THEIR OWN HEALING AND ALLOWING THEMSELVES TO **RECEIVE MORE LOVE IN THEIR LIFE**. THE GREATEST HEALING TOOL THAT WE HAVE IS THE ABILITY TO GIVE AND RECEIVE LOVE. THIS IS WHAT MAKES REIKI SO POWERFUL.

Rolfing®

Structural Integration

What is Rolfing? Rolfing,® otherwise known as Structural Integration, is a scientifically validated system of body restructuring. The theory behind rolfing is that when the physical body is vertically aligned, within the field of gravity, it moves more efficiently. The practitioner uses physical 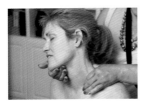 pressure, a distinctive form of deep tissue massage and manipulation, which is applied to the myofascial system - a connective tissue also called fascia, which supports the soft tissues and other connective tissues. Connective tissue wraps and binds all parts of the body including the muscles, bones, organs and the circulatory system.

Imbalanced connective tissue can cause chronic pain, fatigue, headaches, slouching, decreased athletic performance, depression and shallow breathing. Over time, common stressors to the body such as gravity, postural habits, injuries, illness, stress and trauma, cause the connective tissue shorten and bind together. In this state it becomes dehydrated. The result is structural and organ misalignment and compression of the nerves. By lengthening and stretching the connective tissue it facilitates the alignment or proper positioning of the muscles, bones, joints and nerves. Rolfing thus restores the balance of the body.

The usual number of recommended sessions is ten, to create the desired structural changes. At the beginning of the session, the practitioner evaluates the medical history, physical structure, takes notes and photographs to demonstrate problems with alignment. During the session, the client is asked to move and breathe while the practitioner applies pressure to the tense connective tissue.

This helps to further facilitate and release the adhesions of the connective tissue. Practitioners will educate, demonstrate and give physical exercises as homework.

The benefits of Rolfing include increased flexibility; more vitality; the ability to breathe deeply; pain relief; improvement in the level of physical coordination; and it helps the body to move more efficiently, due to the reduced resistance and burden.

Application: Rolfing improves posture, physical and emotional health. It is effective for the relief of chronic pain conditions; speeding up healing and relieves aches and pains; in the case of injuries or trauma, breaks down scar tissue; improves posture; increasing the range of motion; improves the ability to function and perform at jobs that require constant physical activity or repetitive movements; to reach maximum potential for those in sports or creative arts. Rolfing is helpful in relieving digestive problems, constipation, asthma and PMS. Rolfing helps to release traumas stored deep in the tissues and cells of the body. Tension is released layer by layer and emotional trauma are uncovered and dissolved. It is recommended for anyone who wants to be more flexible, energetic and more confident.

Origin and History: The technique of Rolfing was developed in the 1930's by Ida P. Rolf, Ph.D., a biochemist. She discovered that the body's connective tissue could be manipulated and reshaped. Dr. Rolf believed that when the human body works correctly, the force of gravity flows freely through, allowing it to heal.

Cautions: Rolfing has a reputation for being painful. Over the years, practitioners have developed new ways of working gently with the body. It is contraindicated in the case of cancer, severe arthritis and other inflammatory conditions.

Insurance: Rolfing is covered by some insurance plans.

Quick practitioner reference:

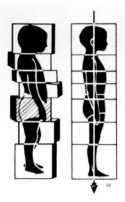
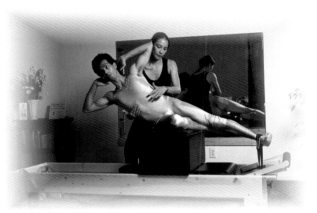
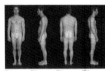
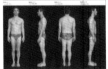
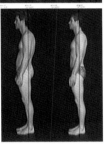
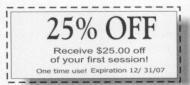
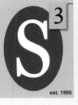

Rolfing Movement Integration
by Anne Sotelo

Rolfing Movement Integration is a system of movement education based on the concepts developed by Ida P. Rolf, Ph.D., the creator of the Rolfing process.

Rolfing Movement focuses on developing balance and support for action in the gravitational field, on learning to move harmoniously with gravity, and on evoking an open and responsive body in which inner strength and centered-ness can be chosen instead of outer tension and armoring. The results are increased grace, ease, and efficiency of movement; a more powerful sense of self; and often the relief of physical stress caused by gravity-resistant movement patterns.

In a series of Rolfing Movement sessions, client and teacher come together to understand the client's present movement patterns. They explore the possibilities for freer, more balanced movement in breathing, walking, standing, sitting and whatever special or daily activities the person is involved in, such as running, desk work, yoga, housework, carpentry, and the like.

They attend to each part of the body, releasing specific holding patterns, and then integrating that part, through movement, with the rest of the body. Over time, the client learns the gentle, simple series of centering movements that can be taken into everyday life to ease pain and stress and to enhance all activities from the workplace to the playing field.

Rolfing Movement can be undertaken by itself or in conjunction with Rolfing sessions. Rolfing Movement Integration and Rolfing combined enhance each other. Rolfing frees and integrates the body's structure so the client has more movement options, and Rolfing Movement teaches the client how to use these possibilities everyday.

The number of Rolfing Movement sessions and their scheduling are flexible according to the individual's needs. Usually, a series of eight private sessions, spaced about a week apart, is recommended.

Rolfers and Rolfing Movement Teachers are trained and certified by the Rolf Institute of Structural Integration in Boulder, Colorado.

See Ad on page 285

Spiritual Psychology

~

What is Spiritual Psychology? Spiritual psychology is a holistic approach to the practice of psychology which includes a body-mind integrative style with an emphasis on spirituality. Therapists are trained in the traditional practices of psychology such as marriage and family therapy, M.F.T, and have undergone university education specifically for the arena of spiritual psychology. Spiritual psychologists understand the transformational spiritual processes which take place on the journey of life.

The goals and skills of spiritual psychologists are quite different from those of traditional therapists, although all therapists assist their patients in moving towards deeper levels of personal truth and authenticity by surrendering their judgments which create blocks to self-love and self-acceptance. It is important to note that all psychologists, regardless of the specific nature of their psychology training, who work with their patients in a holistic manner, are able to facilitate healing, growth and a reconnection to spirit.

Spiritual psychologists help to facilitate healing at the emotional, mental and spiritual levels and use transformational techniques which foster the integration of all aspects of being as a whole. The techniques, methods and language used are unique to the practice of Spiritual Psychology. They help to develop psychological and spiritual growth and maturity; and guide patients in re-awakening or further developing their connection with spirit, while encouraging them to accept life's situations and lessons within the framework of love, wisdom, integrity and compassion. Their guidance helps patients to clearly see their emotional and mental choices or patterns which serve as obstacles to their spiritual growth.

Spiritual psychologists guide their clients and help them to discover their purpose.

They help them recognize and understand the bigger picture - a broader perspective on life, as a whole. They help their clients achieve fulfillment in all areas of life – professionally, creatively, financially and interpersonally - by identifying and healing the emotional and mental blocks within the consciousness that interfere with spiritual growth.

Spiritual psychologists understand that everyone is evolving – at their own pace. They are aware that certain universal patterns are unique to the process and each person will experience similar difficulties in relation to this process. They understand 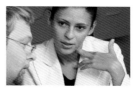 that every issue in our life relates to and is a part of our spirituality. A microcosm of the macrocosm and that nothing is separate. A spiritual psychologist will help clients realize that all experiences, challenges, difficulties and disappointments are supportive to one's growth. They also understand that being joyful, happy, abundant and peaceful is our birthright. They take steps to heal the psyche, and transform their client's outlook so they may adopt a positive nature.

Origin and History: The meaning of the word psyche is "soul." The field of transpersonal psychology emerged in the 1980's. It has a close connection with the founder of analytical psychology, Swiss psychiatrist, Carl Gustav Jung, who's work has a spiritual basis.

Applications: Spiritual psychology is beneficial during times when the assistance of an experienced therapist is needed to facilitate the healing, growth, or a deeper understanding of oneself.

Insurance: Some insurance plans cover visits.

Transitional Healing

~

What is Transitional Healing? Transitional Healing is a profound technique applied to support those making a journey from earthly existence to the afterlife. The time of transition is a time of healing and is supported by this form of therapy. Transitional Healing clears the emotional 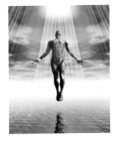 weight or baggage accumulated in one's lifetime. This may include suppressed emotions such as non-forgiveness, trauma, anger, hatred, resentment, sadness, guilt, and most importantly - the fear of letting go and the fear of the beyond. Transitional Healing eases the degree and length of suffering that one experiences during transition. Throughout life, one accumulates personal experiences, both positive and not so positive. Each individual reacts emotionally and mentally to those experiences. The emotional charges are stored in the energy centers and affect one's health. The healer, via special techniques, removes those holding back and preventing the individual in transition from experiencing this uncertain time with a positive frame of mind. This unchartered territory brings up feelings of fear, uncertainty, doubt and resistance for the individual in transition and their loved ones, who do not understand the dying process.

The physical body protects us, to a large degree, from the intensity of strong unwholesome emotions. When the physical body is no longer present, the intensity of the experience felt is much stronger and often painful, hence the teachings of purgatory in many religions. A prayer group of transitional healers is held and is an important part of the healing process. The prayers assist the effortless liberation of the soul's safe journey onward.

A great deal of attention is paid towards healing the low, unrefined astral matter in one's subtle body. The person receiving Transitional Healing is then able to let go of some of their fears and issues, so when the time of physical death comes, the unnecessary pain and suffering is minimized.

The transitional healing service consists of one or more healing sessions and a special prayer group. Mutually agreed upon times are scheduled for the healing sessions between the client and the healer, or the loved one on their behalf. The prayer/meditation session by the healing group is done during and immediately after the time of physical death. Family and loved ones are encouraged to participate via distance at the same time when the prayer/meditation sessions are taking place.

Origin and History: Transitional Healing was developed and taught by Master Choa Kok Sui, who is the modern founder of Pranic Healing. Pranic Healers are trained in the application of this technique.

Applications: Transitional Healing is done several days or weeks before and at the time of physical death. Sometimes individuals will stay on earth through years of painful illness simply because they cannot let go. They may have tremendous guilt and feel responsible for leaving family members and friends, or they may feel that they have unfinished business. Sometimes they stay because of a tremendous fear of moving on. The healing process allows the individual to gracefully let go of the earthly ties and removes the fears and guilt surrounding things that they are no longer able to take care of. Healing may be done in person or via distance-healing.

Insurance: Transitional Healing is not covered by insurance.

Quick practitioner reference:

Workshops 2007

Schedule of Events - Los Angeles

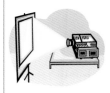

T he following list of events takes place throughout 2007. *Healer's Guide* recommends contacting the presenters by phone or e-mail to ensure available space and to join their mailing list so they may provide you with the current updates on the event location, list of dates, the cost, possible schedule changes and all necessary details.

The Healer's Guide Staff

Ongoing Events - 2007

'Stress = Disease' and the Quality of your Life Matters! Ask, What Can I Do Now?
My Bio Body, Diana Carsola, CBT, www.mybiobody.com, info@mybiobody.com
Ongoing, 2nd Sat. 12-2 pm or 2nd Tues. 6:30-8:30 pm - Sepulveda Blvd. at National
1st hr: Electro Pollution and how to alleviate the cumulative effects of EMFs. Learn about respected energetic modalities of Asia & Europe as safe effective relief for most human maladies. 2nd hr "Hook me Up" - demonstrations along with energetic testing and data-analysis phases of a typical 'Preventative Aging' session. Seating is limited. For more information call:

310-202-0295

In-Treatment Support Group
weSpark - Cancer Support Center, info@wespark.org, www.wespark.org
Ongoing, 13520 Ventura Boulevard, Sherman Oaks, CA
This group is designed for people diagnosed with cancer who are in any stage of treatment. This includes people with impending surgery and those undergoing radiation and/or chemotherapy. This group provides a warm and safe environment and focuses on issues such as medical treatments, clinical trials, fear and anxiety and familial relationships.

818-906-3022

GMCKS Pranic Healing Workshops, Basic and Advanced Certificate Courses
American Institute of Asian Studies, www.pranichealing.com, pranichealing@rocketmail.com
Ongoing, Los Angeles, CA
You will learn how to work with the network of charkas, meridians and auras to accelerate the healing processes of your body; to remove the negative energetic patterns of a disease to prevent it from fully manifesting as a physical ailment. Apply these healing techniques to accelerate your own healing. Also, ongoing Meditation for Peace and Illumination evenings.

888-470-5656

IPSB - Open House, Massage Program
Institute of Psycho-Structural Balancing, www.ipsb.com, massage@ipsb.com
Ongoing, Thursdays - 7:30pm- 9:00pm, 5817 Uplander Way, Culver City, CA
Open House is a great chance for you to meet the teachers, see the school, snack on some tasty treats and if you are one of the lucky volunteers, experience the IPSB massage demo. Classes are beginning all the time. Why wait?
Sign up now. Dates: March 1 & 29, May 3, June 7 & 28, July 26, August 16, September 6 & 27, November 1, December 6.

310-342-7130

Ongoing Events - 2007

Pranic Healing Introductory Workshops and Meditation Nights

Learn2heal, www.learn2heal.com, pranichealing@learn2heal.com

Ongoing, Los Angeles, CA

All are welcome! A 2-hour free introductory Pranic Healing workshop. It is an effective no-touch, painless, healing art which succesfully boosts the body's inborn ability to heal itself and positively affects the most severe illnesses. Learn about your energetic anatomy and how it works. Also, come and join the Meditation for Peace and Illumination evenings.

310-809-2237

Integrated Energy Therapy Basic - Advanced Certification Courses

Energy Well Being, Vicki Frederickson www.energywellbeing.com/classes

Ongoing - Los Angeles, CA

Learn to use the Cellular Memory Map® to target specific areas in the body where these "cellular memories" are stored, helping to release them on all levels – physical, emotional, mental, and spiritual. Massage Therapists can receive National Massage Board CEU Hours for IET Classes. Nurses in California can receive 8 contact hours per class.

818-913-9692

The Art of Living Course & Sri Sri Yoga for Health and Happiness

The Art of Living Los Angeles - www.artoflivingla.org

Ongoing, Los Angeles, CA

The Art of Living Course revives the ancient knowledge and healing power of the breath, with powerful tools and techniques that are easily practiced at home. Over three million course participants around the world have experienced the unconditional joy that is their very nature through this powerful workshop.

310-820-9429

Childbirth Awareness Private Lessons

4wellbeing, Azita Moallef, L.Ac., www.4wellbeing.com

Ongoing - Los Angeles, CA - One-on-one childbirth preparation sessions to cultivate skills & concentration. Transmute the experience of labor pain. Why is there pain and what makes it worse or better? Learn breathing and comfort techniques for coping with labor. How you sit now affects the baby's position in labor. Exercises you can do to help prepare your body. What should you eat and drink in late pregnancy? Be prepared physically, emotionally & spiritually.

310-453-5717

Herbs for Pregnancy, Birth & Beyond

4wellbeing, Azita Moallef, L.Ac., www.4wellbeing.com

Ongoing, Los Angeles, CA - What is the role that herbs can play from conception to birth. How to lessen common prenatal complaints. Herbs to strengthen and tonify the uterus; nourish the mother and developing fetus; and build milk supply for mothers. Which herbs to avoid during pregnancy and lactation. Herbs for common post-partum ailments - such as hemorrhoids, episiotomy - and colic and umbilical cord care for infants.

310-453-5717

Laughter Yoga

weSpark - Cancer Support Center, info@wespark.org, www.wespark.org

Ongoing, 13520 Ventura Boulevard, Sherman Oaks - Laughter is the best medicine. People all over the world are experiencing the healing effects of laughter through laughter yoga, the brainchild of Dr. Madan Kataria from Mumbai. Laughter helps us keep healthy by enriching the blood with ample supplies of oxygen; removes the negative effects of stress; acts as a pain killer and boosts the immune system. Laughter is also anti-aging and tones facial muscles.

818-906-3022

Raj Yog Healing

The Blessings Center, www.gurutej.com

Ongoing, 1310 S. Carmona Avenue, Los Angeles, CA

Using a wonderful array of powerful, penetrating sound & color therapy, we'll break old internal patterns and create new ones, change the energy flow and release disease. This enables us to live as spirit in a healthy energy supporting body. With each session you'll receive specific yoga, meditation or breathing to support this process of change.

323-930-2803

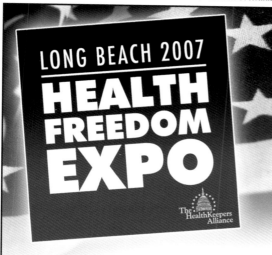

LONG BEACH 2007

HEALTH FREEDOM EXPO

The HealthKeepers Alliance

MARCH 2-4, 2007

Long Beach Convention Center
300 East Ocean Blvd.
Long Beach, CA 90802

JOIN US FOR THIS GREAT EVENT!

The **Long Beach Health Freedom Expo** brings you the latest information, more than 40 outstanding speakers, and 150 exhibitors which support your right to choose and make informed health care decisions. This huge event will share both current legislative issues and new alternative health products and services for you and your family.

Guest Speakers Include:

- ◄ Dr. Julian Whitaker
- • Dr. Earl Mindell
- • Sally Kirkland
- • Jay Kordich
- • Aleta St. James
- ◄ Diane Ladd
- • Jonathan Emord
- • Len Horowitz
- • Dr. Kurt Donsbach
- • and many others!!

Hours:
Friday.............. 10AM to 7PM
Saturday......... 10AM to 7PM
Sunday............ 10AM to 6PM

Admission:
Single Day...................... $10
Weekend $25

DID YOU MISS THE 2007 EVENT? JOIN US NEXT YEAR!

The Health Freedom Expo will be returning to Long Beach on **February 22-24, 2008**. Mark your calendars!

Register Today...
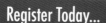

HealthFreedomExpo.com
1-888-658-EXPO

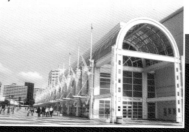

Scheduled Events - 2007

The 2007 Conscious Life Expo
Conscious Life Expo, www.consciouslifeexpo.com
February 9 - 12, LAX Hilton, Los Angeles - 2007 Conscious Life Expo is being held once again. This is the premier show in California bringing together thousands of participants with major national and international speakers and leaders in a four-day Exposition and Conference. This yearly "gathering of the tribes" allows the entire spiritual and progressive community to come together to share, network, learn and celebrate.

800-367-5777

Healing The Light Body
The Four Winds Society, fourwinds@thefourwinds.com, www.thefourwinds.com
March 1 - 7, Joshua Tree, CA
The Healing The Light Body School is a professional training, leading to certification as a practitioner of energy medicine. You become part of a healing community of highly qualified individuals dedicated to their own growth and to healing the earth. Develop a new career path where you can make your contribution and realize your full potential.

888- 437-4077

Health Freedom Expo
Health Freedom Expo, www.healthfreedomexpo.com
March 2 - 4, Long Beach Convention Center, 300 East Ocean Blvd., Long Beach, CA
The Long Beach Health Freedom Expo brings you the latest information, more than 40 outstanding speakers, and 150 exhibitors which support your right to choose and make informed healthcare decisions. This huge event will share both current legislative issues and new alternative health products and services for you and your family. (Fri., Sat.,10am - 7pm, Sun.10am - 6pm)

888-659-3976

Pregnancy Class
4wellbeing, Azita Moallef, L.Ac., www.4wellbeing.com
March 2007, June 2007, September 2007, Santa Monica, CA - With a hectic life style and quick prenatal appointments, pregnant women need nurturing, answers to important questions and time for thoughtful reflection in the first trimester. Make time for this class, to enjoy being pregnant, and to learn: A sound pre-natal diet that insures optimal prenatal health & grows a happy, healthy baby Prenatal Qi gong for relaxation & mindfulness Connect with other new parents.

310-453-5717

Tantric Taster Evenings
Embody Tantra, www.embodytantra.com, charu@embodytantra.com
March 7th, 7:30 - 9pm, Mar Vista, CA
Tantra has the potential to break down our inner walls and re-awaken our sensual nature. Discover Tantra in a supportive and fun environment.
*these are re-occurring classes, call for additional dates
$15 per person/ singles and couples welcome

323-363-3135

Realizing Women's Orgasmic Potential
Embody Tantra, www.embodytantra.com, charu@embodytantra.com
March 27, 7 - 9:30pm, Mar Vista
Tantra offers that when a woman trusts her body, orgasm shifts from a momentary explosion, to an extended state of pleasure that seeps into every aspect of her life.
*all classes are fully clothed with no sexual contact.
$30 in advance/ $40 at the door

323-363-3135

Kriya Shakti - Empowerment for Accelerated Energy Healing
Inner Cosmos, with Satish and Susanna - www.innercosmos.com
April 6th - 8th, Los Angeles, weekend intensive: Fri. Sat. & Sun.
Kriya Shakti is an ancient Indian energy healing technique with a series of abundance manifestation processes. Kriya means action and Shakti means energy. Energy in Action. Apply inner-world formulas for outer-world success.
Learn Kriya Shakti - the science of abundance manifestation. The key to radiant health, true wealth, richer relationship and spiritual growth.

310-470-8150

Scheduled Events - 2007

How To Heal Yourself and Others With Acupressure Massage
Dr Randy Martin, OMD, LAc, PhD, CCH, QME, MUP
May 10, 2007, 8pm - 10pm at Pierce College, Woodland Hills, CA
Learn the basics of Chinese healing as it relates to acupressure massage. This class will focus on specific points to use for problems such as low energy, mental clarity, low back pain, neck & shoulder pain. Learn 16 acupressure points you can perform on yourself or others; the concepts of Chi, Acupressure Meridians, Yin and Yang, 5 Elements, Chinese Tongue diagnosis and more.

818-347-0551

IPSB
INSTITUTE OF PSYCHO-STRUCTURAL BALANCING

IPSB - Skills in Structural Integration - Structural Integration Intro. - Free
Institute of Psycho-Structual Balancing, www.ipsb.com, massage@ipsb.com
June 6, Wednesday - 7:00 pm- 8:30pm, 5817 Uplander Way, Culver City, CA
Structural Integration offers orthopedic and holistic approaches to the restoration and evolution of the human form. Body analysis, structural strategies, practitioner bio-mechanics, palpatory accuracy, joint mobilization and myofascial technique. Structural Integration intro. includes general information on theory and techniques, demonstration and the opportunity for Q&A.

310-342-7130

Professional Clinical Course in Neurofeedback
The EEG Institute, Susan & Siegfried Othmer, www.eeginfo.com/courses
June 7 - 10, Woodland Hills, CA - The professional clinical course is an comprehensive introduction to the theory and clinical application of Neurofeedback, including lecture, demonstration, discussion and hands-on practical experience. You will acquire the knowledge and experience to begin working with this technique for improving self-regulation & brain function. Includes one day introductory to Neurofeedback (qualifies for 8hr CEUs).

877-334-7878

IPSB
INSTITUTE OF PSYCHO-STRUCTURAL BALANCING

IPSB - Craniosacral Unwinding - Cranial Free Intro
Institute of Psycho-Structual Balancing, www.ipsb.com, massage@ipsb.com
September 19, Wed. - 7:00 pm- 9:00pm, 5817 Uplander Way, Culver City, CA
Lecture on Craniosacral unwinding principles and techniques with demonstration how the vertebral spinal fluid expresses itself through connecting tissue and impact the body's healing abilities.

310-342-7130

THE FOUR
WINDS
SOCIETY

Healing The Light Body
The Four Winds Society, fourwinds@thefourwinds.com, www.thefourwinds.com
November 7 - 13, Joshua Tree, CA
The Healing The Light Body School is a professional training leading to certification as a practitioner of energy medicine. You become part of a healing community of highly qualified individuals dedicated to their own growth and to healing the earth. Develop a new career path where you can make your contribution and realize your full potential.

888- 437-4077

Professional Clinical Course in Neurofeedback
The EEG Institute, Susan & Siegfried Othmer, www.eeginfo.com/courses
Dec. 6 - 9, Woodland Hills, CA - The professional clinical course is a comprehensive introduction to the theory and clinical application of Neurofeedback, including lecture, demonstration, discussion and hands-on practical experience. You will acquire the knowledge and experience to begin working with this exciting technique for improving self-regulation and brain function. Includes one day introductory to Neurofeedback. One day Introductory qualifies for 8hr CEUs.

877-334-7878

Health Freedom Expo 2008
Health Freedom Expo, www.healthfreedomexpo.com
February 22-24, 2008, Long Beach Convention Center
The Long Beach Health Freedom Expo brings you the latest information, more than 40 outstanding speakers, and 150 exhibitors which support your right to choose and make informed health care decisions. This huge event will share both current legislative issues and new alternative health products and services for you and your family. (Friday, Saturday,10am - 7pm, Sunday 10am - 6pm)

888-659-3976

293

Readers and Holistic Professionals! Support Healer's Guide 2008

Healer's Guide is an annual, regional project. In order to grow the Los Angeles Healer's Guide and become a strong, driving force in raising awareness to change the future of our healthcare, we value your support. Community participation is the key.

We want to hear from YOU!

Visit

www.HealerGuide.com

anytime and send us

your thoughts.

Healer's Guide 2008 is growing bigger, better and stronger. With over 500 pages of expanded content! We welcome your participation and constructive suggestions, advice, expertise and inspirational stories.

Building a healthy now...

and an even healthier tomorrow

Healing For Body, Mind and Soul

Enter To Win A Healer's Guide

GRAND PRIZE

Valued at $2,600

Our healing gift to you includes a wide variety of complementary sessions & services from the featured Healer's Guide holistic professionals.

- *The Grand Prize Package Includes:*
- *A Hypnotherapy Session - courtesy of LifeWorks*
- *A 2-hour "Healing Your Finance" session - courtesy of Financial Healers*
- *An Acupuncture Treatment and Chinese Herbal prescription - courtesy of 4wellbeing*
- *A Microcurrent Color Light Facial Rejuvenation Treatment - courtesy of Tao of Venus*
- *A Full 'Quantum' Package, includes 2 Full Body, Mind and Spirit Scans for the winner and friend - courtesy of My Bio Body for Quantum Success*
- *A Five Session Package encouraging Balance, Vitality and Overall Wellbeing - courtesy of My Bio Body for Quantum Success*
- *An office visit with a Traditional Naturopathic Doctor to determine what your body nutritional needs are at this stage of your life. Visit includes Neurokinesiology and Sclerology - courtesy of Paramount Herbs*
- *A Full Feng Shui assessment of your home or office with consultation - courtesy of True Feng Shui*
- *An Energy Healing package of 4 Sessions - courtesy of Learn2heal*
- *The "Breakthrough" movie DVD - courtesy of The Garden Diet*
- *A three-year Healer's Guide Subscription*
- *A one-Year Subscription to Whole Life Times Magazine*

Enter to WIN at:
www.healerguide.com/GrandPrize
(must register before
September 31st 2007)

*Healer's Guide Grand Prize
No purchase necessary.*

295

Special Thanks to:

Nzingha Clarke
Jason Love
Master Choa Kok Sui
Master Stephen Co
Eric Robins, M.D.
Susan Bredau
Judy Rossiter
Louise Michaud
Vera Polakova
H. Krejci
Jan Capek
Emil Levin, M.D,
Maria Levin
Craig Rosenthal, D.O.
B. Ctvrtek
Marie Garcia

Thank you to the following companies for their graphics and intellectual properties:

Jason Love - Snapshots Cartoons - www.jasonlove.com
Big Stock Photo - www.bigstockphoto.com
Corel "Copyright (c) 2006, Milan Polak and its licensors. All rights reserved." www.corel.com
Wikipedia - The Free Encyclopedia, www.wikipedia.org

Bibliography
Certain content and topics in the Healer's Guide text were referenced from the following titles.

Adamo, Dr.Peter J.D., *Eat Right for your Type*, Putnam
Bailey Alice A., *Esotheric Healing*, Lucis
Balach A. Phyllis, Ballach F. James.M.D., *Prescription for Nutritional Healing*, Avery
Barney Paul, M.D., *Doctor's Guide to Natural Medicine*, Woodland
Blavatsky H.P., *The Key to Theosophy*,The Theosophical Publishing
Brennan Barbara Ann, *Hands of Light*, Bantam Books
Cedercrans Lucille, *The Nature of The Soul*, Wisdom Impressions
Church Dawson, The Heart of Healing, Church Dawson
Covey Stephen R., *The 7 Habits of Highly Effective People*, Fireside
Encarta, Microsoft, *Encarta World English Dictionary*, St.Martin's Press
Frost Gavin and Yvonne, *Astral Travel*, Samuel Weiser
Grabhorn Lynn, *Excuse Me, Your Life is Waiting, The Astonishing Power of Feelings*, Hampton Roads
Hicks Esther and Jerry, *Ask and It is Given*, Hay House
Krishnamurti J., *Think on These Things*, Perennial Library
Leadbeater C.W., *Clairvoyance*, The Theosophical Publishing House
Leadbeater C.W., *Man Visible and Invisible*, The Theosophical Publishing House
Levine Peter A., *Waking The Tiger*, North Atlantic
Linn Denise, *Sacred Space*, The Random House Ballantine
Maricenko Edward David, *The Business of Medical Practice*, Springer
Master Choa Kok Sui, *Meditation for Soul Realization*, Choa Kok Sui
Master Choa Kok Sui, *Miracles Through Pranic Healing*, Blue Dolphin
Master Choa Kok Sui, *The Spiritual Essence of Man*, Choa Kok Sui
Master Stephen Co and Eric B. Robins, M.D., *Your Hands Can Heal You*, Simon & Schuster
Miller Alice, *The Truth will Set You Free*, Basic Books
Montgomery Kathryn, *How Doctors Think*, Oxford
Powell Arthur E.,*The Astral Body*, Theosophical Publishing House
Powell Arthur E., *The Causal Body and The Ego*, Theosophical Publishing House
Schneider E.L., M.D.,*What Your Doctor Hasn't Told You & the Health Store Clerk Doesn't Know*, Avery
Silva Jose, *The Silva Mind Control Method*, Pocket Books
Stibal Vianna, *Go UP and Work With God*, Rolling Thunder
Tolle Eckhart, *The Power of Now*, New World Library

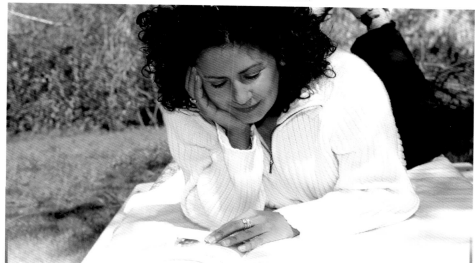

Healer's Guide Book Orders for 2007 & 2008

- **Readers** - A great gift for you, your friends, family members, or business associates. Enjoy the benefits of growing your holistic awareness and knowledge, while accessing quality resources. Discounts from holistic providers. Order online. $14.95 - includes shipping. www.healerguide.com.

- **Retail Locations and Bookstores** - Carry *Healer's Guide* at your business location. Help to introduce your customers to the holistic community and support their healthy lifestyle. For consignment or discount orders contact us at 1.800.495.7106

- **Corporate Wellness Program Coordinators -** Purchasing the *Healer's Guide* for your employees is a smart choice. Support your company's most valuable asset, your loyal staff and take care of their most valuable asset, their health. Preventative holistic care leads to healthier, more productive lives, translating into balance and harmony in the workplace, improved morale and reduced illness. Discounts available for bulk orders. Your company information featured on the cover for orders of 500 or more. *Healer's Guide* corporate wellness educational and experiential days: seminars, workshops and health fairs. Call for details 1.800.495.7106

- **Medical clinics, hospitals, wellness centers, humanitarian or charitable organizations, non-profit or service-oriented healing groups:** Submit your request for complementary copies of *Healer's Guide* for patients and clients. Mail your request to: P.O. Box 6717 Pine Mountain Club, CA, 93222-6717

- **Businesses** – *Healer's Guide* makes a great corporate gift to support and strengthen relationships with your existing clients and new business, throughout the year or at the holiday time. Your company information featured on the cover for orders of 500 or more. Call to order. 1.800.495.7106

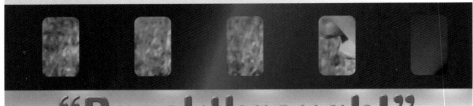
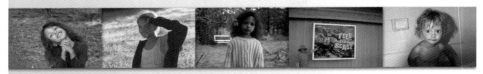
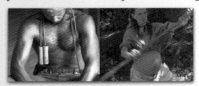
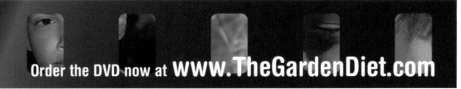